a LANGE medical book

Understanding Health Policy

A Clinical Approach

second edition

a LANGE medical book

Understanding Health Policy

A Clinical Approach

second edition

Thomas S. Bodenheimer, MD
Clinical Professor
Department of Family & Community Medicine
University of California, San Francisco

Kevin Grumbach, MD
Associate Professor
Department of Family & Community Medicine
Institute for Health Policy Studies
University of California, San Francisco
Clinical Faculty
San Francisco General Hospital

Lange Medical Books/McGraw-Hill
Health Professions Division

New York St. Louis San Francisco Auckland Bogotá Caracas Lisbon
London Madrid Mexico City Milan Montreal New Delhi San Juan
Singapore Sydney Tokyo Toronto

McGraw-Hill

A Division of The **McGraw·Hill** *Companies*

4 5 6 7 8 9 0 HAMHAM 0 1 2 3 4 5 6 7 8 9 0

ISBN: 0-8385-9075-6
ISSN: 1080-9465

Acquisitions Editor: Shelley Reinhardt
Development Editor: Cara Lyn Coffey
Production Service: Rainbow Graphics, LLC
Production Editor: Sondra Greenfield
Designer: Libby Schmitz
Associate Art Manager: Maggie Belis Darrow
Illustrator: Gretchen M. Place

ISBN 0-8385-9075-6

90000

9 780838 590751

PRINTED IN THE UNITED STATES OF AMERICA

Contents

Preface

Understanding Health Policy: A Clinical Approach, 2nd edition, is a book about health policy, but it is also about individual patients and care givers and how they interact with each other and with the overall health system.

We, the authors, are practicing primary care physicians, one in a public hospital and clinic and the other in a private practice. We are also analysts of our nation's health care system. In one sense, these two sides of our lives seem quite separate. When treating a patient's illness, health expenditures as a percentage of gross domestic product or variations in surgical rates between one city and another seem remote, if not irrelevant. But they are neither remote nor irrelevant. Health policy affects the patients we see on a daily basis. Managed care referral patterns determine to which specialist we can send a patient, the absence of outpatient medications in the Medicare benefit package affects how we prescribe medications for our elderly patients, and the failure of our nation to legislate universal health insurance influences which patients end up seeing one of us (in the private sector) and which the other (in a public setting). In *Understanding Health Policy,* we hope to bridge the gap separating the microworld of individual patient visits and the macrouniverse of health policy.

The Audience   The book is primarily written for medical students, physicians in training, and practicing physicians, who we feel will benefit from understanding the complex environment in which they work or will work. Because of this choice of audience, physicians feature prominently in the text. In the actual world of clinical medicine, patients' encounters with nurses, physician assistants, nurse practitioners, and other health care givers are an essential part of their health care experience. Physicians would be unable to function without the many other members of the health care team. Patients seldom appreciate the contributions to their well-being made by public health personnel, research scientists, educators, and many other health-related professionals. We hope that the many nonphysician members of the clinical care, public health, and health science education teams, and students aspiring to join these teams, will find the book useful. While the book focuses on physicians, we understand that nothing can be accomplished without the combined efforts of everyone working in the health care field.

The Goal of the Book   *Understanding Health Policy* attempts to explain how the health care system works. We focus on basic principles of health policy in hopes that the reader will come away with a clearer, more systematic way of thinking about health care in the United States, its problems, and the alternatives for managing these problems. Most of the principles also apply to understanding health care systems in other nations.

Given the public's concerns about health care in the United States, the book concentrates on the failures of the system. We spend less time on the successful features because they need less attention. Only by recognizing the difficulties of the system can we begin to fix its problems. The goal of this book, then, is to help all of us understand the health care system, so that we can better work in the system, use the system, and change what needs to be changed.

Clinical Vignettes   In our attempt to unify the overlapping spheres of health policy and health care encounters by individuals, we use clinical vignettes as a central feature of the book. These short descriptions of patients, physicians, and other care givers interacting with the health care system are based on our own experiences as physicians, experiences of colleagues, or cases reported in the medical literature or popular press. Most of the people and institutions presented in the vignettes have been given fictitious names to protect privacy. In three cases that have received widespread publicity, the actual names are retained: Brent McRae and John McGann in Chapter 3 and the Lakeberg twins in Chapter 13. Some names used are emblematic of the occupations, health problems, or attitudes portrayed in the vignettes; most do not have special significance.

Our Opinions   In exploring the many controversial issues of health policy, our own opinions as authors inevitably color and shade the words we use and the conclusions we reach. We present several of our most fundamental values and perspectives here.

The Right to Health Care: We believe that health care should be a right enjoyed equally by everyone. Certain things in life are considered essential. No one gets excited if someone is turned away from a movie or concert because he or she cannot afford a ticket. But sick people who are turned away from an emergency room can make headlines, and rightly so. Legally, health care is not a right in the United States, though many public opinion polls reveal that the great majority of the public believes that health care should be a right. In all other industrialized nations of the world, health care is a right. This right is difficult to translate into reality; it requires the establishment of a network of health care institutions accessible to everyone and a method of financing those institutions that allows everyone to obtain needed services without regard for ability to pay. The right to health care means universal access to health care.

Naturally, this right has limits (see Chapter 13). Were everyone to receive yearly total-body magnetic resonance imaging (MRI) scans, health care costs would go through the roof. A simple statement of the right to health care reads something like this: All people should have equal access to a reasonable level of health services, regardless of ability to pay.

The Imperative to Contain Costs: We believe that limits must be placed on the costs of health care. Cost controls can be imposed in a manner that does relatively little harm to the health of the public.

The rapidly rising costs of health care are in part created by scientific advances that spawn new, expensive technologies. Some of these technologies truly improve health care, some are of little value, and others are of benefit to some patients but are also inappropriately used for patients whom they do not benefit. Eliminating medical services that produce no benefit is one path to "painless" cost control (see Chapter 8).

Reduction in the rapidly rising cost of administering the health care system is another route to painless cost containment. Administrative excess wastes money that could be spent for useful purposes, either within or outside the health care sector. While large bureaucracies do have the advantage of creating jobs, the nation and the health care system have a great need for more socially rewarding and productive jobs (eg, home health aides, drug rehabilitation counselors, childcare workers, and many more) that could be financed from funds currently used for needless administrative tasks.

There is a growing consensus that health care cost increases are bad for the economy. Employers complain that the high cost of health insurance for employees reduces international competitiveness. If government health expenditures continue their rapid rise, other publicly financed programs essential to the nation's economy (eg, education and transportation) will be curtailed because government budgets are limited by the public's willingness to pay taxes.

Rising costs are harmful to everyone because they make health services and health insurance unaffordable. For example, the health care expenses of companies that provide health insurance to their employees increased by about 20% per year in 1988 and 1989. As a result, many companies are shifting more of these costs onto employees. As government health budgets balloon, cutbacks are inevitable, generally hurting the elderly and the poor. Individuals with no health insurance or inadequate coverage have a far harder time paying for care as costs go up. As a general rule, when costs go up, access goes down.

For these reasons, we believe that health care costs should be contained, using strategies that are as painless as possible (ie, that do the least harm to the health of the population).

The Need for Population-Based Medicine: Most physicians, nurses, and other health professionals are trained to provide clinical care to individuals. Yet clinical care is not the only determinant of health status; standard of living and public health measures may have an even greater influence on the health of a population (see Chapter 3). Health care, then, should have another dimension: concern for the population as a whole. Individual physicians may be first rate in caring for their patients' heart attacks, but may not worry enough about the prevalence of hypertension, smoking, elevated cholesterol levels, uncontrolled diabetes, and lack of exercise in their city, in their neighborhood, or among the group of patients enrolled in their practices. For years, clinical medicine has divorced itself from the public health community, which does concern itself with the health of the population.

Currently, health maintenance organizations (HMOs) see themselves as responsible for their enrollees who seek health care; an expanded orientation would broaden that responsibility to the provision of comprehensive preventive health care services to the entire population enrolled in that HMO. We believe that health care givers should be trained to add a population orientation to their current role of caring for individuals.

Acknowledgments We could not have written this book by ourselves. The circumstances encountered by hundreds of our patients provided the insights we needed to understand and describe the health care system. Moreover, numerous health care professionals and academics read parts of our manuscript, made wise and helpful suggestions, and encouraged us to proceed. Any inaccuracies in the book are entirely our responsibility.

Our warmest thanks go to Dr. Drummond Rennie, without whose enthusiasm the entire project would not have taken place, and to our families, who provided both encouragement and patience. We are also most grateful for the excellent suggestions of Ginger Ayala, Trude Bennett, Andrew Bindman, Paula Braveman, Troyen Brennan, David Colfax, Joan Gill, Charlene Harrington, David Himmelstein, Marek Koperski, Donald Light, John Luce, Charles Miller, Victor Sidel, Sara Syer, Milton Terris, the participants in the writing seminar at the University of California, San Francisco Institute for Health Policy Studies, and our editor at Appleton & Lange, Shelley Reinhardt. The assistance of Michelle Won with manuscript preparation was invaluable.

Finally, Chapters 2, 4–6, 8, 9, and 16 were published serially as articles in the Journal of the American Medical Association (1994;272:634–639, 1994;272:971–977, 1994;272:1458–1464, 1995;273:160–167, 1995;274:85–90, and 1996;276:1025–1031) and are published here with permission (copyright, 1994, 1995, and 1996, American Medical Association).

Conclusion This is a book about health policy. As such, we will cite technical studies and will make cross-national generalizations. We will take matters of profound personal meaning—sickness, health, providing of care to individuals in need—and discuss them using the detached language of "inputs and outcomes," "providers and consumers," and "cost-effectiveness analysis." As practicing physicians, however, we are daily reminded of the human realities of health policy. *Understanding Health Policy: A Clinical Approach* is fundamentally about the people we care for: the uninsured janitor enduring the pain of a gallbladder attack because surgery might leave him in financial ruin; or the retired university professor who sustains a stroke and whose life savings are disappearing in nursing home bills uncovered by her Medicare or private insurance plans.

Almost every person, whether a mother on public assistance, a working father, a well-to-do physician, or a millionaire insurance executive, will someday become ill, and all of us will die. Everyone stands to benefit from a system in which health care for all people is accessible, affordable, appropriate in its use of resources, and of high quality.

Thomas S. Bodenheimer
Kevin Grumbach

May 1998
San Francisco, California

a LANGE medical book

Understanding
Health Policy

A Clinical Approach

second edition

Introduction: The Changing US Health Care System

1

When we wrote the introduction to the first edition of *Understanding Health Policy: A Clinical Approach* in the early 1990s, we characterized the health care system in the United States as a "paradox of excess and deprivation," borrowing this phrase from a published article of that period (Enthoven and Kronick, 1989). Excess and deprivation refers to the observation that people with comprehensive health insurance may receive unnecessary and inappropriate health services while those without insurance, or with inadequate insurance, may be deprived of needed care. We saw "excess and deprivation" as a paradigm—an overview within which many particular observations could be fitted.

As history progresses, paradigms shift. Unexpected phenomena occur, or new discoveries change how humans understand their world. In the past few years, the United States health care system has experienced a paradigm shift. A new overarching concept now helps to describe and influence the events dominating United States health care. That concept is "managed care."

Managed care expresses a new relationship between the payers, insurers, and providers of care in the United States. Traditionally, organized payers of health care (especially employers who pay for the health care of their employees) sent a premium to a health insurer, and the insurer paid the health care provider (physician, hospital, home care agency, nursing home, or pharmacy). Under this system, a patient's physician decided how much care a patient would receive, of what kind, and by which providers; and the providers often unilaterally decided how much to charge. The insurers simply paid the bills and, if the bills were too high, the insurers would charge higher premiums to the payers the following year.

Under managed care, organizations that foot the bill for a patient's care have taken on the role of managing that patient's care. Payers and insurers no longer simply write checks; they become involved in decisions about how much care a patient receives, of what kind, and by which providers. In addition, payers and insurers are deciding how much money providers will receive and how that money is paid.

It is no exaggeration to state that managed care represents a revolution in the health care system. In the past, providers, particularly physicians, were able to make most health care decisions and to determine their own compensation with minimal interference. Under managed care, physicians must share, and sometimes give up, decision making to insurers and payers. It is truly a paradigm shift in the health care system, a shift of major proportions.

Understanding the new paradigm requires knowledge of many basic elements of health policy discussed in this book. Particularly relevant to managed care are Chapters 4 and 5 (explaining how physicians and hospitals are paid), Chapters 6 and 7 (describing changes in the organization of health services), Chapter 9 (analyzing how managed care has an impact on health care costs), and Chapter 16 (offering a historical account of the managed care revolution). Managed care, then, is a concept that pervades all aspects of health care financing and organization. One cannot simply say that managed care is a new way of paying physicians—or a new way of organizing health services—or a new power relationship between payers, insurers, and providers. Managed care is all of these and more.

Managed care is a bit like the blind person and the elephant. To the blind person, from the front, the elephant feels like sharp tusks. Under the trunk, the elephant feels like a swaying hose. Near the rear leg, the elephant feels like a tree trunk. Depending on one's vantage point, managed care appears in different ways to different people.

Just because there is a new paradigm—managed care—within which many events in the health care system can be explained, does this mean that the old paradigm— excess and deprivation—is invalid or inaccurate? In physics, the theory of relativity explains more than the Newtonian theories, but the Newtonian laws are still accurate. Similarly, within the paradigm of managed care, the paradox of excess and deprivation continues to describe many elements of the health care system.

EXCESS AND DEPRIVATION

> Louise Brown was an accountant with a 25-year history of diabetes. Her physician taught her to monitor her glucose at home, and her nutritionist helped her follow a diabetic diet. Her diabetes was brought under good control. Diabetic retinopathy was discovered at yearly eye examinations, and periodic laser treatments to her retina prevented loss of vision. Ms. Brown lived to the age of 83, a success of the United States health care system.

> Angela Martini grew up in an inner-city housing project, never had a chance for a good education, became pregnant as a teenager, and has been on public assistance while caring for her four children. Her Medicaid card allows her to see her family physician for yearly physical examinations. A breast examination located a suspicious lesion, which was found to be cancer on biopsy. She was referred to a surgical breast specialist, underwent a mastectomy, was treated with tamoxifen, and has been healthy for the past 15 years.

For people with private or public insurance who have access to health care services, the melding of high-quality primary and preventive care with appropriate specialty treatment can produce the best medical care in the world.

The United States is blessed with thousands of well-trained physicians, nurses, pharmacists, and other health care givers who compassionately provide up-to-date medical attention to patients who seek their assistance. This is the face of the health care system in which we can take pride. Success stories, however, are only part of the reality of health care in the United States.

Too Little Care   Some persons receive too little care because they are uninsured, inadequately insured, or have Medicaid coverage that many physicians will not accept.

James Jackson's Medicaid benefits were terminated because of state cutbacks. At age 34 years, he developed abdominal pain but did not seek care for 10 days because he had no insurance and feared the cost of treatment. He began to vomit, became weak, and was finally taken to an emergency room by his cousin. The physician diagnosed a perforated ulcer with peritonitis and septic shock. The illness had gone on too long; Mr. Jackson died on the operating table. Had he received prompt medical attention, his illness would likely have been cured.

Betty Yee was a 68-year-old woman with angina, high blood pressure, and diabetes. Her total bill for medications, which were not covered under her Medicare plan, came to $200 per month. She was unable to afford the medications, her blood pressure went out of control, and she suffered a stroke. Ms. Yee's final lonely years were spent in a nursing home; she was paralyzed on her right side and unable to speak.

Mary McCarthy became pregnant but could not find an obstetrician who would accept her Medicaid card. After 7 months, she began to experience severe headaches, went to the emergency room, and was found to have hypertension and preeclampsia. She delivered a stillborn baby.

Over 40 million people in the United States have no health insurance (Schroeder, 1996). Many are victims of the changing economy, which has shifted from a manufacturing economy based on highly paid, full-time jobs with good fringe benefits toward a service economy with lower paid jobs that are often part-time and have poor or no benefits (Renner and Navarro, 1989). Two-thirds of the uninsured are in families with an employed adult. Lack of insurance is not simply a problem of the poor but has also become a middle class phenomenon, particularly for families of people who are self-employed or work in small establishments.

Underinsurance is also a major issue. Medicare covers only 45% of the health care costs of the elderly (Aaron and Reischauer, 1995). In 1994, 19% of the privately insured population under age 65 had health insurance coverage so inadequate that a major illness would create severe financial hardship (Short and Banthin, 1995).

Too Much Care   In contrast to the deprivation created by absent or inadequate health insurance, the health care sector is beset by two varieties of excess: administrative and medical. Administrative costs are rising more rapidly than the costs of the medical care being administered. In the words of Steffie Woolhandler and David Himmelstein (1991):

Medicine is increasingly a spectator sport. Doctors, patients, and nurses perform before an enlarging audience of utilization reviewers, efficiency experts, and cost managers. A cynic viewing the uninflected curve of rising health care spending might wonder whether the cost-containment experts cost more than they contain . . . (Excerpted from information appearing in the New England Journal of Medicine: Woolhandler S, Himmelstein DU: The deteriorating administrative efficiency of the US health care system. N Engl J Med 1991;324:1253.)

The price tag for administrative costs in the United States comes to an extraordinary 19–24% of the total dollars spent on health care. The US General Accounting Office (1991) estimated that 9% of all 1991 health care costs consisted of unnecessary administrative spending.

Some people receive too much care that is costly and may be harmful.

> At age 66, Daniel Taylor noticed that he was getting up to urinate twice each night. It did not bother him much. His family physician sent him to a urologist, who found that his prostate was enlarged (though with no signs of cancer) and recommended surgery. Mr. Taylor did not want surgery. He had a friend with the same symptoms whose urologist had said that surgery was not needed. Since Mr. Taylor never questioned doctors, he went ahead with the procedure anyway. After the surgery he became incontinent of urine.

> Consuelo Gonzalez had a minor pain in her back, which was completely relieved by over-the-counter acetaminophen. She went to the doctor just to make sure the pain was nothing serious, and it was not. The physician gave Ms. Gonzalez a stronger medicine, indomethacin, 3 times a day. The indomethacin caused a bleeding ulcer, requiring a 9-day hospital stay at a cost of $17,000 to her health insurer.

According to health services expert Robert Brook (1989):

> . . . almost every study that has seriously looked for overuse has discovered it, and virtually every time at least double-digit overuse has been found. If one could extrapolate from the available literature, then perhaps one-fourth of hospital days, one-fourth of procedures, and two-fifths of medications could be done without. (Copyright 1989 American Medical Association: Brook RH: Practice guidelines and practicing medicine. JAMA 1989;262:3027.)

Concern about the plight of the uninsured dominated discourse about health care reform during the early 1990s. By 1996, in the aftermath of defeat of legislative efforts to expand insurance coverage, growing controversy over managed care eclipsed public concern about the unsolved problems of the medically deprived. This paradigm shift has not changed the fundamental reality for tens of millions of uninsured people in the United States, but it has reduced their priority in the political arena. Increasingly, attention has been focused on the medical excess that managed care was designed to cure.

MANAGED CARE

> Kathy Fine was glad when her employer enrolled her in a managed care plan, Apple a Day HMO. Her previous insurance had failed to cover preventive services such as Pap smears and mammograms, and the HMO covered these

items. For the first time in her life, her prescriptions were largely paid by the HMO. She had previously gone to several physicians in an uncoordinated fashion, and she now had a primary care provider who coordinated her services. Her employer was also happy because employee health care costs had not risen in the past 2 years.

Ken Madden was angry. Under his old insurance, he went to a good orthopedist for his back pain, and now Dollar a Day HMO, his new insurer, had no contract with the orthopedist and wanted to send him to see a specialist way across town. Worse yet, Dollar a Day was denying him the physical therapy he needed for his back pain. When Ken read that Dollar a Day was siphoning off 26% of its income to administrative costs, high executive pay, and profits, he got even more angry.

Health maintenance organizations (HMOs), a rapidly growing form of managed care covering over 60 million people in the United States, are controversial. Most HMOs cover a broad array of services including preventive care, and many coordinate the care of their enrollees through a primary care physician (PCP). From 1994 through 1996, many employers have enjoyed relatively stable premiums for their employees enrolled in HMOs.

On the other hand, the number of complaints against HMOs is growing because some patients are denied services, especially care by specialists, which they feel they need. Since HMOs, and sometimes PCPs, may increase their profits and income by withholding services (see Chapter 5), patients are expressing growing unease over a conflict between physicians' desire to make money and their responsibility to provide care (Anders, 1996; Bodenheimer, 1996). The increase in administrative excess described above is in part related to the expensive authorization processes of managed care organizations.

THE PUBLIC'S VIEW OF THE HEALTH CARE SYSTEM

Health care in the United States encompasses a wide spectrum (Fuchs, 1992), ranging from the highest-quality, most compassionate treatment of a complex illness to the turning away of a sick person because of lack of ability to pay; from well-designed protocols for prevention of illness to inappropriate high-risk surgical procedures performed on uninformed patients. Despite the recent upheavals in health care, one fundamental truth remains. The United States still has the least universal, most costly health care system in the industrialized world.

Many people view the high costs of care and the lack of universal access as indicative of serious failings in the health care system. In 1994, only 18% of people in the United States felt that the system worked well; 81% felt that the system needed fundamental changes or a complete overhaul. Fifty-five percent believed that the wealthy always get better care than those who are less well off. Twenty percent of Americans had a problem paying medical bills during the previous year, compared with 6% of Canadians and 3% of West Germans. Only 29% of Americans had confidence in their health care institutions, compared with 45% of Canadians and 53% of West Germans (Blendon et al, 1995).

Understanding the Crisis In order to correct the weaknesses of the health care system while maintaining its strengths, it is necessary to understand how the system works. How is health care financed? What are the causes and consequences of incomplete access to care? How are physicians paid, and what is the effect of their mode of reimbursement on health care costs? How are health care services organized and quality of care enhanced? Is sufficient attention paid to the prevention of ill health, and what are different strategies for preventing illness?

How can the problems of health care be solved? Is managed care the answer? Can costs be controlled in a manner that does not reduce access? Can access be expanded in a manner that does not increase costs? How have other nations done it—or attempted to do it? How might the health care system look in the United States of the twenty-first century?

REFERENCES

Aaron HJ, Reischauer RD: The Medicare reform debate: What is the next step? Health Aff 1995;14(4):8.

Anders G: Health Against Wealth: HMOs and the Breakdown of Medical Trust. Houghton Mifflin Company, 1996.

Blendon RJ et al: Who has the best health care system? A second look. Health Aff 1995;14(4):220.

Bodenheimer T: The HMO backlash: Righteous or reactionary? N Engl J Med 1996;335:1601.

Brook RH: Practice guidelines and practicing medicine. JAMA 1989;262:3027.

Enthoven A, Kronick R: A consumer-choice health plan for the 1990s. N Engl J Med 1989;320:29.

Fuchs VR: The best health care system in the world? JAMA 1992;268:916.

Renner C, Navarro V: Why is our population of uninsured and underinsured persons growing? The consequences of the "deindustrialization" of the United States. Int J Health Serv 1989;19:433.

Schroeder S: The medically uninsured: Will they always be with us? N Engl J Med 1996;334:1130.

Short PF, Banthin JS: New estimates of the underinsured younger than 65 years. JAMA 1995;274:1302.

U.S. General Accounting Office: Canadian Health Insurance: Lessons for the United States. 1991.

Woolhandler S, Himmelstein DU: The deteriorating administrative efficiency of the US health care system. N Engl J Med 1991;324:1253.

Paying for Health Care

Health care is not free. Someone must pay. But how? Does each person pay when receiving care? Do people contribute small amounts in advance so that their care will be paid for when they need it? When a person contributes in advance, might the contribution be used for care given to someone else? If so, who should pay how much?

Health care financing in the United States evolved to its current status as a series of social interventions. Each intervention solved a problem but in turn created its own problems requiring further intervention. This chapter will discuss the historical process of health care financing as solution-creating-new-problem-requiring-new-solution.

MODES OF PAYING FOR HEALTH CARE

The four basic modes of paying for health care are out-of-pocket payment, individual private insurance, employment-based group private insurance, and government financing (Table 2–1). These four modes can be viewed both as a historical progression and as a categorization of current health care financing.

Out-of-Pocket Payments

> Fred Farmer broke his leg in 1892. His son ran 4 miles to get the doctor, who came to the farm to splint the leg. Fred gave the doctor a couple of chickens to pay for the visit. His great-grandson, Ted, who is uninsured, broke his leg in 1992. He was driven to the emergency room, where the physician ordered an x-ray and called in an orthopedist who placed a cast on the leg; the cost was $580.

In the nineteenth century, people like Fred Farmer paid physicians and other health care practitioners in cash or through barter. In the first half of the twentieth century, out-of-pocket cash payment was the most common method of reimbursement. This is the simplest mode of financing—direct purchase by the consumer of goods and services (Figure 2–1).

People in the United States purchase most consumer items, from VCRs to haircuts, through direct out-of-pocket payments. This is not the case with health care, and one may ask why this is so. Economists such as Robert Evans (1984) and Kenneth Arrow (1963) have discussed some reasons why health care is not considered just another typical consumer item.

Need Versus Luxury: Whereas a VCR is considered a luxury, health care is regarded as a basic human need by most people.

> For 2 weeks, Marina Perez has had vaginal bleeding and has felt dizzy. She has no insurance and is terrified that medical care might eat up her $250 in savings. She scrapes

Table 2–1. Health care financing in 1994.[1]

Type of Payment	Percentage of Personal Health Care Expenditures
Out-of-pocket payment	20%
Individual private insurance	3%
Employment-based private insurance	35%[2]
Government financing	43%
Total	101%[3]

Principal Source of Coverage	Percentage of Population
Uninsured	15%
Individual private insurance	4%
Employment-based private insurance	58%
Government financing	23%
Total	100%

[1] Data extracted from Cowan CA et al: Business, households, and government: Health spending 1994. Health Care Fin Rev 1996;17:157; U.S. Department of Health and Human Services: Health United States 1995. 1996; and U.S. General Accounting Office: Private Health Insurance. (GAO/HEHS-97-8). 1996.

[2] This includes private insurance obtained by federal, state, and local employees, which is in part purchased by tax funds.

[3] Total expenditures add up to 101% due to rounding error.

NOTE: For out-of-pocket payments, the percentage of expenditures is greater than the percentage of the uninsured population because out-of-pocket dollars are paid not only by the uninsured but also by the insured in the form of deductibles and copayments and payments for uncovered services. Because private insurance tends to cover healthier people, the percentage of expenditures is far less than the percentage of population covered. Public expenditures are far higher per population because the elderly and disabled are concentrated in the public Medicare and Medicaid programs.

up $30 to see her doctor, who finds that her blood pressure falls to 90/50 mm Hg upon standing and that her hematocrit is 26%. The doctor calls her sister, Juanita, to drive her to the hospital. Marina gets into the car and tells Juanita to take her home.

If health care is a basic human right, then people who are unable to afford health care must have a payment mechanism available that is not reliant on out-of-pocket payments.

Unpredictability of Need and Cost: Whereas the purchase of a VCR is a matter of choice and the price is known to the buyer, the need for and cost of health care services are unpredictable. Most people do not know if or when they may become severely ill or injured or what the cost of care will be.

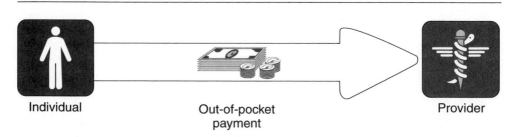

Individual   Out-of-pocket payment   Provider

Figure 2–1. Out-of-pocket payment is made directly from patient to provider.

> Jake has a headache and visits the doctor, but he does not
> know whether the headache will cost $45 for a physician
> visit plus the price of a bottle of aspirin, $1200 for an MRI,
> or $70,000 for surgery and irradiation for a brain tumor.

The unpredictability of many health care needs makes it difficult to plan for these expenses. The medical costs associated with serious illness or injury usually exceed a middle class family's savings.

Patients' Need to Rely on Physicians' Recommendations: Unlike the purchaser of a VCR, a person in need of health care may have little knowledge of what he or she is buying at the time when care is needed.

> Jenny develops acute abdominal pain and goes to the hospi-
> tal to purchase a remedy for her pain. The physician tells
> her that she has acute cholecystitis or a perforated ulcer and
> recommends hospitalization, an abdominal sonogram, and
> upper endoscopic studies. Will Jenny, lying on a gurney in
> the emergency room and clutching her abdomen with one
> hand, use her other hand to leaf through a textbook of inter-
> nal medicine to determine whether she really needs these
> services, and should she have brought along a copy of Con-
> sumer Reports to learn where to purchase them at the
> cheapest price?

Health care is the foremost example of asymmetry of information between providers and consumers (Evans, 1984). A patient with abdominal pain is in a poor position to question a physician's ordering of laboratory tests, x-rays, or surgery. When health care is elective, patients can weigh the pros and cons of different treatment options, but even so, recommendations may be filtered through the biases of the physician providing the information. Compared with the voluntary demand for VCRs (the influence of advertising notwithstanding), the demand for health services is partially involuntary and is often physician- rather than consumer-driven.

For these reasons, among others, out-of-pocket payments are flawed as a dominant method of paying for health care services. Because the direct purchase of health services became increasingly difficult for consumers and was not meeting the needs of hospitals and physicians to be paid, health insurance came into being.

Individual Private Insurance

> Bud Carpenter is self-employed. He recently purchased a
> health insurance policy from his insurance broker for his
> family. To pay the $250 monthly premium, he had to work
> some extra jobs on weekends, and the $2000 deductible
> meant he would still have to pay quite a bit of his family's
> medical costs out of pocket. Mr. Carpenter preferred to pay
> these costs rather than take the risk of spending the money
> saved for his children's college education on a major illness.
> When his son became ill with leukemia and the hospital bill
> reached $50,000, Mr. Carpenter appreciated the value of
> health insurance. Nonetheless, he had to feel disgruntled
> when he read a newspaper story listing his insurance com-
> pany among those that paid out on average less than 50 cents
> on health services for every dollar collected in premiums.

With private health insurance, a third party, the insurer, is added to the patient and the health care provider, who are the basic two parties of the health care transaction. While the out-of-pocket mode of payment is limited to a single financial transaction, private insurance requires two transactions—a premium payment from individual to insurance plan (sometimes called health plan), and a reimbursement payment from insurance plan to provider (Figure 2–2). (With indemnity insurance, the process requires three transactions—the premium from individual to insurer, the payment from individual to provider, and the reimbursement from insurer to individual. For simplicity's sake, health insurance will be treated here as reimbursement from insurance plan to provider.) In nineteenth century Europe, voluntary benefit funds were set up by guilds, industries, and mutual societies. In return for paying a monthly sum, people received assistance in case of illness. This early form of private health insurance was slow to develop in the United States. In the early twentieth century, European immigrants set up some small benevolent societies in United States cities to provide sickness benefits for their members. During the same period, two commercial insurance companies, Metropolitan Life and Prudential, collected 10–25 cents per week from workers for life insurance policies that also paid for funerals and the expenses of a final illness. The policies were paid for by individuals on a weekly basis, so large numbers of insurance agents had to visit their clients to collect the premiums as soon after payday as possible. Because of the huge administrative costs, individual health insurance never became a dominant method of paying for health care (Starr, 1982). Currently, individual policies provide health insurance for only 4% of the United States population (see Table 2–1).

Employment-Based Private Insurance

Betty Lerner and her schoolteacher colleagues paid $6 per year to Prepaid Hospital in 1929. Ms. Lerner suffered a heart attack and was hospitalized at no cost. The following year, Prepaid Hospital built a new wing and raised the teachers' prepayment to $12.

Rose Riveter retired in 1961. Her health insurance premium for hospital and physician care, formerly paid by her employer, had been $25 per month. When she called the insurance company to obtain individual coverage, she was told that premiums at age 65 cost $70 per month. She could not

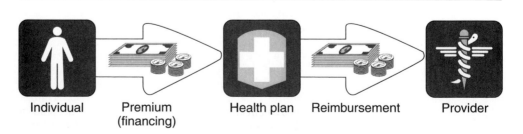

Individual   Premium   Health plan   Reimbursement   Provider
(financing)

Figure 2–2. Individual private insurance. A third party, the insurance plan (health plan), is added, dividing payment into a financing component and a reimbursement component.

afford the insurance, and wondered what would happen if
she became ill.

The development of private health insurance in the United States was impelled by
the increasing effectiveness and rising costs of hospital care. Hospitals became places
not only in which to die but also in which to get well. Many patients were unable to
pay for hospital care, however, and this meant that hospitals were unable to attract
"customers."

In 1929, Baylor University Hospital agreed to provide up to 21 days of hospital
care to 1500 Dallas schoolteachers such as Betty Lerner if they paid the hospital $6
per person per year. As the Great Depression deepened and private hospital occupancy in 1931 fell to 62%, similar hospital-centered private insurance plans spread.
These plans (anticipating more modern health maintenance organizations [HMOs])
restricted care to a particular hospital. The American Hospital Association built on
this prepayment movement and established statewide Blue Cross hospital insurance
plans allowing free choice of hospital. By 1940, 39 Blue Cross plans, controlled by
the private hospital industry, had enrolled over 6 million people. The Great Depression reduced the amount patients could pay physicians out of pocket, and in 1939, the
California Medical Association set up the first Blue Shield plan to cover physician
services. These plans, controlled by state medical societies, followed Blue Cross in
spreading across the nation (Starr, 1982; Fein, 1986).

In contrast to the consumer-driven development of health insurance in European nations, coverage in the United States was initiated by health care providers seeking a
steady source of income. Hospital and physician control over the "Blues," a major sector of the health insurance industry, guaranteed that reimbursement would be generous
and that cost control would remain on the back burner (Starr, 1982; Law, 1974).

The rapid growth of employment-based private insurance was spurred by an accident of history. During World War II, wage and price controls prevented companies
from granting wage increases but allowed the growth of fringe benefits. With a labor
shortage, companies competing for workers began to offer health insurance to employees such as Rose Riveter as a fringe benefit. After the war, unions picked up on
this trend and negotiated for health benefits. The results were dramatic. Enrollment in
group hospital insurance plans grew from 12 million in 1940 to 142 million in 1988.

With employment-based health insurance, employers usually pay all or part of the
premium that purchases health insurance for their employees (Figure 2–3). This flow
of money is not as simple as it looks, however. The federal government views employer premium payments as a tax-deductible business expense. The government
does not treat the health insurance fringe benefit as taxable income to the employee,
even though the payment of premiums could be interpreted as a form of employee income. Because each premium dollar of employer-sponsored health insurance results
in a reduction in taxes collected, the federal government is in essence subsidizing employer-sponsored health insurance. This subsidy is enormous, estimated at $75 bil-
lion in 1991 (Reinhardt, 1993).

The growth of employment-based health insurance attracted commercial insurance
companies to the health care field to compete with the Blues for customers. The commercial insurers changed the entire dynamic of health insurance. The new dynamic was
called **experience rating.** (The following discussion of experience rating can be applied to individual as well as employment-based private insurance.)

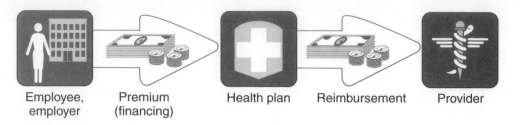

Employee, employer   **Premium (financing)**   **Health plan**   **Reimbursement**   **Provider**

Figure 2–3. Employment-based private insurance. In addition to the direct employer subsidy, indirect government subsidies occur through the tax-free status of employer contributions for health insurance benefits.

Healthy Insurance Company insures three groups of people—a young healthy group of bank managers, an older healthy group of truck drivers, and an older group of coal miners with a high rate of chronic illness. Under experience rating, Healthy sets its premiums according to the experience of each group in using health services. Because the bank managers rarely use health care, each pays a premium of $100 per month. Because the truck drivers are older, their risk of illness is higher, and their premium is $300 per month. The miners, who have high rates of black lung disease, are charged a premium of $500 per month. The average premium income is $300 per member per month.

Blue Cross insures the same three groups and needs the same $300 per member per month to cover health care plus administrative costs for these groups. Blue Cross sets its premiums by the principle of community rating. For a given health insurance policy, all subscribers in a community pay the same premium. The bank managers, truck drivers, and mine workers all pay $300 per month.

Health insurance provides a mechanism to distribute health care more in accordance with human need rather than exclusively on the basis of ability to pay. To achieve this goal, funds are redistributed from the healthy to the sick, a subsidy that helps pay the costs of those unable to purchase services on their own.

Community rating achieves this redistribution in two ways:

(1) Within each group (bank managers, truck drivers, and mine workers), people who become ill receive benefits in excess of the premiums they pay, while people who remain healthy pay premiums while receiving few or no health benefits.

(2) Among the three groups, the bank managers, who use less health care than their premiums are worth, help pay for the miners, who use more health care than their premiums could buy.

Experience rating is far less redistributive than community rating. Within each group, those who become ill are subsidized by those who remain well, but among the different groups, healthier groups (bank managers) do not subsidize high-risk groups (mine workers). Thus, the principle of health insurance, which is to distribute health care more in accordance with human need rather than exclusively on the ability to pay, is weakened by experience rating (Light, 1992).

In the carly years, Blue Cross plans set insurance premiums by the principle of community rating, whereas commercial insurers used experience rating as a "weapon" to compete with the Blues (Fein, 1986). Commercial insurers such as Healthy Insurance Company could offer cheaper premiums to low-risk groups such as bank managers, who would naturally choose a Healthy commercial plan at $100 over a Blue Cross plan at $300. Experience rating helped commercial insurers overtake the Blues in the private health insurance market. While in 1945 commercial insurers had only 10 million enrollees, compared with 19 million for the Blues, by 1955 the score was commercials 54 million and the Blues 51 million (Health Insurance Association of America, 1990).

Many commercial insurers would not market policies to such high-risk groups as minc workers, leaving Blue Cross with high-risk patients who were paying relatively low premiums. To survive the competition from the commercial insurers, Blue Cross had no choice but to seek younger, healthier groups by abandoning community rating and reducing the premiums for those groups. In this way, most Blue Cross and Blue Shield plans switched to experience rating. Without community rating, older and sicker groups became less and less able to afford health insurance.

From the perspective of the elderly and those with chronic illness, experience rating is discriminatory. Healthy persons, however, might have another viewpoint on the situation, and might ask why they should voluntarily transfer their wealth to sicker people through the insurance subsidy? The answer lies in the unpredictability of health care needs. When purchasing health insurance, an individual does not know if he or she will suddenly change from a state of good health to one of illness. Thus, *within a group,* people are willing to risk paying for health insurance, even though they may not use it. *Among different groups,* however, healthy people have no economic incentive to voluntarily pay for community rating and subsidize another group of sicker people. This is why community rating cannot survive in a laisscz faire competitive private insurance system (Aaron, 1991).

The most positive aspect of health insurance —that it assists people with serious illness to pay for their care—has also become one of its main drawbacks—the difficulty in controlling costs in an insurance environment. With direct purchase, the "invisible hand" of each individual's ability to pay holds down the price and quantity of health care. If a patient is well insured, however, and the cost of care causes no immediate fiscal pain, the patient will use more services than someone who must pay for care out of pocket. In addition, particularly before the advent of HMOs, health care providers could increase fees far more easily if a third party was available to foot the bill.

Health insurance, then, was originally an attempt by society to solve the problem of unaffordable health care under an out-of-pocket payment system; but its very capacity to make health care more affordable created a new problem. If people no longer had to pay out of their own pockets for health care, they would use more health care; and if health care providers could charge insurers rather than patients, they could more easily raise prices, especially during the era when the major insurers (the Blues) were controlled by hospitals and physicians. The solution of insurance fueled the problem of rising costs. As private insurance became largely experience rated and employment based, persons who had low incomes, were chronically ill, or were elderly found it increasingly difficult to afford private insurance.

Government Financing

> In 1984, Rose Riveter, age 74, developed colon cancer. She was now covered by Medicare, which had been enacted in 1965. Even so, her Medicare premium, hospital deductible expenses, physician copayments, short nursing home stay, and uncovered prescriptions cost her $2700 the year she became ill with cancer.

Employment-based private health insurance grew rapidly in the 1950s, helping working people and their families to afford health care. But two groups in the population received little or no benefit: the poor and the elderly. The poor were usually unemployed or employed in jobs without the fringe benefit of health insurance; they could not afford insurance premiums. The elderly, who needed health care the most and whose premiums had been partially subsidized by community rating, were hard hit by the trend toward experience rating. In the late 1950s, less than 15% of the elderly had any health insurance (Harris, 1966). Only one program could provide affordable care for the poor and the elderly—tax-financed government health insurance.

Government entered the health care financing arena long before the 1960s through such public programs as municipal hospitals and dispensaries to care for the poor and through state-operated mental hospitals. But only with the 1965 enactment of Medicare (for the elderly) and Medicaid (for the poor) did public insurance payments for privately operated health services become a major feature of health care in the United States.

Medicare Part A (Table 2–2) is a hospital insurance plan for the elderly financed largely through social security taxes from employers and employees. Medicare Part B (Table 2–3) insures the elderly for physicians' services and is paid for by federal taxes and monthly premiums from the beneficiaries. Medicaid (Table 2–4) is a program run by the states, funded from federal and state taxes, which pays for the care of certain low-income groups. Because Medicare has large deductibles, copayments, and gaps in coverage, many Medicare beneficiaries also have supplemental ("Medigap") private insurance, Medicaid, or Medicare HMO coverage. Most HMOs that enroll Medicare beneficiaries eliminate the deductibles and other large patient payments required under traditional Medicare. Some Medicare HMO plans pay part of a patient's pharmacy expenses, but Medicare HMOs minimally cover nursing home care. Many states are requiring Medicaid recipients to receive their care through HMOs.

Government health insurance for the poor and the elderly added a new factor to the health care financing equation: the taxpayer (Figure 2–4). With government-financed health plans, the taxpayer can interact with the health care consumer in two distinct ways:

(1) The social insurance model, exemplified by Medicare, allows only those who have paid a certain amount of social security taxes to be eligible for Part A and only those who pay a monthly premium to receive benefits from Part B. As with private insurance, social insurance requires people to make a contribution in order to receive benefits.

(2) The contrasting model is the Medicaid public assistance model, in which those who contribute (taxpayers) may not be eligible for benefits (Bodenheimer and Grumbach, 1992).

It must be remembered that private insurance contains a subsidy: redistribution of funds from the healthy to the sick. Tax-funded insurance has the same subsidy and usually adds another: redistribution of funds from the wealthy to the poor. Under this double subsidy, exemplified by Medicare and Medicaid, healthy middle-income employees generally pay more in social security payments and other taxes than they receive in health services, whereas unemployed, disabled, and lower-income elderly persons tend to receive more in health services than they contribute in taxes.

The advent of government financing improved financial access to care for some people but in turn aggravated the problem of rising costs. The federal government and state governments, faced with chronic budgetary crises and unwilling to enact major tax increases, are responding by channeling Medicare and Medicaid patients into lower-cost HMOs and by reducing payments to physicians and hospitals. At the same time, the high costs of private insurance are placing employment-based coverage out of the fiscal reach of more and more employers.

Table 2–2. Summary of Medicare Part A, 1997.

Who is eligible?

Upon reaching the age of 65 years, people who are eligible for Social Security are automatically enrolled in Medicare Part A whether or not they are retired. A person who has paid into the Social Security System by earning $3000 or more per year for 10 years and that person's spouse are eligible for Social Security. People who are not eligible for Social Security can enroll in Medicare Part A by paying a monthly premium.

People under the age of 65 who are totally and permanently disabled may enroll in Medicare Part A after they have been receiving Social Security disability benefits for 24 months. People with chronic renal disease requiring dialysis or a transplant may also be eligible for Medicare Part A without a 2-year waiting period.

How is it financed?

Financing is through the Social Security system. Employers and employees each pay to Medicare 1.45% of wages and salaries. Self-employed people pay 2.9%.

What services are covered?

Services	Benefit	Medicare Pays
Hospitalization	First 60 days[1]	All but a $760 deductible per spell of illness
	61st to 90th day[1]	All but $190/day
	91st to 150th day[2]	All but $380/day
	Beyond 90 days if lifetime reserve days are used up	Nothing
Skilled nursing facility	First 20 days	All
	21st to 100th day	All but $95/day
	Beyond 100 days	Nothing
Home health care	As long as a person requires skilled care as defined by Medicare requirements	100% for skilled care; 80% of approved amount for medical equipment
Hospice care	As long as a doctor certifies person suffers from a terminal illness	100% for most services
Nursing home care	Care that is mainly custodial is not covered	Nothing

[1] Part A benefits are provided by each "spell of illness" rather than for each year. A "spell of illness" begins when a beneficiary enters a hospital and ends 60 days after discharge from the hospital or from a skilled nursing facility.
[2] Beyond 90 days, Medicare pays for 60 additional days only once in a lifetime ("lifetime reserve days").

Table 2–3. Summary of Medicare Part B, 1997.

Who is eligible?

People who are eligible for Medicare Part A who elect to pay the Medicare Part B premium of $43.80 per month.

How is it financed?

Financing is in part by general federal revenues (personal income and other federal taxes) and in part by Part B monthly premiums.

What services are covered?

Services	Benefit	Medicare Pays

Medical expenses
   Physician services
   Physical, occupational,
     and speech therapy
   Medical equipment
   Diagnostic tests
	All medically necessary services	80% of approved amount after a $100 annual deductible

Preventive care	Some Pap smears; some mammograms; hepatitis B, pneumococcal, and influenza vaccinations	Included in medical expenses
Outpatient medications	Not covered	Nothing

Eye refractions, hearing
   evaluations, dental
   services
	Not covered	Nothing

Table 2–4. Summary of Medicaid, 1997.

Who is eligible?

Medicaid covers about one-half of all Americans with incomes below the federal poverty level (about $13,000 for a family of three); the federal government requires only certain categories of low-income people to be enrolled in state Medicaid programs:

(1) Families who in 1996 received welfare assistance through Aid to Families with Dependent Children (AFDC). Even though AFDC was phased out in the welfare reform legislation of 1996 and replaced by Temporary Assistance for Needy Families (TANF), families who received AFDC in 1996 remain eligible for Medicaid even if they no longer receive welfare payments under TANF.

(2) Most people over 65, the blind, and the totally disabled who receive cash assistance under the federal Supplemental Security Income (SSI) program.

(3) Pregnant women (for pregnancy-related services), children under age 6 with family incomes up to 133% of the federal poverty line, and some older children.

Some states have received federal waivers to cover more people under Medicaid. For example, Oregon covers everyone below the federal poverty line and Tennessee covers many low-income people not in these three categories. Under the 1997 legislation to expand health insurance for children, states will receive federal grants that can be used to expand Medicaid eligibility to more children.

How is it financed?

Through federal and state (and sometimes local) taxes. The federal government pays between 50 and 83% of total Medicaid costs; the federal contribution is greater for states with lower per capita incomes.

What services are covered?

The federal government requires the following services to be provided: hospital, physician, laboratory, x-ray, prenatal, and preventive care services; nursing home and home health care; and medically necessary transportation. Medicaid programs are required to pay the Medicare premiums, deductibles, and copayments for certain low-income people on Medicare.

States can add services to this list and can place certain limitations on these federally mandated services.

Most states have received federal waivers to require some or all of their Medicaid enrollees to join managed care plans. The managed care plans can deny services they deem to be medically inappropriate.

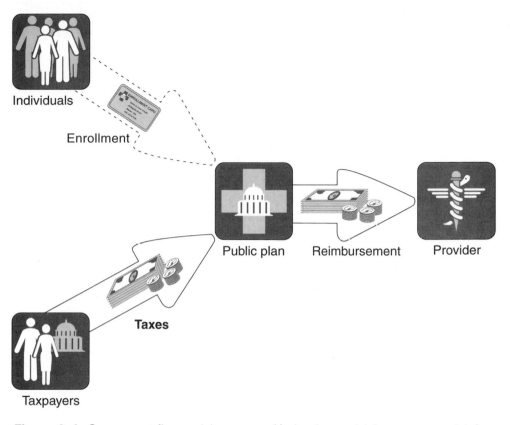

Figure 2–4. Government-financed insurance. Under the social insurance model (eg, Medicare Part A), only individuals paying taxes into the public plan are eligible for benefits. In other models (eg, Medicaid), an individual's eligibility for benefits may not be directly linked to payment of taxes into the plan.

THE BURDEN OF FINANCING HEALTH CARE

Different methods of financing health care place different burdens on the various income levels of society. Payments are classified as **progressive** if they take a rising percentage of income as income increases, **regressive** if they take a falling percentage of income as income increases, and **proportional** if the ratio of payment to income is the same for all income classes (Pechman, 1985).

What principle should underlie the choice of revenue source for health care? A central purpose of the health care system is to maintain and improve the health of the nation's population. As is discussed in Chapter 3, rates of mortality and disability are far higher for low-income people than for the wealthy. Burdening low-income families with high levels of payments for health care (ie, regressive payments) reduces their disposable income, amplifies the ill effects of poverty, and thereby worsens their health. It makes little sense to finance a health care system—whose purpose is to improve health—with payments that worsen health. Regressive payments, then, could be considered "unhealthy."

> Rita Blue earns $10,000 per year for her family of four. She develops pneumonia, and her out-of-pocket health costs come to $1000, 10% of her family income.

> Cathy White earns $100,000 per year for her family of four. She develops pneumonia, and her out-of-pocket health costs come to $1000, 1% of her family income.

Out-of pocket payments are a regressive mode of financing. The National Medical Care Expenditure Survey confirms that in 1987, out-of-pocket payments took 12% of the income of families in the nation's lowest-income quintile, compared with 1.2% for families in the wealthiest 5% of the population (Bodenheimer and Sullivan, 1997). Many economists and health policy experts would consider this regressive burden of payment as unfair, yet out-of-pocket payments make up fully 20% of total health care payments (Levit et al, 1996). Aggravating the regressivity of out-of-pocket payments is the fact that lower-income people tend to be sicker and thus have more out-of-pocket payments than the wealthier and healthier.

> Jim Hale is a young, healthy, self-employed accountant, whose monthly income is $6000, with a health insurance premium of $200, or 3% of his income.

> Jack Hurt is a disabled mine worker with black lung disease. His income is $1800 per month of which $400 (22%) goes for his health insurance.

Experience-rated private health insurance is a regressive method of financing health care because increased risk of illness tends to correlate with reduced income. If Jim Hale and Jack Hurt were enrolled in a community-rated plan, each with a premium of $300, they would, respectively, pay 5% and 17% of their incomes for health insurance. With community rating, the burden of payment is regressive but less so than with experience rating.

Most private insurance is not individually purchased but rather obtained through employment. How is the burden of employment-linked health insurance premiums distributed?

> Jill is an assistant hospital administrator. To attract her to the job, the hospital offered her a package of salary plus health insurance of $5250 per month. She chose to take $5000 in salary, leaving the hospital to pay $250 for her health insurance.

> Bill is a nurse's aide, whose union negotiated with the hospital for a total package of $1750 per month; of this, $1500 is salary and $250 pays his health insurance premium.

Do Jill and Bill pay nothing for their health insurance? Not exactly. Employers generally agree on a total package of wages and fringe benefits; if Jill and Bill did not receive health insurance, their pay would probably go up by nearly $250 per month. That is why employer-paid health insurance premiums are generally considered deductions from wages or salary (Cantor, 1990; Reinhardt, 1988). For Jill, health insurance amounts to only 5% of her income, but for Bill, it is 17%. The National Medical Expenditure Survey corroborates the regressivity of employment-based health insurance; in 1987, premiums took about 6% of the income of families in the lowest-income decile, compared with about 2% for those in the highest-income decile (Bodenheimer and Sullivan, 1997).

> Larry Lowe earns $10,000 and pays $410 in federal and state income taxes, or 4.1% of his income.

> Harold High earns $100,000 and pays $12,900 in income taxes, or 12.9% of his income.

The progressive income tax is the largest tax providing money for government-financed health care. Most other taxes are regressive (eg, sales and social security taxes), and the combined burden of all taxes that finance health care is roughly proportional (Pechman, 1985).

In 1994, 57% of health care was financed through out-of-pocket payments and premiums, which are regressive, while 43% was funded through government revenues (Levit et al, 1996), which are proportional. The sum total of health care financing is regressive. Data from 1989 reveal that the poorest decile of households spent 20% of income on health care while the highest-income decile spent only 8% (Holahan and Zedlewski, 1992). Overall, the United States health care system is financed in a manner that is unhealthy.

CONCLUSION

Neither Fred Farmer nor his great-grandson Ted had health insurance, but the modern-day Mr. Farmer's predicament differs drastically from that of his ancestor. Third-party financing of health care has fueled an expansive health care system that offers treatments unimaginable a century ago but at tremendous expense.

Each of the four modes of financing health care developed historically as a solution to the inadequacy of the previous modes. Private insurance provided protection to patients against the unpredictable costs of medical care as well as protection to providers of care against the unpredictable ability of patients to pay. But the private insurance solution created three new, interrelated problems:

(1) The opportunity for health care providers to increase fees to insurers caused health services to become increasingly unaffordable for those with inadequate insurance or no insurance.

(2) The employment-based nature of group insurance placed people who were unemployed, retired, or working part-time at a disadvantage for the purchase of insurance and partially masked the true costs of insurance for employees who did receive health benefits at the workplace.

(3) Competition inherent in a deregulated private insurance market gave rise to the practice of experience rating, which made insurance premiums unaffordable for many elderly people and other medically needy groups.

To solve these problems, government financing was required, but government financing fueled an even greater inflation in health care costs.

As each "solution" was introduced, health care financing improved for a time. By the 1990s, however, rising costs had jeopardized private and public coverage for many people and made services unaffordable for those without a source of third-party payment. The problems of each financing mode, and the problems created by each successive solution, had accumulated into a complex crisis characterized by inadequate access for some and high costs for everyone.

REFERENCES

Aaron HJ: Serious and Unstable Condition: Financing America's Health Care. Brookings Institution, 1991.

Arrow KJ: Uncertainty and the welfare economics of medical care. Am Econ Rev 1963;53:941.

Bodenheimer T, Grumbach K: Financing universal health insurance: Taxes, premiums, and the lessons of social insurance. J Health Polit Policy Law 1992;17:439.

Bodenheimer T, Sullivan K: The logic of tax-based financing for health care. Int J Health Services 1997;27:409.

Cantor JC: Expanding health insurance coverage: Who will pay? J Health Polit Policy Law 1990;15:755.

Cowan CA et al: Business, households, and government: Health spending 1994. Health Care Fin Rev 1996;17:157.

Evans RG: Strained Mercy. Butterworths, 1984.

Fein R: Medical Care, Medical Costs. Harvard Univ Press, 1986.

Harris R: A Sacred Trust. New American Library, 1966.

Health Insurance Association of America: Source Book of Health Insurance Data, 1990.

Holahan J, Zedlewski S: Who pays for health care in the United States? Implications for health system reform. Inquiry 1992;29:231.

Law SA: Blue Cross: What Went Wrong? Yale Univ Press, 1974.

Levit KR et al: Health care spending in 1994: Slowest in decades. Health Aff 1996;15(2):130.

Light DW: The practice and ethics of risk-rated health insurance. JAMA 1992;267:2503.

Pechman JA: Who Paid the Taxes, 1966–1985. Brookings Institution, 1985.

Reinhardt UE: Are mandated benefits the answer? Health Manage Q 1988;10(1):10.

Reinhardt UE: Reorganizing the financial flows in U.S. health care. Health Aff 1993;12 (Suppl):172.

Starr P: The Social Transformation of American Medicine. Basic Books,1982.

U.S. Department of Health and Human Services: Health United States 1995. 1996.

U.S. General Accounting Office: Private Health Insurance. (GAO/HEHS-97-8). 1996.

Access to Health Care
3

Access to health care is the ability to obtain health services when needed. Lack of adequate access for millions of people is a serious crisis in the United States.

Access to health care has two major components. First, and most frequently discussed, is ability to pay. Second is the availability of health care personnel and facilities that are close to where people live, accessible by transportation, culturally acceptable, and capable of providing appropriate care in a timely manner and in a language spoken by those who need assistance. The first and longest portion of this chapter dwells on financial barriers to care. The second portion touches on nonfinancial barriers. The final segment explores the influences other than health care (in particular, income and race) that are important determinants of the health status of a population.

FINANCIAL BARRIERS TO HEALTH CARE

Lack of Insurance

> Ernestine Newsome, who lived in South Central Los Angeles, was 5 years old in 1960. She had never seen a doctor and had received no immunizations. In 1962, her mother began working for the telephone company, and this provided the family with health insurance. Ernestine went to a neighborhood physician for regular checkups. When she reached 19, she left home and began work as a part-time secretary. She was no longer eligible for her family's health insurance coverage, and her new job did not provide insurance. She has not seen a physician since starting her job.

Health insurance coverage, whether public or private, is a key factor in making health care accessible. In 1990, 35 million people were uninsured, but by 1995, the number had increased to over 40 million (Table 3–1), or nearly one in six people in the United States (U.S. Congress, Office of Technology Assessment, 1992; Bennefield, 1996a). The particular pattern of uninsurance is related to the employment-based nature of health care financing. Most people, like Ernestine Newsome, obtain health insurance when employers voluntarily decide to provide coverage to employees and their families. People whose employers choose not to provide health insurance, and many who are unemployed, are left without health insurance. Often, people without employment-based insurance are not eligible for public programs such as Medicare and Medicaid, and are unable to purchase individual private coverage because they cannot afford the premiums.

Between the 1930s and mid-1970s, because of the growth of private health insurance and the 1965 passage of Medicare and Medicaid, the number of uninsured persons declined steadily, but since 1976, the number has been growing (Figure 3–1). This trend can be explained by limitations in the system of employment-based private

Table 3–1. Principal source of health insurance, 1994.[1]

	Number of People (millions)	% of Population
Medicare[2]	31	12
Medicaid	24	9
Employment-based private insurance	151	58
Individual private insurance	11	4
CHAMPUS, VA, or military[3]	4	2
Uninsured	40	15
Total United States population	261	100

[1] Data extracted from U.S. General Accounting Office: Private Health Insurance. (GAO/HEHS-97-8), 1996; and U.S. Department of Health and Human Services: Health United States 1995. 1996.

[2] For people with Medicare plus private insurance or Medicaid, Medicare is considered the principal source of insurance. The Medicaid and private insurance figures do not count Medicare beneficiaries who also have Medicaid or private insurance.

[3] CHAMPUS is the Civilian Health and Medical Program of the Uniformed Services. VA is the U.S. Department of Veterans Affairs.

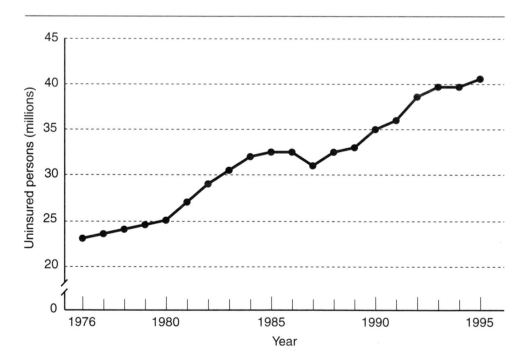

Figure 3–1. Number of uninsured persons in the United States 1976–1995. (Data extracted from Himmelstein DU, Woolhandler S, Wolfe SM: The vanishing health care safety net: New data on uninsured Americans. Int J Health Serv 1992;22:381; and Bennefield RL: Health insurance coverage: 1995. U.S. Dept of Commerce: Economics and Statistics Administration, P60-195, September 1996a.)

health insurance. The number of people covered by Medicare and Medicaid has grown substantially since 1976. The number covered by private health insurance has fallen, however, dropping by 10 million between 1980 and 1990, a decade during which the number of uninsured rose by 10 million. During the 1990s, the number of people with employment-based insurance fell by several million more (Schroeder, 1996). Many of the newly uninsured are employed or are dependents of employed persons (Himmelstein et al, 1992).

Why People Lack Insurance

> Jean Irons worked for US Steel as a clerk, and her fringe benefits included health insurance. The plant moved to another state, and she found a job as a food service worker in a small restaurant; her pay decreased by 25%, and the restaurant did not provide health insurance.

Why has private health insurance coverage declined since the early 1980s, creating the uninsurance crisis? There are several explanations:

(1) During the past 2 decades, the economy in the United States has undergone a major transition. The number of highly paid, largely unionized, full-time manufacturing workers with employer-provided health insurance has declined, and the work force has shifted toward a larger number of low-wage, increasingly part-time, nonunionized service and clerical workers whose employers are less likely to provide insurance (Renner and Navarro, 1989). From 1989 to 1992, the economy experienced a loss of 639,000 full-time jobs while adding 894,000 part-time jobs (Morrisey et al, 1994). During each of the years 1992 through 1995, almost 3.5 million workers were laid off from their jobs. Two-thirds of these ended up unemployed, in part-time work, or in jobs with less pay or fewer benefits (New York Times, 1996).

(2) The high cost of health insurance has made it unaffordable for many businesses and individuals (Friedman, 1991). Insurance premiums went from 2.1% of disposable income in 1960 to 4.7% by 1986. From 1989 to 1991, group insurance premiums rose by about 50% for the average employer.

(3) The experience rating practices and administrative costs of the health insurance industry (see Chapter 2) make insurance premiums more costly and less predictable for small employers and individuals.

> Ben Wing was an engineer in an aircraft plant; he developed leukemia, was unable to work, and lost his health insurance. His disease went into remission and he started his own consulting business but was unable to obtain health insurance because his chronic illness made the cost of his insurance prohibitive.

> Sally Lewis worked as a receptionist in a physician's office; she received health insurance through her husband, who was a construction worker. They got divorced, she lost her health insurance, and her physician employer told her he could not provide her with health insurance because of the cost.

> When Hazel Booker retired from her job as a librarian at age 59, she converted her group insurance to an individual policy. After 3 years, she missed one monthly payment, at which time her insurance was canceled. When she reapplied for coverage, the insurance company had doubled her premium because of her high blood pressure.

Because of its link with employment, health insurance may be a fleeting benefit. In 1993, 54 million people lacked insurance for at least 1 month during the calendar year, and 67 million lacked coverage at some point during the 2-year period 1992–1993, substantially more than the 40 million uninsured during the entire year (Bennefield, 1996b). In a given year, 10.8% of employees change jobs and may lose their insurance temporarily or permanently (Light, 1992). People who are laid off from their jobs or who leave jobs because of illness may lose their insurance. Nearly half of workers with an interruption in their employment during the year experience a lapse in their insurance coverage (Bennefield, 1996b). Family members insured through the workplace of a husband or wife may lose their insurance in the case of divorce, job loss, or death of the working family member. And those who retire before age 65 may be uninsured before they become eligible for Medicare. People who leave their employment may be eligible to pay for coverage at group insurance rates for 18 months, as stipulated in the Consolidated Omnibus Budget Reconciliation Act of 1985 (COBRA); however, many people cannot afford the premiums (Pepper Commission, 1990).

Almost all uninsured individuals desire health insurance. Fewer than 10% of the uninsured polled in 1995 stated that they "didn't need or want insurance." Most cited the unaffordability of insurance as the main obstacle to coverage (Donelan et al, 1996).

> Randy Fisher was a commercial fisherman and felt an obligation to obtain health insurance for his seven employees. Five private insurers offered policies with extremely high premiums. He finally gave up.

> Spud Bennett, owner of a small potato farm in Idaho, developed a brain tumor, which was successfully excised. A few months later, the health insurer for Mr. Bennett and his employees announced that the monthly rate would increase from $1300 to $10,000. The farm was forced to drop the policy; Mr. Bennett and his employees had no health insurance.

Loss or change of employment is not the only trigger for loss of health insurance. Certain categories of jobs, usually in the small business sector, may be offered unaffordable premiums by insurance companies because persons holding those jobs tend to use health services more often. In some cases, these jobs are stereotypically characterized as "gay" (eg, beauty shop employees and entertainers) and in others, there are inherent health risks (eg, commercial fishermen like Randy Fisher, construction workers, and loggers) (Pepper Commission, 1990). Individuals who develop a chronic health condition, or small groups including such individuals (eg, Spud Bennett), are often charged higher premiums. Chronic conditions include such diagnoses as coronary artery disease, diabetes, allergies, back strain, obesity, and arthritis. Insurers may raise insurance premiums for small employers by several hundred percent in 1 year, thereby forcing employers to cancel coverage for their employees. In the small business market, the "inverse coverage law" is operative: "The more people need coverage, the less coverage they are likely to get or the more they are likely to pay for what they get" (Light, 1992).

Who Are the Uninsured?   In 1995, 14% of whites were uninsured, compared with 21% of African-Americans and 33% of Latinos. The rate of uninsurance decreases as income rises. Nearly one-quarter of individuals with annual household incomes of less than $25,000 are uninsured, compared with 7% of individuals with household incomes of $75,000 or more (Bennefield, 1996a). Fewer than half of the poor are covered by Medicaid. The uninsured population contains a somewhat smaller share of people in good health than is found among those with health insurance. People who are poor and a member of a minority group are four times as likely to be uninsured as higher-income white persons (Valdez et al, 1993; Friedman, 1991) (Figures 3–2 and 3–3).

> Morris works for a corner grocery store that employs five people. Morris once asked the owner whether the employees could receive health insurance through their work, but the owner said it was too expensive. Morris, his wife, and their three kids are uninsured.
>
> A shipyard worker, Norris, was laid off 3 years ago, and at age 60 is unable to get another job. He lives on county general assistance at $400 per month, but is ineligible for Medicaid because he is not a parent, not over 65, and not disabled. He is uninsured.

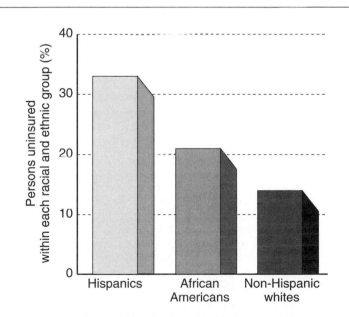

Figure 3–2. Percentage of population lacking health insurance by race and ethnicity in 1995. (Data extracted from Bennefield RL: Health insurance coverage: 1995. U.S. Dept of Commerce: Economics and Statistics Administration, P60-195, September 1996a.)

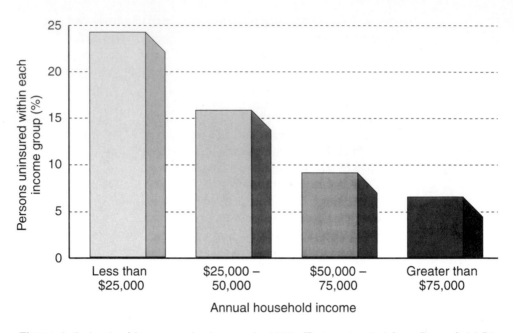

Figure 3–3. Lack of insurance by income in 1995. (Data extracted from Bennefield RL: Health insurance coverage: 1995. U.S. Dept of Commerce: Economics and Statistics Administration, P60-195, September 1996a.)

The uninsured can be divided into two major categories: the employed uninsured (Morris) and the unemployed uninsured (Norris). About three-fourths of the uninsured are considered employed uninsured: they are in families like Morris's with at least one working adult. Most of the jobs held by the employed uninsured are low paying and in small firms and may be part time. The other one-fourth of the uninsured are unemployed, often with incomes below the poverty line but, like Norris, ineligible for Medicaid (Figures 3–4 and 3–5).

Does Health Insurance Make a Difference?

> Two United States senators are debating the issue of access to health care. One decries the stigma of uninsurance and claims that people without insurance receive less care and suffer worse health than those with insurance. The other disagrees, claiming that hospitals and doctors deliver large amounts of charity care, which allows uninsured people to receive the services they need.

To resolve this debate, the U.S. Congress Office of Technology Assessment (1992) conducted a comprehensive review to determine whether health insurance makes a difference in the use of health care and in health outcomes. The findings proved that in spite of a certain amount of unpaid care received by the uninsured, people lacking health insurance receive less care and have worse health outcomes.

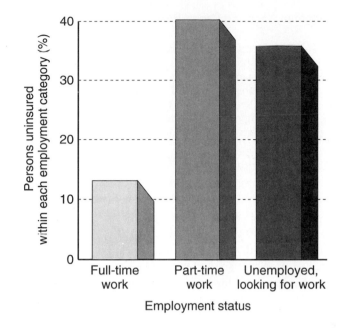
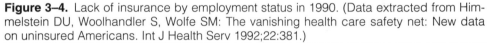

Figure 3–4. Lack of insurance by employment status in 1990. (Data extracted from Himmelstein DU, Woolhandler S, Wolfe SM: The vanishing health care safety net: New data on uninsured Americans. Int J Health Serv 1992;22:381.)

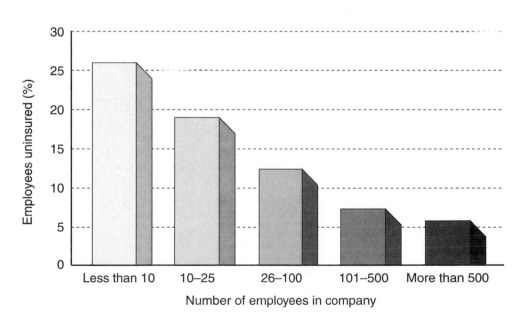

Figure 3–5. Lack of insurance by size of employer in 1987. (Data extracted from National Medical Expenditure Survey: A Profile of Uninsured Americans. Rockville, Maryland: Department of Health and Human Services, 1989.)

Health Insurance and Use of Health Services

> Percy, a child whose parents were both employed but not insured, was refused admission by a private hospital for treatment of an abscess. Outpatient treatment failed, and his mother attempted to admit Percy to other area hospitals, who also refused care. Finally, an attorney arranged for the original hospital to admit the child; the parents then owed the hospital $4000.

Access to health care is most simply measured by the number of times a person uses health care services. Commonly used are numbers of physician visits, hospital days, and preventive services received. In addition, access can be quantified by surveys in which respondents report whether or not they failed to seek care or delayed care when they felt they needed it.

Compared with insured people, the uninsured are less likely to have a regular source of medical care and more likely to report delays in receiving health care. The insured in poor health see a physician 70% more often than the uninsured in poor health. Despite the common perception that the uninsured receive hospital care through charity, adults who are insured in fact receive 90% more hospital services than the uninsured (Hadley et al, 1991). Sick newborns with insurance receive far more hospital services than comparably ill newborns without insurance (Braveman et al, 1989). In 1992, 67% of the uninsured reported postponing health care because they could not afford it and 19% said they or a member of their family had been refused care for financial reasons. These figures are far higher than those reported for people with private insurance (Smith et al, 1992).

People without insurance, who are frequently poor, are more likely than privately insured people to receive care in the emergency rooms or clinics of underbudgeted public hospitals, often enduring 7- or 8-hour waits before receiving service (Grumbach et al, 1993). Higher rates of hypertension and cervical cancer and lower survival rates for breast cancer among the uninsured, compared to those with insurance, are associated with less frequent blood pressure screenings, Pap smears, and clinical breast examinations (Woolhandler and Himmelstein, 1988).

The influence of health insurance on access is complicated by the factor of income, because lack of insurance is correlated with low income (Franks et al, 1993a). Historical data strongly suggest that lack of insurance rather than low income is the main barrier to using health services; after the passage of the Medicaid program, lower-income people began seeing physicians more frequently than those with higher incomes (Freeman et al, 1990).

Health Insurance and Health Outcomes

> Dan Sugarman noticed that he was urinating a lot and feeling weak. His friend told him that he had diabetes and needed medical care, but lacking health insurance, Mr. Sugarman was afraid of the cost. Eight days later, his friend found him in a coma. He was hospitalized for diabetic ketoacidosis.

> Penny Evans worked in a Nevada casino. She was uninsured and ignored a growing mole on her chest. After many

months of delay, she saw a dermatologist and was diagnosed with malignant melanoma, which had metastasized. She died 2 years later at the age of 44.

Leo Morelli, a hypertensive patient, was doing well until his company relocated to Mexico and he lost his job. Lacking both paycheck and health insurance, he became unable to afford his blood pressure medications. Six months later, he collapsed with a stroke.

A variety of indicators are used to measure health outcomes, including avoidable hospitalizations (admissions that could have been avoided if ambulatory care had been provided in a timely manner), severity of illness at the time of hospitalization, mortality rates, control of blood pressure among hypertensives, and adverse outcomes for newborns (eg, low birth weight, long hospital stays, and neonatal death).

The uninsured suffer worse health outcomes than those with insurance. Compared with insured persons, the uninsured, like Mr. Sugarman, have more avoidable hospitalizations; like both Mr. Sugarman and Ms. Evans, they tend to be diagnosed at later stages of life-threatening illnesses; and they are on the average more seriously ill when hospitalized. Uninsured patients with appendicitis are much more likely than insured patients to have their appendix rupture as a result of a delay in surgical treatment (Braveman et al, 1994). Adults who lost their Medicaid coverage in 1983 were found to have worse control of blood pressure than those who retained Medicaid. Uninsured newborns have a higher rate of adverse outcomes, including death, when compared with insured newborns. Uninsured adults have higher rates of in-hospital mortality compared with privately insured adults, even after adjusting for severity of illness on admission. Severe uncontrolled hypertension, as in the case of Mr. Morelli, is associated with lack of a primary care physician (PCP) and also lack of health insurance (U.S. Congress, Office of Technology Assessment, 1992; Lurie et al, 1984; Braveman et al, 1989; Hadley et al, 1991; Shea et al, 1992). Most significantly, people who lack health insurance suffer a higher overall mortality rate than those with insurance. A study that followed mortality rates between 1971 and 1987 found that by the end of the follow-up period, 9.5% of the insured and 18.4% of the uninsured had died. After adjusting for other factors that might have contributed to this difference (eg, age, sex, education, lower initial health status, and smoking), it was concluded that lack of insurance by itself increased the risk of dying by 25% (Franks et al, 1993b).

Does Medicaid Make a Difference? Medicaid, the federal and state public insurance plan for some low-income people, was designed to alleviate the problem of access for those in poverty, and it has made great strides in doing so. For example, in 1982, low-income residents of Arizona, the only state with no Medicaid program, saw physicians 20% less often than low-income people in the rest of the country. Poor Arizona children had 40% fewer physician visits.

But Medicaid has its limitations. Between 1975 and 1983, the proportion of low-income people insured by Medicaid fell from 63% to 46% because of stricter eligibility requirements (Blendon et al, 1986). Even with the rapid increase in the number of Medicaid recipients between 1988 and 1994, only half of low-income persons (income under 150% of the federal poverty level) received Medicaid in 1994 (Kaiser Commission on the Future of Medicaid, 1996).

Medicaid and Use of Health Services

> An urban hospital has a service to refer patients without physicians to doctors on the hospital staff. The hospital receives 50 calls each week from Medicaid patients looking for a doctor; the referral service is unable to find any physician who will accept these patients.

For those people with Medicaid coverage, access to care is by no means guaranteed. Medicaid pays physicians far less than does Medicare or private insurance, with the result that in 1991, 26% of the nation's physicians did not accept Medicaid patients and an additional 35% limited the number of Medicaid patients served.

As a rule, people with Medicaid have a level of access to medical care that is intermediate between those without insurance and those with private insurance. Compared with uninsured people, those with Medicaid are more likely to have a regular source of medical care, receive more preventive services, and are less likely to report delays in receiving care. Compared with uninsured children, children receiving Medicaid have much higher use of preventive services and, among those with chronic illness and disability, greater use of treatment services (Newacheck et al, 1995). But compared with privately insured people, Medicaid recipients are less likely to have a regular source of care, receive fewer preventive services, and are more likely to report delays in receiving care. In a 1992 survey, 18% of Medicaid beneficiaries under the age of 65 reported that doctors or hospitals had refused to accept their coverage (U.S. Congress, Office of Technology Assessment, 1992; Blendon et al, 1993).

> Concepcion Ortiz lived in a town of 25,000 persons. When she became pregnant, her sister told her that she was eligible for Medicaid, which she obtained. She called each obstetrician in town and none would take Medicaid patients. When she reached her sixth month, she became desperate.

Many pregnant women have trouble finding an obstetrician who will accept Medicaid. A 1990 study in California demonstrated that pregnant women with Medicaid coverage tended to initiate prenatal care later than did those without insurance or with private insurance; once prenatal care had been initiated, Medicaid recipients made more prenatal visits than those lacking insurance but fewer visits than the privately insured (Braveman et al, 1993).

Medicaid and Health Outcomes: Health outcomes for Medicaid recipients lag behind those for privately insured people (U.S. Congress, Office of Technology Assessment, 1992). In some studies (Lurie et al, 1984), Medicaid recipients have health outcomes better than those of uninsured people, but as the following example shows, this is not always the case.

> Maureen Patterson, a 38-year-old woman with Medicaid coverage, noticed a mass in her breast and thought she should see a doctor to have it checked. But she did not have a regular doctor and heard that the best doctors did not accept Medicaid. So she worried that she might fall into the hands of someone she could not trust. She asked some friends about their doctors, but still could not make up her mind to go. A year later, she decided that the lump was

Table 3–2. Stage of breast cancer at time of initial diagnosis, New Jersey, 1985–1987.[1]

	Local[2]	Regional	Distant
Privately insured	54%	39%	7%
Uninsured	45%	43%	12%
Medicaid	46%	37%	17%

[1] Data extracted from Ayanian JZ et al: The relation between health insurance coverage and clinical outcomes among women with breast cancer. N Engl J Med 1993; 329:326.
[2] Local disease: cancer is confined to the breast. Regional disease: cancer has spread to the regional lymph nodes. Distant disease: cancer has spread to other parts of the body.

> quite a bit larger, and made an appointment with her cousin's doctor. She was terrified when she found that she had breast cancer, which had spread to her axillary nodes.

In a highly disturbing finding, uninsured women and women with Medicaid, like Ms. Patterson, had on the average significantly more advanced breast cancer at initial diagnosis than privately insured women, and survival rates were markedly lower among uninsured and Medicaid patients. Differences between those without insurance and those with Medicaid were not significant (Tables 3–2 and 3–3). In another study, Medicaid patients, compared with the privately insured, had a higher hospitalization rate for conditions that can often be treated outside of the hospital or avoided altogether; rates of avoidable hospitalizations were similar for Medicaid patients and the uninsured (Weissman et al, 1992). Persons with Medicaid are sometimes relegated, with the uninsured, to the lowest tier of the health care system.

Underinsurance   Private health insurance does not guarantee financial access to care. Many people are underinsured, ie, their health insurance coverage has limitations that restrict access to needed services (Bodenheimer, 1992). The landscape of underinsurance in the United States is a varied one (Table 3–4).

Lack of Coverage for Catastrophic Expenses

> Janet Lim, a nurse's aide insured by an HMO, suffered a severely fractured femur following a hit-and-run automobile accident; weight bearing was not allowed for 3 months. After weeks in the hospital, the HMO's benefits ran out.

Table 3–3. Adjusted relative risk of death[1] from breast cancer, New Jersey, 1985–1987.[2]

Privately insured	1
Uninsured	1.49
Medicaid	1.40

[1] Relative risk of death is adjusted for age, race, marital status, income, and stage of disease at time of diagnosis.
[2] Data extracted from Ayanian JZ et al: The relation between health insurance coverage and clinical outcomes among women with breast cancer. N Engl J Med 1993; 329:326.

Table 3–4. Categories of underinsurance.

Lack of coverage for catastrophic expenses
Exclusion of coverage for preexisting illnesses
Services not covered
Insurance deductibles and copayments
Gaps in Medicare coverage
Lack of coverage for long-term care

> Though unable even to sit up in a chair, Ms. Lim became responsible for all her health care costs.

An estimated 29 million people have private health insurance that leaves major expenses uncovered in the event of a serious illness (Short and Banthin, 1995). Fourteen percent of insurance plans have a maximum lifetime benefit of $250,000 or less. Costs for a child with congenital heart disease or anoxic brain damage may exceed this threshold within a few years. Two-thirds of plans limit lifetime costs to $1 million or less; thousands of motor vehicle accidents each year cause head injuries whose medical care exceeds such limits (Pepper Commission, 1990).

Exclusion of Coverage for Preexisting Illnesses

> Two months after changing jobs, Brent McRae [actual name], age 27, developed colon cancer. He thought he was insured, but "Five weeks into the chemotherapy, I walk into my oncologist's office, and he sits me down, puts his hand on my knee, and tells me there's been no payment because John Hancock is denying coverage, saying the cancer was a preexisting condition, even though it hadn't been diagnosed when the coverage began." The chemotherapy was stopped because of Mr. McRae's inability to pay. "At one point in the middle of the whole thing, I hit bottom, between having cancer and being told I had no insurance, and I tried to commit suicide." (High medical costs hurt growing numbers in U.S. New York Times, April 28, 1991.)

In 1990, over 60% of group health insurance plans contained exclusions for preexisting conditions, clauses that deny benefits for any illness present at the time of enrollment in an insurance plan (Sullivan and Rice, 1991). Nine months is the average waiting period before a newly insured person receives coverage for a preexisting condition. The Health Insurance Portability and Accountability Act of 1996 placed limits on the amount of time insurance companies can deny coverage for preexisting illnesses. An estimated 81 million people under age 65 have medical problems (eg, hypertension, diabetes, asthma, chronic back pain) that insurance companies may consider to be preexisting conditions (Citizens Fund, 1991).

Services Not Covered

> Flora Dos Santos was a single mother who gave birth to twins; her insurance plan did not cover childhood vaccinations. She paid $75 for the babies' first set of vaccinations but did not have the money to pay for more shots. One of the twins developed a serious case of measles and nearly died.

In 1989, 55% of employment-based health insurance plans failed to include coverage for basic childhood vaccinations, and 58% did not cover well-baby care. According to Donald Henderson, former dean of the Johns Hopkins School of Hygiene and Public Health, "It has been very difficult to get third-party payers to pay for mammograms, Pap smears, or other preventive services" (Skolnick, 1991). Health maintenance organizations (HMOs) do cover these preventive services, but many traditional insurers do not.

Insurance Deductibles and Copayments

> Eva Stefanski works as a legal secretary and has a Blue Cross policy with a $500 deductible. Last year, she failed to show up for her mammogram appointment because she did not have $120 to pay for the test. This year, she decides to forego her annual gynecologic checkup altogether.

In 1987, 75% of group health insurance plans featured a deductible and 20% or more copayments for physician services. In 1990, employer-sponsored health insurance recipients experienced increases in deductibles, copayments, and out-of-pocket maximums. For plans that were not preferred provider organizations (PPOs) or HMOs (see Chapter 4), the mean 1990 deductible was over $170. HMOs do not require deductibles but do charge copayments for physician visits and medications.

Gaps in Medicare Coverage

> Corazon Estacio suffers from angina, congestive heart failure, and high blood pressure, in addition to diabetes. She takes 17 pills per day: four each of glyburide and isosorbide, three captopril, two potassium chloride, and one each of nifedipine, aspirin, digoxin, and furosemide. Her Medicare HMO does not cover outpatient medications; her yearly medication bill comes to $3840.
>
> In 1997, Ferdinand Foote was covered by Medicare and had no Medigap, HMO, or Medicaid coverage. He was hospitalized for peripheral vascular disease caused by diabetes and a nonhealing infected foot ulcer. He spent 4 days in the acute hospital and 1 month in the skilled nursing facility, and made weekly physician visits following his discharge. The costs of the illness uncovered by Medicare included a $760 deductible for acute hospital care, a $95 per day copayment for days 21–31 of the skilled nursing facility stay, a $100 physician deductible, and a 20% ($8) physician copayment per visit for 12 visits. The total came to $1906, not including the cost of outpatient medications.

Medicare covers only 45% of the medical expenses of the elderly. Almost 20% of Medicare recipients have no supplemental private "Medigap," HMO, or Medicaid coverage. Out-of-pocket expenses among the 10% of the Medicare population with the highest health care costs were about $5600 per beneficiary in 1996. Even individuals with Medigap and HMO policies often pay hundreds of dollars per year for prescription drugs (Pepper Commission, 1990; Physician Payment Review Commission, 1997).

Lack of Coverage for Long-Term Care

> Victoria and Gus Pappas had $80,000 in the bank when Gus had a stroke. After his hospitalization, he was still paralyzed on the right side and unable to speak or to swallow. After 18 months in the nursing home, most of the $80,000 was gone. At that point, Medicaid picked up the nursing home costs.

Medicare pays only 9% of the elderly's nursing home bills, and private insurance policies pick up only an additional 3% (see Chapter 10). Many elderly families spend their life's savings on long-term care, qualifying for Medicaid only after becoming impoverished.

Insecurity About Insurance Coverage

> John McGann [actual name] worked for a music store in Houston for 6 years; the employer served as the insurer. His policy had a $1 million lifetime maximum. Mr. McGann contracted AIDS. Soon after he filed his first claim for medical care, the company set a $5000 lifetime limit on AIDS-related employee health benefits. The courts upheld the company's decision. Mr. McGann's policy had become useless, and he was uninsurable through any other private insurer. (A health insurance horror. New York Times, Nov 16, 1992.)

While not a category of underinsurance in the strict sense, fear of losing health insurance is a pervasive problem. Thirty percent of people surveyed in a 1991 poll reported that someone in their household remained in an unwanted job to avoid losing health benefits (Eckholm, 1991). In small group and individual insurance markets, people found to have chronic conditions face the possibility of large premium increases. Use of screening tests for chronic illnesses among job and health insurance applicants contributes to fear of uninsurability. A 1991 federal appeals court ruling held in the case of John McGann that self-insured employers have the right to reduce maximum lifetime benefits to as low as $5000 for employees who develop AIDS; the average lifetime health care cost for a person with AIDS has been estimated at $85,000 (Hellinger, 1991). For many, health insurance is an uncertain benefit: "If you use it, you lose it."

The Effects of Underinsurance: Does underinsurance represent a serious barrier to the receipt of medical care? The Rand Health Insurance Experiment compared nonelderly individuals who had health insurance plans with no out-of-pocket costs and those who had plans with varying amounts of patient cost sharing (deductibles or copayments). The study found that cost sharing reduces the rate of ambulatory care use, especially among the poor, and that patients with cost-sharing plans demonstrate a reduction in both appropriate and inappropriate medical visits. For low-income adults, the cost-sharing groups received Pap smears 65% as often as the free-care group. Hypertensive adults in the cost-sharing groups had higher diastolic pressures, and children had higher rates of anemia and lower rates of immunization (Lohr et al, 1986; Lurie et al, 1987; Brook et al, 1983).

Hayward et al (1988) studied access to care for adults with chronic or serious medical problems. Eight percent of Medicare recipients and 12% of privately insured working-age adults reported that their illness had caused a major financial problem. The authors concluded that the elderly and privately insured people under 65 years of age face serious access problems because of gaps in Medicare and private insurance coverage.

The percentage of children 1–4 years of age immunized against measles dropped from 66% in 1976 to 61% in 1985, and the number of measles cases rose from 2800 in 1985 to 26,500 in 1990. According to the National Vaccine Advisory Committee, one factor contributing to this epidemic was the reluctance of insurers to include childhood immunizations in their benefit structures (Skolnick, 1991).

In a 1981 survey, 36.5% of uncontrolled hypertensives reported difficulty paying for their medications, compared with 15.5% of those whose blood pressure was controlled; the study concluded that cost of prescriptions contributed to inadequate hypertensive control (Shulman et al, 1986). In 1987, 700,000 insured people were unable to obtain needed emergency services, and over 1 million insured people were unable to obtain needed prescription medications; 60% of these cited cost (inadequate insurance) as the main factor blocking access to these services (Himmelstein and Woolhandler, 1995). In summary, lack of comprehensive insurance reduces access to health care services and may contribute to poorer health outcomes.

NONFINANCIAL BARRIERS TO HEALTH CARE

Nonfinancial barriers to health care include long distances between patients and health care facilities, language and cultural incompatibilities between patients and health care givers, and factors of gender and race. Two of these problems will be discussed here: gender and race.

Gender & Access to Health Care

> Olga Madden is angry. Her male physician had not listened. He told her that her incontinence was from too many childbirths and she'd have to live with it. She had questions about the hormones he was prescribing, but he always seemed too busy, so she never asked. Ms. Madden calls her HMO and gets the names of two women physicians, a female physician assistant, and a nurse practitioner. She calls them. The receptionist tells her that none of them is accepting new patients; they are all too busy.

Studies comparing interactions between female patients and male or female physicians suggest that male physicians often give unsatisfactory answers to patient questions. In one study, male physicians were shown to perform more extensive diagnostic workups for men than for women with the same complaints; a later study failed to confirm these findings (Muller, 1990). Female health care providers are often told by their female patients that male physicians, as in the case of Olga Madden, appear too busy to answer their questions. In fact, female health care providers who do take time with their patients are often busier than their "busy" male colleagues. Women were 50% more likely than men to report leaving a physician because of dissatisfaction with their care, and they were over twice as likely to report that their physician "talked down" to them or told them their problems were "all in their head" (Leiman et al, 1997).

The gender of the physician has been shown in some studies to influence the provision of preventive services for women. In a 1990 study of patients with insurance coverage for Pap smears and mammograms, the patients of female physicians were almost twice as likely to receive a Pap smear and 1.4 times as likely to have a mammogram than the patients of male physicians (Lurie et al, 1993).

Although women are more likely than men to have some form of health insurance coverage, they are more likely to be insured by Medicaid or to be underinsured. Women are 25% more likely than men to report not being able to obtain needed health care (Clancy and Massion, 1992; Berk et al, 1995). Women spend far more out of pocket for their health care than do men.

Millions of privately insured women have plans that exclude coverage for maternity care and for routine preventive health services such as Pap smears. Cost remains the single most common reason women cite for not obtaining preventive screening tests (Leiman et al, 1997). For those women who wish to terminate a pregnancy, access to abortions is limited in many areas of the country. A 1995 poll concluded that only one-third of gynecologists performed abortions (Henry J. Kaiser Family Foundation, 1996). No abortion services were available in 21% of metropolitan areas and 91% of nonmetropolitan counties (Muller, 1990).

For at least two highly technical procedures, women have less access than men. Women with end-stage renal disease are less likely to receive a kidney transplant than men (AMA Council on Ethical and Judicial Affairs, 1991). Most (but not all) studies that have investigated sex differences in treatment of coronary artery disease have found that women are less likely to receive procedures such as coronary angiography, bypass surgery, and angioplasty; these differences are not explained by differences in illness severity or insurance status (Stone et al, 1996; Ayanian and Epstein, 1991; Udvarhelyi et al, 1992; Krumholz et al, 1992). The differences in rates for these cardiac procedures were not, however, reflected in differences in subsequent mortality rates (Udvarhelyi et al, 1992). One large study of hospital care for Medicare patients found that the process of care was similar for men and women. Of the 88 services examined, men and women received an equivalent number of procedures for 72%; for 15% of services, men received more procedures, and for 3%, women received more than men (Pearson et al, 1992).

While women have reduced access to certain kinds of care, an equally serious problem may be instances of inappropriate care. Many hysterectomies are of questionable need even by conservative standards; one-third of women in the United States have had hysterectomies by age 60 years. Many cesarean section deliveries are inappropriately performed (Muller, 1990). Women are prescribed tranquilizers 2.5 times as often as men (Society for the Advancement of Women's Health Research, 1994).

Race & Access to Health Care

> Jose is suffering. The pain from his fractured femur is excruciating, and the emergency room doctor has given him no pain medication. In the next room, Joe is asleep. He has received 10 mg of morphine for his femur fracture.

At a California emergency room during 1990 and 1991, 55% of Latino patients with extremity fractures received no pain medication, compared with 26% of non-Latino whites. This marked difference in treatment was attributable not to insurance status but to ethnicity (Todd et al, 1993).

Because a far higher proportion of minorities than whites is uninsured, has Medicaid coverage, or is poor, access problems are amplified for these groups. African-Americans and Latinos in the United States receive fewer physician visits, preventive services, and surgical procedures than white non-Latino patients. In some instances, such as access to primary care services for children, much of these disparities appear to be explained by the less extensive insurance coverage among nonwhite groups (Halfon, 1997). But racial and ethnic differences in access to care are not always simply a matter of differences in financial resources and insurance coverage. Many studies have shown that African-Americans and Latinos receive fewer services even when compared with non-Latino whites who have the same level of health insurance and income.

Patterns of care for patients with coronary artery disease insured by Medicare, for example, differ according to patient race. Despite similar insurance coverage and clinical status, white Medicare patients are 30–50% more likely than African-American patients to undergo procedures such as coronary angiography, bypass surgery, and angioplasty (Ford and Cooper, 1995). Similar differences exist in treatment patterns for coronary artery disease among African-Americans and whites eligible for the same health benefits in Veterans Administration medical facilities. Latino patients hospitalized for cardiac disease in Los Angeles have also been found to be 20% less likely than non-Latino whites to receive coronary angiography or bypass surgery, even after controlling for income and type of insurance (Carlisle et al, 1995). Studies have also detected such disparities in the receipt of primary care services. African-Americans insured by Medicare are 25% less likely to receive mammograms and 40% less likely to receive influenza vaccines than white Medicare beneficiaries with comparable incomes (Gornick et al, 1996). Satisfaction with health care, as well as rates of service use, differs according to race. Compared with whites, African-Americans surveyed in 1992 were twice as likely to rate the quality and responsiveness of health services as only fair or poor (Blendon et al, 1995).

Neighborhoods that have high proportions of African-American or Latino residents have far fewer physicians practicing in these communities. Even among communities that are not low income, neighborhoods with high proportions of white residents have a greater supply of PCPs than do minority communities. African-American and Latino PCPs are more likely than white physicians to locate their practices in underserved communities (Komaromy et al, 1996).

What explains these disparities in access to care across racial and ethnic groups that are not fully accounted for by differences in insurance coverage and socioeconomic status? Several hypotheses have been proposed. Cultural differences may exist in patients' beliefs about the value of medical care and attitudes toward seeking treatment for their symptoms. One study found that African-Americans were less likely than whites to agree to coronary artery bypass surgery when recommended by their physician (Maynard et al, 1986), although differences in patient preferences do not appear to account for racial variations in cardiac surgery rates in all studies. Latinos and non-Latino whites have been found to have different attitudes and knowledge about cancer, with Latinos being more likely to have a fatalistic view of cancer. However, these differences in beliefs were not found to lead to differences in the use of cancer-screening services among Latinos and non-Latinos (Perez-Stable et al, 1995). A related factor may be ineffective communication between patients and care givers of differing races, cultures, and language. African-Americans are more likely than whites to report that their physician did not properly explain their illness and its treatment (AMA Council, 1990). Access barriers related to communication problems may be particularly acute for the subset of Latino patients for whom Spanish is the primary language. However, language issues clearly do not fully account for access barriers faced by Latinos. In the study of emergency room pain medication cited previously, even Latinos who spoke English as their primary language were much less likely than non-Latino whites to receive pain medication.

Because many of these hypotheses do not satisfactorily explain the observed racial disparities in access to care, an important consideration is whether racism may also contribute to these patterns. Medicine in the United States has not escaped the nation's legacy of institutionalized racism toward many minority groups. Many hospitals—including institutions in the North—were for much of the twentieth century either completely segregated or had segregated wards, with inferior facilities and services available to nonwhites. Explicit segregation policies persisted in many hospitals until a few decades ago. Racial barriers to entry into the medical profession gave rise to the establishment of black medical schools, such as the Howard, Morehouse, and Meharry schools of medicine. Although such overt racism is a diminishing feature of medicine in the United States, more insidious and often unconscious forms of discrimination continue to color the interactions between patients and their care givers and influence access to care for minorities.

THE RELATION BETWEEN HEALTH CARE & HEALTH STATUS

Access to health care does not by itself guarantee good health. A complex array of factors, one of which is health care, determines whether a person is healthy or not.

> Ace Banks is 48, an executive vice president, with four grandparents who lived past 90 years of age and parents alive and well in their late 70s. Mr. Banks went to an Ivy League college, where he was a star athlete. He has never seen a physician, except for a sprained ankle.

> Keith Cole is a coal miner, and at age 48, he developed pneumonia. He had excellent health insurance through his union, and went to see the leading pulmonologist in the state. He was hospitalized but became less and less able to breathe because the pneumonia was severely complicated by black lung disease, which he contracted through his job. He received high-quality care in the intensive care unit at a fully insured cost of $65,000, but he died.

> Bill Downes, an African-American male, knew that his father was killed by high blood pressure and his mother died of diabetes. Mr. Downes spent his childhood in poverty, living with eight children at his grandmother's house. He had little to eat except what was provided at the school

lunch program, a diet heavily laden with cheese and butter. To support the family, he left school at age 15 and got a job. At age 24, he was diagnosed with high blood pressure and diabetes. He did not smoke and was meticulous in following the diet prescribed by his physician. He had private health insurance through his job as a security guard, and was cared for by a professor of medicine at the medical school. In spite of excellent medical care, his glucose and cholesterol levels and blood pressure were difficult to control, and he developed retinopathy, kidney failure, and coronary heart disease. At age 48, he collapsed at work and died of a heart attack.

The achievement of a healthy population requires not only health care—preventive care and medical treatment—but also

full employment and adequate family income; improved working conditions; decent housing, including the elimination of urban and rural slums and the grim spectacle of homeless Americans; effective protection from environmental discomforts such as excessive heat and cold, smog, noise and noxious odors; good nutrition that will foster optimal physical and mental development; increased financial support to public education and elimination of financial barriers to higher education; improved opportunities for rest, recreation, and cultural development; greater participation in community activities and decision-making; an end to discrimination . . . based on race, gender, age, social class, religious belief, national background or sexual preference; and freedom from the pervasive fear of violence, war, and nuclear annihilation. (Terris M: What is health promotion? J Public Health Policy 1986;7:146.)

Health Status & Income As the stories of Ace Banks, Keith Cole, and Bill Downes suggest, the health of an individual or a population is influenced less by medical care than by broad socioeconomic factors. One-seventh of people in the United States and one-fourth of children under age 6 years live in a family with an income below the federal poverty level. In 1986, people in the United States with a yearly income of less than $9000 had a death rate three to six times higher than those with a yearly income of $25,000 or more (Table 3–5). The mortality rate for heart

Table 3–5. Income, race, and mortality rates (1986 age-adjusted deaths per 1000 for ages 25–64).*

	Men		Women	
Income	White	African-American	White	African-American
Under $9000	16.0	19.5	6.5	7.6
$9000–14,999	10.2	10.8	3.4	4.5
$15,000–18,999	5.7	9.8	3.3	3.7
$19,000–24,999	4.6	4.7	3.0	2.8
$25,000 or more	2.4	3.6	1.6	2.3

* Data extracted from Terris M: Determinants of health: A progressive political platform. J Public Health Policy 1994;15(1):5.

Table 3–6. Limitation of activity caused by chronic illness, 1994.*

	% of Population With Limited Activity
Total population	14.3
African-American	18.0
White	14.0
Family income under $14,000	26.4
$14,000–24,999	16.5
$25,000–34,999	13.6
$35,000–49,999	11.5
$50,000 or more	9.2

* Data extracted from U.S. Department of Health and Human Services, Health United States 1995. 1996.

disease among laborers is more than twice the rate for managers and professionals. The incidence of cancer increases as family income decreases, and survival rates are lower for low-income cancer patients. Higher infant mortality rates are linked to low income and low educational level. In 1994, people in families with incomes of less than $14,000 per year were almost three times as likely as those with incomes of $50,000 or more to be limited in their normal daily activities as a result of chronic illness (Table 3–6). Similarly, children in poor households are twice as likely as those who are not poor to have limitations in school and play activities because of illness (Newacheck et al, 1995). Over 20% of people with incomes below $14,000 reported themselves to be in fair or poor health, compared with 3.9% of those with incomes over $50,000 (U.S. Department of Health and Human Services, 1996; Angell, 1993; Navarro, 1991).

Health Status & Race African-Americans experience dramatically worse health than white Americans. Life expectancy is far lower for African-Americans than for other racial and ethnic groups in the United States (Table 3–7). African-American men living in Harlem, New York, have less chance of surviving to age 65 years than men living in Bangladesh, and this trend appears to be worsening over time (McCord and Freeman, 1990; Geronimus et al, 1996). In 1993, African-American men had a life expectancy that was 2 years shorter than the life expectancy for white men half a century ago (Table 3–7). Infant mortality rates among African-Americans are double those for whites, and the relative disparity in infant mortality has widened during the

Table 3–7. Life expectancy in years.[1]

	Women	Men
In 1950		
White	72.2	66.5
African-American	62.7	58.9
In 1993		
White	79.5	73.1
African-American	73.7	64.6

[1] Data extracted from U.S. Department of Health and Human Services. Health United States 1995. 1996.

Table 3–8. Infant mortality, 1991 (per 1000 live births).[1]

White, non-Latino	7.0
African-American	16.6
Latino	7.1
Asian American	5.8
Native American	11.3

[1] Data extracted from U.S. Department of Health and Human Services. Health United States 1995. 1996.

past decade (Table 3–8). Mortality rates for African-Americans exceed those for whites for 8 of the 10 leading causes of death in the United States. Although deaths resulting from AIDS and homicide are relatively higher among African-Americans, most of the excess mortality among African-Americans is attributable to the common "killers" in the U.S. population: heart disease, strokes, and cancer (Geronimus et al, 1996; Secretary's Task Force on Black and Minority Health, 1985). For example, African-American men under 45 years have 10 times the likelihood of dying of hypertension than white men in the same age group. Although the incidence of breast cancer is lower in African-American women than in white women, in African-American women this disease is diagnosed at a more advanced stage of illness, and they are more likely to die of breast cancer (Ayanian et al, 1993; U.S. Department of Health and Human Services, 1996). Death rates for African-Americans are higher across a variety of different diseases characterized by differing causes, and this makes it unlikely that these racial disparities reflect a genetic disposition toward premature mortality among African-Americans.

African-Americans have an excess burden of morbidity as well as mortality. African-Americans are 30% more likely than whites to have a chronic illness that limits their activity (Table 3–6), and are nearly twice as likely to report that they are in poor or fair health (U.S. Department of Health and Human Services, 1996).

American Indians are another ethnic group with far poorer health than that of whites. American Indians under age 45 years have far higher death rates than whites of comparable age, and the American Indian infant mortality rate is 1.6 times the rate of whites (U.S. Department of Health and Human Services, 1996).

Latinos and Asian and Pacific Islanders are minority groups characterized by great diversity. Health status varies widely between Cuban Americans, who tend to be more affluent, and poor Mexican-American migrant farm workers; between Japanese families, who are more likely to be middle class, and Laotians, who are often indigent. Compared with whites, Latinos have three times the risk of diabetes, an increased prevalence of hypertension, and higher rates of tuberculosis and AIDS (AMA Council on Scientific Affairs, 1991). Overall, Latinos have lower age-adjusted mortality rates than whites because of less cardiovascular disease in Latino men, and mortality rates from cancer are lower in Puerto Rican and Mexican immigrants. Asians in the United States have lower death rates than whites for all age groups (Fingerhut and Makuc, 1992).

Some of the differences in mortality rates between African-Americans and American Indians compared with whites are related to the higher rates of poverty among these minority peoples. In 1994, the white poverty rate was 12%, compared with 31% for African-Americans. In 1994, 43% of African-American children lived in households with incomes below the poverty line, compared with 16% of white children. The African-American unemployment rate has been twice that of whites for over 30 years. One-fourth of American Indian families have incomes below the poverty level (U.S. Department of Health and Human Services, 1996).

Even compared with whites in the same income class, African-Americans appear to have inferior health status. Although mortality rates decline with rising income among both African-Americans and whites, at any given income level the mortality rate for African-Americans is consistently higher than the rate for whites (Table 3–5). Thus, social factors and stresses related to race itself seem to contribute to the relatively poorer health of African-Americans. A portion of the inferior health outcomes among African-Americans, such as lower survival for women with breast cancer, is also probably explained by the lower access to health services among this group described earlier in this chapter. However, in some cases this relationship may not be so direct. For example, despite less use of invasive coronary procedures in African-Americans, African-Americans and whites with coronary artery disease appear to have similar functional status and survival after diagnosis (Ayanian, 1994; Stone et al, 1996).

If lower income is associated with poorer health, and if Latinos tend to be poorer than non-Latino whites (poverty rate of 29%) in the United States, then why do Latinos have overall lower mortality rates than non-Latino whites? This is probably related to the fact that many Latinos are immigrants, and foreign-born people often have lower mortality rates than people born in the United States at the same level of income. This phenomenon is often referred to as the "healthy immigrant" effect. If this is the case, mortality rates for Latinos may rise as a higher proportion of their population is born in the United States. The "healthy immigrant" effect may also occur among African-American groups in the United States. For example, Caribbean-born blacks residing in New York have lower rates of cardiovascular disease than both whites and American-born blacks in New York (Fang et al, 1996).

Access to Health Care & Health Status To what degree is the poorer health among low-income people caused by their reduced access to health care? Considerable evidence exists that socioeconomic status (income, education, and occupation) rather than access to health care may be the dominant determinant of health status.

(1) It is not just poverty but any variation in socioeconomic status that is a strong, consistent predictor of morbidity and premature mortality rates. In the United States, differences in mortality rates among census tracts are associated with the median family income of the census tract. In the United Kingdom, mortality rates in 1981 were inversely related to occupational status, being the highest for unskilled workers, second highest for semiskilled workers, third highest for skilled workers, fourth highest for managers, and lowest for professionals (Susser, 1993).

Were health status in the United States largely determined by access to health care, one would expect that the poor (uninsured and Medicaid patients) would have a poorer health status but that the association between health status and socioeconomic status would disappear for middle- and higher-income people with private insurance, whose access to health care would likely be similar (Adler et al, 1993). In fact, health status improves as one ascends the socioeconomic ladder through the entire range of incomes, thereby making it less likely that differences in access to care fully explain differences in health status.

(2) If access to care accounted for most of the differences in health status, mortality rates from illnesses amenable to treatment should show a strong association with socioeconomic status, and untreatable illnesses should show a weaker association. In fact, the association of health status with socioeconomic status is just as strong for illnesses not amenable to treatment (Adler et al, 1993).

(3) Nations with universal health insurance systems that have greatly reduced the disparity in access to care between lower- and higher-income people (eg, the United Kingdom and Canada) continue to have disparities in health status among socioeconomic classes (Angell, 1993; Susser, 1993; Adler et al, 1993; Badgley, 1991).

(4) Though access to care in the United States for millions of lower-income people improved markedly from 1960 to 1986 because of Medicaid, the gap in mortality rates between lower- and higher-income people widened during that period, which was characterized by increasing income inequality (Pappas et al, 1993).

This discussion might lead to the belief that medical care does not matter, and that only by reducing the gap between rich and poor can people be made healthier. Such a belief would err in dismissing a valuable role for health care. While socioeconomic status may be the dominant influence on health status, medical care and public health interventions are extremely important. The advent of the polio vaccine markedly reduced the number of paralytic polio cases. From 1970 to 1983, death rates from stroke decreased by about 50%, a successful result of hypertension diagnosis and treatment. Early prenatal care can prevent low birth weights and infant deaths. Irradiation and chemotherapy have transformed the prognosis of some cancers (eg, Hodgkin's disease) from a certain fatal outcome toward complete cure. A 1980 study of mortality rates in 400 counties in the United States found that after controlling for income, education, cigarette consumption, and prevalence of disability, a 10% increase in per capita medical care expenditures was associated with a reduced average mortality rate of 1.57% (Roemer, 1991). Moreover, the health care system provides patients with chronic disease welcome relief from pain and suffering and helps them to cope with their illnesses. Access to health care does not guarantee good health, but without such access, health is certain to suffer.

REFERENCES

Adler NE et al: Socioeconomic inequalities in health. JAMA 1993;269:3140.

AMA Council on Ethical and Judicial Affairs: Black-white disparities in health care. JAMA 1990;263:2344.

AMA Council on Ethical and Judicial Affairs: Gender disparities in clinical decision making. JAMA 1991;266:559.

AMA Council on Scientific Affairs: Hispanic health in the United States. JAMA 1991;265:248.

Angell M: Privilege and health: What is the connection? N Engl J Med 1993;329:126.

Ayanian JZ: Race, class, and the quality of medical care. JAMA 1994;271:1207.

Ayanian JZ, Epstein AM: Differences in the use of procedures betwen women and men hospitalized for coronary heart disease. N Engl J Med 1991;325:221.

Ayanian JZ et al: The relation between health insurance coverage and clinical outcomes among women with breast cancer. N Engl J Med 1993;329:326.

Badgley RF: Social and economic disparities under Canadian health care. Int J Health Serv 1991;21:659.

Bennefield RL: Health insurance coverage: 1995. U.S. Dept of Commerce: Economics and Statistics Administration, P60-195, September 1996a.

Bennefield RL: Who loses coverage and for how long? U.S. Dept of Commerce: Economics and Statistics Administration, P70-54, May 1996b.

Berk ML, Schur CL, Cantor JC: Ability to obtain health care: Recent estimates from the Robert Wood Johnson Foundation national access to care survey. Health Aff 1995; 14(3):139.

Blendon RJ et al: How White and African Americans view their health and social problems. JAMA 1995;273:341.

Blendon RJ et al: Medicaid beneficiaries and health reform. Health Aff 1993;12(1):132.

Blendon RJ et al: Uncompensated care by hospitals or public insurance for the poor: Does it make a difference? N Engl J Med 1986;314:1160.

Bodenheimer T: Underinsurance in America. N Engl J Med 1992;327:274.

Braveman P et al: Access to prenatal care following major Medicaid eligibility expansions. JAMA 1993;269:1285.

Braveman P et al: Adverse outcomes and lack of health insurance among newborns in an eight-county area of California, 1982 to 1986. N Engl J Med 1989;321:508.

Braveman P et al: Insurance-related differences in the risk of ruptured appendix. N Engl J Med 1994;331:444.

Brook RH et al: Does free care improve adults' health? N Engl J Med 1983;309:1426.

Carlisle DM, Leake BD, Shapiro MF: Racial and ethnic differences in the use of invasive cardiac procedures among cardiac patients in Los Angeles County, 1986 through 1988. Am J Public Health 1995;85:352.

Clancy CM, Massion CT: American women's health care. JAMA 1992;268:1918.

Donelan K et al: Whatever happened to the health insurance crisis in the United States? Voices from a national survey. JAMA 1996;276:1346.

Eckholm E: Health benefits found to deter job switching. New York Times, Sept 26, 1991.

Fang J, Madhavan S, Alderman MH: The association between birthplace and mortality from cardiovascular causes among Black and White residents of New York City. N Engl J Med 1996;335:1545.

Fingerhut LA, Makuc DM: Mortality among minority populations in the United States. Am J Public Health 1992;82:1168.

Ford ES, Cooper RS: Racial/ethnic differences in health care utilization of cardiovascular procedures: A review of the evidence. Health Serv Res 1995;30(1):237.

Franks P, Clancy CM, Gold MR: Health insurance and mortality. JAMA 1993b;270:737.

Franks P et al: Health insurance and subjective health status: Data from the 1987 National Medical Expenditure Survey. Am J Public Health 1993a;83:1295.

Freeman HE et al: Americans report on their access to health care. In: The Nation's Health. Lee PR, Estes CL (editors). Jones & Bartlett, 1990.

Friedman E: The uninsured: From dilemma to crisis. JAMA 1991;265:2491.

Geronimus AT et al: Excess mortality among Blacks and Whites in the United States. N Engl J Med 1996;335:1552.

Gornick ME et al: Effects of race and income on mortality and use of services among Medicare beneficiaries. N Engl J Med 1996;35:791.

Grumbach K, Keane D, Bindman A: Primary care and public emergency department overcrowding. Am J Public Health 1993;83:372.

Hadley J, Steinberg EP, Feder J: Comparison of uninsured and privately insured hospital patients. JAMA 1991;265:374.

Halfon N et al: Medicaid enrollment and health services access by Latino children in inner-city Los Angeles. JAMA 1997;277:636.

Hayward RA et al: Inequities in health services among insured Americans. N Engl J Med 1988;318:1507.

A health insurance horror. New York Times, Nov 16, 1992.

Hellinger FJ: Forecasting the medical care costs of the HIV epidemic: 1991–1994. Inquiry 1991;28:213.

The Henry J. Kaiser Family Foundation: Making sense of health care; meeting health care needs. 1996 Report.

High medical costs hurt growing numbers in U.S. New York Times, April 28, 1991.

Himmelstein DU, Woolhandler S: Care denied: US residents who are unable to obtain needed medical services. Am J Public Health 1995;85:341.

Himmelstein DU, Woolhandler S, Wolfe SM: The vanishing health care safety net: New data on uninsured Americans. Int J Health Serv 1992;22:381.

The Kaiser Commission on the Future of Medicaid: Medicaid Expenditures and Beneficiaries, 1984–1994. Nov 1996.

Komaromy M et al: The role of Black and Hispanic physicians in providing health care for underserved populations. N Engl J Med 1996;334:1305.

Krumholz HM et al: Selection of patients for coronary angiography and coronary revascularization early after myocardial infarction: Is there evidence for a gender bias? Ann Intern Med 1992;116:785.

Leiman JM et al: Selected facts on U.S. women's health: A chart book. The Commonwealth Fund, March 1997.

Light DW: The practice and ethics of risk-rated health insurance. JAMA 1992;267:2503.

Lohr KN et al: Use of medical care in the Rand Health Insurance Experiment. Med Care 1986(Suppl);24:S1.

Lohr S. Though upbeat on the economy, people still fear for their jobs. New York Times, Dec 29, 1996, p 1.

Lurie N et al: Preventive care: Do we practice what we preach? Am J Public Health 1987;77:801.

Lurie N et al: Preventive care for women: Does the sex of the physician matter? N Engl J Med 1993;329:478.

Lurie N et al: Termination from MediCal: Does it affect health? N Engl J Med 1984;311:480.

Maynard C et al: Blacks in the coronary artery surgery study (CASS): Race and clinical decision making. Am J Public Health 1986:76:1446.

McCord C, Freeman HP: Excess mortality in Harlem. N Engl J Med 1990;322:173.

Morrisey MA et al: Small employers and the health insurance market. Health Aff 1994;13(5):149.

Muller CF: Health Care and Gender. Russell Sage Foundation, 1990.

Navarro V: Race or class or race and class: Growing mortality differentials in the United States. Int J Health Serv 1991;21:229.

Newacheck PW et al: The effect on children of curtailing Medicaid spending. JAMA 1995;274:1468.

Pappas G et al: The increasing disparity in mortality between socioeconomic groups in the United States, 1960 and 1986. N Engl J Med 1993;329:103.

Pearson ML et al: Differences in quality of care for hospitalized elderly men and women. JAMA 1992;268:1883.

Pepper Commission: A Call for Action. U.S. Government Printing Office, 1990.

Perez-Stable EJ, Sabogal F, Otero-Sabogal R: Use of cancer-screening tests in the San Francisco Bay area: Comparison of Latinos and Anglos. J Natl Cancer Inst 1995;18:147.

Physician Payment Review Commission: Annual Report to Congress. 1997.

Renner C, Navarro V: Why is our population of uninsured and underinsured persons growing? The consequences of the "deindustrialization" of the United States. Int J Health Serv 1989;19:433.

Roemer MI: National Health Systems of the World. Oxford Univ Press, 1991.

Schroeder SA: The medically uninsured: Will they always be with us? N Engl J Med 1996;334:1130.

Secretary's Task Force on Black and Minority Health: Report. U.S. Department of Health and Human Services, 1985.

The seven warning signs: Health insurance at risk. Citizens Fund, 1991.

Shea S et al: Predisposing factors for severe, uncontrolled hypertension in an inner-city minority population. N Engl J Med 1992;327:776.

Short PF, Banthin JS: New estimates of the underinsured younger than 65 years. JAMA 1995;274:1302.

Shulman NB et al: Financial cost as an obstacle to hypertension therapy. Am J Public Health 1986;76:1105.

Skolnick A: Should insurance cover routine immunizations? JAMA 1991;265:2453.

Smith MD et al: Taking the public's pulse on health reform. Health Aff 1992;11(2):125.

Society for the Advancement of Women's Health Research: Toward a women's health research agenda. In: Health Policy and Nursing. Harrington C, Estes CL (editors). Jones & Bartlett, 1994.

Stone PH et al: Influence of race, sex, and age on management of unstable angina and non-Q-wave myocardial infarction. JAMA 1996;275:1104.

Sullivan CB, Rice T: The health insurance picture in 1990. Health Aff 1991;10(2):104.

Susser M: Health as a human right: An epidemiologist's perspective on the public health. Am J Public Health 1993;83:418.

Terris M: Determinants of health: A progressive political platform. J Public Health Policy 1994;15(1):5.

Terris M: What is health promotion? J Public Health Policy 1986;7:147.

Todd KH, Samaroo N, Hoffman JR: Ethnicity as a risk factor for inadequate emergency department analgesia. JAMA 1993;269:1537.

Udvarhelyi IS et al: Acute myocardial infarction in the Medicare population. JAMA 1992;268:2530.

U.S. Congress, Office of Technology Assessment: Does Health Insurance Make a Difference? OTA-BP-H-99. U.S. Government Printing Office, 1992.

U.S. Department of Health and Human Services: Health United States 1995. 1996.

U.S. General Accounting Office: Private Health Insurance. (GAO/HEHS-97-8), 1996.

Valdez RB et al: Insuring Latinos against the costs of illness. JAMA 1993;269:889.

Weissman JS, Gatsonis C, Epstein AM: Rates of avoidable hospitalization by insurance status in Massachusetts and Maryland. JAMA 1992;268:2388.

Woolhandler S, Himmelstein DH: Reverse targeting of preventive care due to lack of health insurance. JAMA 1988;259:2872.

Reimbursing Health Care Providers

4

Chapter 2 described the different modes of financing health care: out-of-pocket payments, individual health insurance, employment-based health insurance, and government financing. Each of these mechanisms attempted to solve the problem of unaffordable care for certain groups, but each "solution" in turn created new problems by stimulating rapid rises in health care costs. One of the factors contributing to this inflation was reimbursement of physicians and hospitals by insurance companies and government programs. Therefore, new methods of reimbursement are now being promoted as one way of lowering the growth rate in health care costs; these new methods are a central feature of managed care.

> Dr. Mary Young has recently finished her family practice residency and joined a small group practice, PrimaryCare. On her first day, she has the following experiences with health care financing: her first patient is insured by Blue Shield; PrimaryCare is paid a fee for the physical examination and for the EKG performed. Dr. Young's second patient requires the same services, for which PrimaryCare receives no payment but is forwarded $10 for each month that the patient is enrolled in the practice. In the afternoon, a hospital utilization review physician calls Dr. Young, explains the DRG payment system, and suggests that she send home a patient hospitalized with pneumonia. In the evening, she goes to the emergency room, where she has agreed to work two shifts per week for $55 per hour.

During the course of a typical day, many physicians will be involved with four or five distinct types of reimbursement. This chapter will describe the different ways in which physicians and hospitals are paid. Although reimbursement has many facets, from the setting of prices to the processing of claims, this discussion will focus on one of its most basic elements: establishing the unit of payment. This basic principle must be grasped before one can understand the key managed care concept of physician-borne "risk."

UNITS OF PAYMENT

Methods of payment can be placed along a continuum that extends from the least to the most aggregated unit. The methods range from the simplest (one fee for one service rendered) to the most complex (one payment for many types of services rendered), with many variations in between (Table 4–1) (Lee et al, 1990).

Definitions of Methods of Payment

Fee-for-Service Reimbursement: The unit of payment is the visit or procedure: The physician or hospital is paid a fee for each office visit, EKG, intravenous fluid, or

Table 4–1. Units of payment.

| | Least Aggregated ◀──────────────────────────────────▶ Most Aggregated | | | | |
	Procedure	Day	Episode of Illness	Patient	Time
Physician	Fee-for-service	—	Surgical or obstetric fee Physician DRG[1]	Capitation	Salary
Hospital	Fee-for-service	Per diem	Hospital DRG	Capitation	Global budget

[1] DRG = diagnosis-related group.

other service or supply provided. This is the only form of payment that is based on individual components of health care. All other reimbursement modes aggregate or group together several services into one unit of payment.

Reimbursement by Episode of Illness: The physician or hospital is paid one sum for all services delivered during one illness, as is the case with global surgical fees for physicians and diagnosis-related groups (DRGs) for hospitals.

Per Diem Payments to Hospitals: The hospital is paid for all services delivered to a patient during 1 day.

Capitation Payment: One payment is made for each patient's treatment during a month or year; this method is closely associated with managed care.

Payment for All Services Delivered to All Patients Within a Certain Time Period: This includes global budget reimbursement of hospitals and salaried payment of physicians.

Managed Care Plans Traditionally, physicians and hospitals have been paid on a fee-for-service basis. During the 1980s, more and more people enrolled in managed care plans, which often change the methods by which hospitals and physicians are paid, for the purpose of controlling costs. Managed care organizations are discussed in more detail in Chapter 7; in this chapter, only those aspects needed to understand physician and hospital reimbursement will be considered.

There are three major forms of managed care organizations: fee-for-service practice with utilization review, preferred provider organizations (PPOs), and health maintenance organizations (HMOs).

Fee-for-Service Reimbursement With Utilization Review: This is the traditional type of reimbursement, with the addition that the third-party payer (whether private insurance company or government agency) assumes the power to authorize or deny payment for expensive medical interventions such as hospital admissions, extra hospital days, and surgeries.

PPOs: PPOs are loose-knit organizations in which insurers contract with a limited number of physicians and hospitals who agree to care for patients, usually on a discounted fee-for-service basis with utilization review.

HMOs: HMOs are organizations whose patients are required (except in emergencies) to receive their care from providers within that HMO. There are several types of HMOs, which are discussed in Chapter 7. HMOs tend to pay physicians and hospitals by more highly bundled units of payment (eg, per diem, capitation, or salary).

METHODS OF PHYSICIAN PAYMENT

Payment Per Procedure: Fee-for-Service

> Roy Sweet, a patient of Dr. Weisman, is seen for recent on-set of diabetes. Dr. Weisman spends 20 minutes performing an examination, finger-stick blood glucose test, urinalysis, and EKG. Each service has a fee set by Dr. Weisman: $62 for a complex visit, $8 for a finger-stick glucose test, $12 for a urinalysis, and $60 for an EKG. Because Mr. Sweet is uninsured, Dr. Weisman reduces the total bill from $142 to $70.

> In 1988, Dr. Lenz requested that Dr. Weisman do a medical consultation for Gertrude Rales, who developed congestive heart failure and arrhythmias following cataract surgery. Dr. Weisman took 90 minutes to perform the consultation and was paid $100 by Medicare. Dr. Lenz had spent 90 minutes on the surgery plus pre- and postoperative care and received $1600 from Medicare. In 1995, Dr. Weisman did a similar consultation for Dr. Lenz and received $130; Dr. Lenz was sent $900 for the operation.

> Melissa High, a Medicaid recipient, makes three visits to Dr. Weisman for hypertension. He bills Medicaid $62 for one complex visit and $32 each for two shorter visits. He is paid $16 per visit, less than 40% of his total charges. Under Medicaid, Dr. Weisman may not bill Ms. High for the balance of his fees.

> Dr. Weisman contracted with Blue Cross to care for its PPO patients at 70% of his normal fee. Rick Payne, a PPO patient, comes in with a severe headache and is found to have left arm weakness and hyperreflexia; Dr. Weisman is paid $43.40 for a complex visit. Before an MRI scan can be ordered, the PPO must be called for authorization.

Traditionally, private physicians have been reimbursed by patients and insurers through the fee-for-service mechanism. Before the passage of Medicare and Medicaid, physicians often discounted fees for elderly or poor patients, and even afterward, many physicians have continued to assist uninsured people in this way.

Private insurers, as well as Medicare and Medicaid in the early years, usually reimbursed physicians according to the usual, customary, and reasonable (UCR) system, which allowed physicians a great deal of latitude in setting fees (Langwell and Nelson, 1986).

With cost containment becoming a priority in the past decade, the UCR approach to fees has been largely supplanted by payer-determined fee schedules. An example of this is Melissa High's three visits, which incurred charges of $126 of which Medicaid paid only $48 ($16 per visit).

In the early 1990s, Medicare moved to a fee schedule determined by a resource-based relative-value scale (RBRVS). With this system, fees (which vary by geographic area) are set for each service by estimating the time, mental effort and judgment, technical skill, physical effort, and stress typically related to that service (Lee et al, 1989). The RBRVS system attempts to correct the bias of physician payment that has historically paid for surgical and other procedures at a far higher rate than primary care and cognitive services. In 1995, Dr. Weisman was paid nearly 15% of Dr. Lenz's surgery fee, compared with only 6% of that fee in 1988, before the advent of RBRVS.

PPO managed care plans often pay contracted physicians on a discounted fee-for-service basis and require prior authorization for expensive procedures.

With fee-for-service payments, physicians have an economic incentive to perform more services because more services bring in more payments (see Chapter 12). The fee-for-service incentive to provide more services contributed to the rapid rise in health care costs in the United States (Relman, 1983).

Payment Per Episode of Illness

> Dr. Nick Belli removes Tom Stone's gallbladder and is paid $1300 by Blue Cross. Besides performing the cholecystectomy, Dr. Belli sees Mr. Stone three times in the hospital and twice in his office for postoperative visits. Because surgery is paid by means of a global fee, Dr. Belli may not bill separately for the visits, which are included in his $1300 cholecystectomy fee.

> Joan Flemming complains of having had coughing, fever, and green sputum for 1 week. Dr. Violet Gramm analyzes a sputum smear and orders a chest x-ray and makes the diagnosis of pneumonia. She treats Ms. Flemming as an outpatient with a cephalosporin, checking her twice a week for 3 weeks. With the experimental ambulatory DRG system, Dr. Gramm is paid one fee for all services and procedures involved in Ms. Flemming's pneumonia.

Surgeons usually receive a single payment for several services (the surgery itself and postoperative care) that have been grouped together, and obstetricians are paid in a similar manner for a delivery plus pre- and postnatal care. This bundling together of payments is often referred to as reimbursement at the unit of the case or episode.

With payment by episode, surgeons have an economic incentive to limit the number of postoperative visits because they do not receive extra payment for extra visits. On the other hand, they continue to have an incentive to perform more surgeries, as with the traditional fee-for-service system. Some health care experts recommend paying physicians through a DRG system (see below) similar to that used by Medicare for hospital reimbursement (Langwell and Nelson, 1986). Under such a system, which is currently experimental, one fee would be paid for one episode of illness, no matter how many times the patient visited the physician.

At this point, it is helpful to introduce the important concept of risk. Risk refers to the potential to lose money, earn less money, or spend more time without additional payment on a reimbursement transaction. With the traditional fee-for-service system, the payer (insurance company, government agency, or patient) absorbs all the risk; if Dr. Weisman sees Rick Payne 10 times rather than five times for his headaches, Blue Cross pays more money and Mr. Payne spends more in copayments. Bundling of services transfers a portion of the risk from the payer to the physician; if Dr. Belli sees Tom Stone 10 times rather than five times for follow-up after cholecystectomy, he does not receive any additional money. Similarly, if Dr. Gramm sees Joan Flemming

10 times rather than six times for her pneumonia, the insurer spends no additional money and the physician does not receive additional payments for the additional time spent with the patient. Payment by episode of illness transfers a portion of the risk from the payer to the physician. As a general rule, the more services bundled into one payment, the larger the share of financial risk that is shifted from payer to provider.

Payment Per Patient: Capitation With Two-Tiered Structures

> Jennifer is a young woman in England who develops an ear infection; her general practitioner, Dr. Walter Liston, sees her and prescribes antibiotics. Jennifer pays no money at the time of the visit and receives no bill. Dr. Liston is paid the British equivalent of $5 per month to care for Jennifer, no matter how many times she requires care. When Jennifer develops appendicitis and requires an x-ray and surgical consultation, Dr. Liston sends her to the local hospital for these services; payment for these referral services is incorporated into the hospital's operating budget paid for separately by the National Health Service.

British System: Capitation payments (ie, per capita payments, or payments "by the head") to physicians in the United States are complicated, as will shortly be seen. But in the United Kingdom, they have traditionally been relatively simple (see Chapter 14). Under the traditional British National Health Service, each person enrolls with a general practitioner, who becomes the primary care physician (PCP). For each person on the general practitioner's list, the physician receives a monthly capitation payment. The more patients on the list, the more money the physician earns. Patients are required to route all nonemergency medical needs through the general practitioner "gatekeeper," who, when necessary, makes referrals for specialist services or hospital care. Patients can freely change from one general practitioner to another (Grumbach and Fry, 1993). This simple arrangement, illustrated in Figure 4–1A, is referred to as a two-tiered capitation structure. One tier is the health plan and the other tier the individual PCP or a small number of physicians in group practice (Welch et al, 1990). Traditionally, the National Health Service has paid for referral services (eg, specialist physician care, radiologic studies, and laboratory tests) through a separate funding channel.

United States System: In the United States, approximately 20% of HMO plans have two-tiered structures, with HMOs paying capitation fees directly to PCPs (Welch et al, 1990). However, unlike the traditional British system, HMOs may subsume payments for referral services under the primary care capitation payment (Figure 4–1B). Rather than the HMO plan paying for these services separately, the HMO shifts the financial risk to the PCP for these expenses.

> Andy, who lives in the United States, is 14 years old and has severe acne. His family has insurance through the Stay Fit health plan, which pays Andy's pediatrician, Dr. Ursula Kinderhoff, a monthly capitation fee. When Andy's acne fails to respond to topical treatments, his family requests a referral to a dermatologist. Dr. Kinderhoff agrees to the referral, but under the Stay Fit plan, Dr. Kinderhoff knows that she will have to pay for the dermatologist's fee out of the capitation funds she receives from Stay Fit.

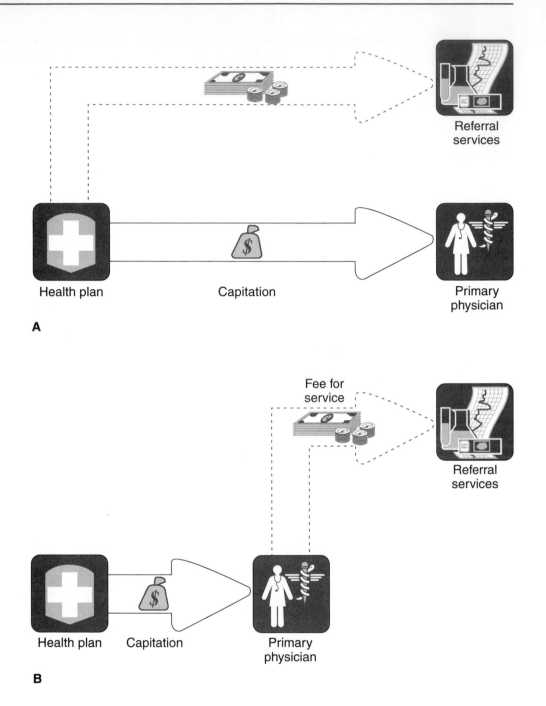

Figure 4–1. Two-tiered capitated payment structures. **A:** The health plan pays the primary care physician by capitation and pays for referral services (eg, x-rays and specialist consultations) through a different reimbursement stream (as in the traditional British National Health Service). **B:** Under some United States HMO contracts, the primary physician is at risk for paying for referral services out of the physician's capitation income.

Comparison of Risk Between the Two Systems: The nature of risk is quite different when comparing the traditional British and United States capitation arrangements. In the case of Dr. Liston, only the primary care physician's (PCP's) time is at risk. For example, if 1500 patients choose Dr. Liston as their general practitioner, he earns $7500 per month (ie, $5 × 1500) in gross income from capitated payments. If 2000 patients choose Dr. Liston, he receives $10,000 monthly. If Dr. Liston has chronically ill patients who must be seen each week, he earns no more than if he has healthy patients who are seen once a year. Thus, Dr. Liston bears the nonmonetary "risk" of doing more work with no additional pay. Extensive use of laboratory tests and specialist consultations will not jeopardize Dr. Liston's income, however.

Dr. Kinderhoff, in contrast, is at much greater financial risk. Let's examine her situation in more detail.

> Stay Fit pays Dr. Kinderhoff's practice $30 per month for each patient such as Andy who is enrolled in the practice, whether or not the patient visits Dr. Kinderhoff. Andy twists his knee playing basketball and is unable to bear weight on his leg. Dr. Kinderhoff examines Andy's knee, prescribes a knee immobilizer, ice packs, rest, and anti-inflammatory medications. After 2 weeks, Andy's knee has not improved. Dr. Kinderhoff considers sending Andy to an orthopedist. She anticipates that four visits with the orthopedist will cost $400, and an MRI of the knee an additional $900. She will have to pay these charges out of her Stay Fit capitation income.

In this example, Dr. Kinderhoff would receive $360 per year for Andy's care but would spend $1300 for specialty care for his knee injury. That is the real meaning of "at risk!" This risk may be balanced by the fact that many enrolled patients rarely visit Dr. Kinderhoff; for these patients, $360 per year in capitation payments may yield a generous profit for her practice. But the potential remains for high-cost patients to erode Dr. Kinderhoff's take-home earnings. Usually, a dollar limit is placed on the physician's risk, so that excessive costs for an extremely sick patient are covered by a stop-loss insurance policy (see Chapter 5).

Payment Per Patient: Capitation With Three-Tiered Structures Although some HMOs in the United States pay capitation fees directly to individual physicians or small group practices, many plans have developed an intermediary administrative structure for processing these payments (Robinson and Casalino, 1995). In one variety of such three-tiered structures (Figure 4–2A), physicians remain in their own private offices but join together into physician groups called independent practice associations (IPAs).

> George is enrolled through his employer in SmartCare, an HMO run by Smart Insurance Company. SmartCare has contracted with two IPAs to provide physician services for its enrollees in the area where George lives. George has chosen to receive his care from Dr. Bunch, a PCP affiliated with one of these IPA groups, CapCap Associates IPA. SmartCare pays CapCap Associates a $40 monthly capitation fee on George's behalf for all physician and related outpatient services. CapCap Associates in turn pays Dr.

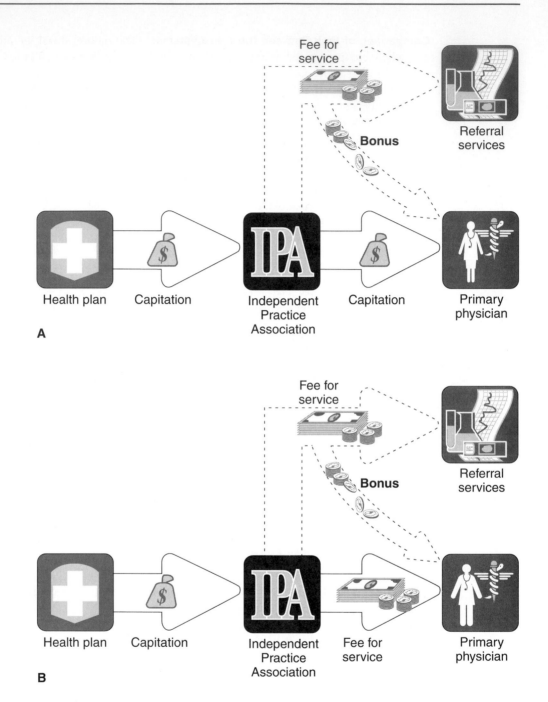

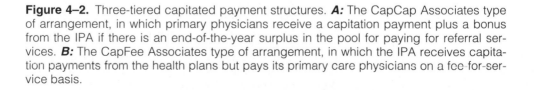

Figure 4–2. Three-tiered capitated payment structures. *A:* The CapCap Associates type of arrangement, in which primary physicians receive a capitation payment plus a bonus from the IPA if there is an end-of-the-year surplus in the pool for paying for referral services. *B:* The CapFee Associates type of arrangement, in which the IPA receives capitation payments from the health plans but pays its primary care physicians on a fee-for-service basis.

Bunch a $10 monthly capitation fee to serve as George's primary physician and "gatekeeper."

George develops symptoms of urinary obstruction consistent with benign prostatic hyperplasia. Dr. Bunch orders some laboratory tests and refers George to a urologist for cystoscopy. The laboratory and the urologist bill CapCap Associates on a fee-for-service basis and are paid by the IPA from a pool of money (called a risk pool) that the IPA has set aside for this purpose from the capitation payments CapCap Associates receives from SmartCare. At the end of the year, CapCap Associates has money left over in this diagnostic and specialist services risk pool. CapCap Associates distributes this surplus revenue to its PCPs as a bonus.

Sorting out the flow of payments and nature of risk sharing becomes difficult in this type of three-tiered capitation structure. In most three-tiered HMOs, the financial risk for diagnostic and specialist services is borne by the overall IPA organization and spread among all the participating PCPs in the IPA. This eliminates some of the high-stakes risk that occurs when only one or a few PCPs accept a full-risk capitation contract, as in the case of Dr. Kinderhoff (see Figure 4–1B). The CapCap Associates type of IPA usually provides financial incentives to PCPs to limit the use of diagnostic and specialist services by returning to these physicians any surplus funds that remain at the end of the year. This method of reimbursement is known as capitation-plus-bonus payment (see Chapter 5). The less frequent the use of diagnostic and specialist services, the higher the year-end bonus for IPA physician gatekeepers. Some people feel that this arrangement represents a conflict of interest for PCPs because their personal income is increased by denying diagnostic and specialty services to their patients (Rodwin, 1993). Because year-end bonuses are usually based on the collective performance of IPA PCPs, financial risk in an IPA setting presents less of a conflict of interest than financial incentives in a two-tiered setting that are directly indexed to an individual physician's use of ancillary services (eg, the case of Dr. Kinderhoff) (Hillman, 1991).

A considerable price must be paid for setting up a three-tiered structure because administrative costs are substantial for both the health plan and the IPA.

George's brother Steve works for the same company as George and also has SmartCare insurance. Steve, however, obtains his primary care from a physician in the other SmartCare IPA plan, CapFee Associates. Like CapCap Associates, CapFee Associates is an IPA that receives $40 per month in capitation fees for every patient enrolled. Unlike CapCap Associates, CapFee Associates pays its PCPs on a fee-for-service basis.

Three-tiered IPA structures become even more confusing when the unit of reimbursement differs across tiers. In the CapCap Associates model, capitation is the basic payment method for both the IPA as a whole and its constituent physicians. In the CapFee Associates model, however, the IPA receives capitation payments from the health insurance plan but then reimburses its participating PCPs on a fee-for-service basis (Figure 4–2B). Under this arrangement, the fees billed by the IPA physicians may well exceed the amount of money the IPA has received from the insurance plan on a capitated basis to pay for physician and related outpatient services. To reduce this risk, many IPAs of the CapFee Associates type pay their physicians only a portion, perhaps 60%, of a predetermined fee schedule and withhold the other 40%. If money is left over at the end of the year, the physicians receive a portion of the withheld money as a bonus.

With the CapFee system, the IPA is the main entity at risk because provision of more services can cause the IPA to lose money. But individual physicians are also partially at risk because if expenditures by the IPA are high, there will be no year-end bonus. The economic incentive for individual primary physicians is a mixed one. It is to the physician's financial advantage to schedule as many patient visits as possible because the physician receives a fee for each visit. But a large number of visits overall by IPA patients, as well as high use of laboratory and x-ray studies and specialist services, will deplete the IPA budget, thereby reducing the possibility of a large year-end bonus.

Payment Per Time: Salary

> Dr. Joyce Parto is employed as an obstetrician-gynecologist by a large staff model HMO. She considers the financial security and lack of business worries in her current work setting an improvement over the stresses she faced as a solo, fee-for-service practitioner before joining the HMO. She has some concerns, however, that the other obstetricians are allowing the hospital's obstetric house staff to manage most of the deliveries during the night, and wonders if the lack of financial incentives to attend deliveries may be partly to blame. She is also annoyed by the bureaucratic "hoops" she has to jump through to cancel an afternoon clinic to attend her son's school play.

In contrast with traditional private physicians, physicians in the public sector (municipal, Veterans Affairs and military hospitals, state mental hospitals, and community clinics) are usually paid by salary. Salaried practice aggregates payment for all services delivered during a month or year into one lump sum. Managed care has brought salaried practice to the private sector, sometimes with a salary-plus-bonus arrangement, particularly in integrated medical groups and group and staff model HMOs (see Chapter 7). Group and staff model HMOs bring physicians and hospitals under one organizational roof.

The distinction between staff and group model HMOs is analogous to the difference between the two- and three-tiered IPA model HMOs discussed previously. The staff model HMO is essentially a two-tiered payment structure, with an HMO insurance plan directly employing physicians on a salaried basis (Figure 4–3A). In the group model HMO, the HMO insurance plan contracts on a capitated basis with an intermediary physician group, which in turn pays its individual physicians a salary (Figure 4–3B).

HMO physicians paid purely by salary usually bear little, if any, individual financial risk, and instead the HMO or the physician group is at risk if expenses are too great. To manage risk, administrators at group and staff model HMOs may place

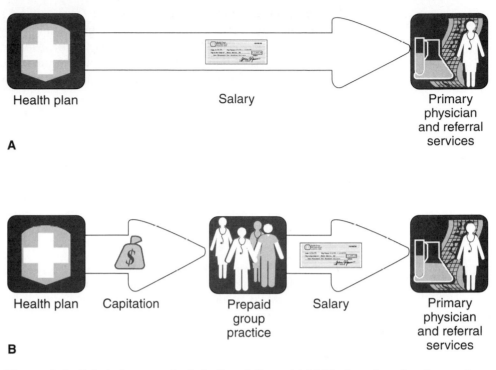

Figure 4–3. Salaried payment. **A:** In the staff model HMO, the plan directly employs physicians. **B:** In the group model HMO, a "prepaid group practice" receives capitation payments from the plan and then reimburses its physicians by salary.

constraints upon their physician employees, such as scheduling them for a high volume of patient visits or limiting the number of available specialists. Salaried physicians are mainly at risk of not getting extra pay for extra work hours. For a physician paid an annual salary without allowances for overtime pay, a high volume of complex patient visits may turn an 8-hour day into a 12-hour day with no increase in income. HMOs and medical groups may offer year-end bonuses to salaried physicians if overall expenses are less than the amounts budgeted for these expenses. Physicians paid salary plus bonus, like those paid capitation plus bonus, are at risk of earning less income.

METHODS OF HOSPITAL PAYMENT

Payment Per Procedure: Fee-for-Service

> Kwin Mock Wong is hospitalized for a bleeding ulcer. At the end of his 4-day stay, the hospital sends a $8,600, seven-page itemized hospital bill to Blue Cross, Mr. Wong's insurer.

The traditional method of payment for private hospitals is fee-for-service. Until recently, Blue Cross paid hospitals on the principle of "reasonable cost," a system under which hospitals had a great deal of influence in determining the level of payment.

Because the American Hospital Association and Blue Cross played a strong role in writing reimbursement regulations for Medicare, that program initially paid hospitals according to a similar reasonable cost formula (Law, 1974). More recently, private and public payers concerned with cost containment have begun to question hospital charges and negotiate lower payments, or to shift financial risk toward the hospitals by using per diem, DRG, or capitation payments.

Payment Per Day: Per Diem

> John Johnson, an HMO patient, is admitted to the hospital with a severe headache. During his 3-day stay, he undergoes MRI scanning, lumbar puncture, and cerebral arteriography, procedures that are all costly to the hospital in terms of personnel and supplies. The hospital receives $3000, or $1000 per day from the HMO; Mr. Johnson's stay costs the hospital $5400.

> Tom Thompson, in the same HMO, is admitted for congestive heart failure. He receives intravenous furosemide for 3 days, and his condition improves. Diagnostic testing is limited to a chest x-ray, EKG, and basic blood work. The hospital receives $3000; the cost is $2400.

Many HMOs contract with hospitals for per diem payments rather than paying a fee for each itemized service (room charge, MRI, arteriogram, chest x-ray, EKG). The hospital receives a lump sum for each day the HMO patient is in the hospital. The HMO sends a utilization review nurse to the hospital to review the charts of its patients, and if the nurse decides that a patient is not acutely ill, the HMO stops paying for additional days.

Per diem payments represent a bundling of all services provided for one patient on a particular day into one payment. With traditional fee-for-service payment, if the hospital performs several expensive diagnostic studies, it makes more money because it charges for each study, whereas with per diem payment, the hospital receives no additional money for expensive procedures. Per diem bundling of services into one fee reverses the hospital's financial incentive because it loses, rather than profits, by performing expensive studies.

With per diem payment, the HMO continues to be at risk for the number of days a patient stays in the hospital because it must pay for each additional day. However, the hospital is at risk for the number of services performed on any given day because it incurs more costs without additional payment by providing more services. It is in the HMO's interest to conduct utilization review to reduce the number of hospital days, but the HMO is less concerned about how many services are performed within each day; that fiscal concern has been transferred to the hospital.

Payment Per Episode of Hospitalization: Diagnosis-Related Groups

> Bill is a 67-year-old man who enters the hospital for acute pulmonary edema. He is treated with furosemide and oxygen in the emergency room, spends 36 hours in the hospital, and is discharged. The cost to the hospital is $2400. On the basis of DRG 127 (congestive heart failure), the hospital receives $4000 from Medicare.

> Will is an 82-year-old man who enters the hospital for acute pulmonary edema. In spite of repeated treatments with furosemide, captopril, digoxin, and nitrates, he remains in heart failure. He requires telemetry, daily blood tests, several chest x-rays, electrocardiograms, and an echocardiogram, and is finally discharged on the ninth hospital day. His hospital stay costs $18,000. On the basis of DRG 127, the hospital receives $4000 from Medicare.

The DRG method of payment for Medicare patients started in 1983. Rather than pay hospitals on a fee-for-service basis, Medicare pays a lump sum for each hospital admission, with the size of the payment dependent on the patient's diagnosis. The DRG system has gone one step further than per diem payments in bundling services into one payment. While per diem payment lumps together all services performed during one day, DRG reimbursement lumps together all services performed during one hospital episode. (Although an episode of illness may extend beyond the boundaries of the acute hospitalization, eg, there may be an outpatient evaluation preceding the hospitalization and transfer to a nursing facility for rehabilitation afterward, the term "episode" under the DRG system refers only to the portion of the illness actually spent in the acute care hospital.)

With the DRG system, the Medicare program is at risk for the number of admissions, but the hospital is at risk for the length of hospital stay and the resources used during the hospital stay. Accordingly, Medicare conducts utilization review of the actual admission and has the authority to deny payment for admissions it deems unnecessary, but Medicare has no financial interest in the length of stay, which (except in unusually long "outlier" stays) does not affect Medicare's payment. The hospital, in contrast, has an acute interest in the length of stay and in the number of expensive procedures performed; a long, costly hospitalization such as Will's produces a financial loss for the hospital, whereas a short stay yields a profit. Hospitals therefore conduct internal utilization review to reduce the costs incurred by Medicare patients.

Payment Per Patient: Capitation

> Jane is enrolled in Blue Cross HMO, which contracts with Upscale Hospital to care for Jane if she requires hospitalization. Upscale receives $40 per month as a capitation fee for each patient enrolled in the HMO. Jane is healthy, and during the 36 months that she is an HMO member, the hospital receives $1440, even though Jane never sets foot in the hospital.

> Wayne is also enrolled in Blue Cross HMO. Twenty-four months following his enrollment, he contracts *Pneumocystis carinii* pneumonia, and in the following 12 months, he spends 6 weeks in Upscale Hospital at a cost of $35,000. Upscale receives a total of $1440 (the $30 capitation fee per month for 36 months) for Wayne's care.

With capitation payment, hospitals are at risk for admissions, length of stay, and resources used; in other words, hospitals bear all the risk and the insurer, usually an HMO, bears no risk. Capitation payment to hospitals is not common; most HMOs pay hospitals on a per diem basis, as described in Chapter 5.

Payment Per Institution: Global Budget

> Don Samuels, a member of the Kaiser Health Plan, suffers a sudden overwhelming headache and is hospitalized for 1 week at Kaiser Hospital in Oakland, California, for an acute cerebral hemorrhage. He goes into a coma and dies. No hospital bill is generated as a result of Mr. Samuels' admission, and no capitation payments are made from any insurance plan to the hospital.

Kaiser Health Plan is a large HMO that in some regions of the United States operates its own hospitals. Kaiser hospitals are paid by the Kaiser Health Plan through a global budget: a fixed payment is made for all hospital services for 1 year. Global budgets are also used in Veterans Affairs and Department of Defense hospitals in the United States, as well as being a standard payment method in Canada and many European nations. In managed care parlance, one might say that the hospital is entirely at risk because no matter how many patients are admitted and how many expensive services are performed, the hospital must figure out how to stay within its fixed budget. Global budgets represent the most extensive bundling of services: Every service performed on every patient during 1 year is aggregated into one payment.

CONCLUSION

As cost containment becomes a priority for those who pay for health care in the United States, payments to physicians and hospitals are changing in two regards.

(1) Fee-for-service payment, which encourages use of more services, is being replaced with new reimbursement mechanisms that place economic pressure on physicians and hospitals to limit the number and cost of services offered. The bundling of services into one payment tends to shift financial risk away from payers toward physicians and hospitals.

One of the challenges in designing an optimal payment system is striking the right balance between economic incentives for "overtreatment" and "undertreatment" (Casalino, 1992). The British National Health Service has traditionally mixed units of payment for general practitioners, paying a global budget for overhead costs (eg, office rent and staff), a capitation payment for each patient enrolled in the practice, and fee-for-service payments selectively for preventive services (eg, vaccinations and Pap tests) and some home visits in order to encourage provision of these items.

(2) Whereas levels of payment were formerly set largely by providers themselves (reasonable cost reimbursement for hospitals and usual, customary, and reasonable fees for physicians), payment levels are increasingly determined by negotiation between payers and providers or by fee schedules set by payers.

In Chapter 5, details of reimbursement under managed care will be discussed.

REFERENCES

Casalino LP: Balancing incentives: How should physicians be reimbursed? JAMA 1992;267:403.

Grumbach K, Fry J: Managing primary care in the United States and in the United Kingdom. N Engl J Med 1993;328:940.

Hillman AL: Managing the physician: Rules versus incentives. Health Aff 1991;10(4):138.

Langwell KM, Nelson LM: Physician payment systems: A review of history, alternatives, and evidence. Med Care Rev 1986;43:5.

Law SA: Blue Cross: What Went Wrong? Yale Univ Press, 1974.

Lee PR, Grumbach KL, Jameson WJ: Physician payment in the 1990s: Factors that will shape the future. Ann Rev Public Health 1990;11:297.

Lee PR et al: The Physician Payment Review Commission report to Congress. JAMA 1989;261:2382.

Relman A: The future of medical practice. Health Aff 1983;2(2):5.

Robinson JC, Casalino LP: The growth of medical groups paid through capitation in California. N Engl J Med 1995;333:1684.

Rodwin MA: Medicine, Money, and Morals: Physicians' Conflicts of Interest. Oxford University Press, 1993.

Welch WP, Hillman AL, Pauly MV: Toward new typologies for HMOs. Milbank Q 1990;68:221.

Capitation Payment in Managed Care 5

> Dr. Violet Fairbanks is disgusted. The meeting, a negotiating session for a physician-hospital managed care agreement, has degenerated into mutual name-calling. Dr. George Capwell accuses the hospital of picking his pocket and sending him into financial ruin. Jack Powers, hospital administrator, fingers the physicians as the cause of the hospital's fiscal problems. The meeting ends in chaos.
>
> The next morning, the physician leadership of the CapCap independent practice association (IPA) meets. Until now, Dr. Fairbanks has steered clear of managed care politics. Now, curiosity and mistrust of the hospital and of some physician leaders has brought her to meetings as a spectator. As the CapCap IPA leaders plan their negotiating tactics, Dr. Fairbanks timorously raises her hand. "Does it have to be like this? Can't we give in a bit, ask them to give in a bit, get this behind us, and go back to practicing medicine?" She leaves the room at 8:30 AM to finish her hospital rounds. At 9 AM a message is left on her voicemail: "We'd like you to become the IPA's new negotiator. Good luck."

The centerpiece of managed care, 1990s style, can be summed up in one word: capitation. Touted as the magic answer to many of health care's pressing problems, capitation is expected to slow rising costs, reduce unnecessary medical services, and correct the imbalance between specialty and primary care. This chapter examines some practical aspects of how capitation payments are structured in the managed care marketplace.

Health maintenance organizations (HMOs) increasingly rely on capitation to pay physicians. In markets with high HMO penetration, capitation is the method of paying primary care physicians (PCPs) for 63% of enrollees. For 46% of HMO enrollees in large markets, specialists are receiving capitation checks as well (Interstudy, 1995a).

The shift from fee-for-service to capitation has sent physicians and other providers scampering to figure out how to cope with the new economic realities of health care. Physicians flock to weekend seminars where consultants instruct attendees on how to reconfigure their practices and negotiate capitated contracts. Busy clinicians finish their day's patient care duties and face the prospect of long evenings locked in negotiating sessions. In these sessions, specialists argue with PCPs and physicians vie with hospital administrators over how to divvy up capitation revenues. Understanding the nuances of capitation payment is not simply the prerogative of entrepreneurial physicians seeking to stay one step ahead of the market, but a necessity of economic survival for most practitioners. As Dr. Fairbanks realized, clinicians do not have the luxury of leaving capitation expertise to a small handful of hospital, insurance, and physician executives.

CAPITATION: SHIFTING THE RISK

> Dr. Fairbanks might as well be attending a conference held in Russian. At her first negotiating session, she cannot understand what anyone is saying. "With 50,000 lives and a cap split of 60-40, we can relieve the risk pool at $850 as long as our commercial days per thousand fall below 150." "If you cap ancillary we'll give you an exclusive, and the risk pool will be divided 35-50-15 with 10% physician downside risk."
>
> Lives? Cap split? Risk pool? Days per thousand? Dr. Fairbanks phones James Jefferson, CapCap IPA's executive director, and schedules a meeting on the ABCs of capitation.

As described in Chapter 4, the essence of capitation is a shift in financial risk from insurers to providers. Under fee-for-service, patients who require expensive health services cost their health plan more than they pay the plan in insurance premiums; the insurer is at risk and loses money. Physicians and hospitals, who provide the care, earn more money for treating ill people.

In a 180-degree role reversal, capitation frees insurers of risk by transferring risk to providers. An HMO that pays physicians and hospitals via capitation has little to fear in the short run from patients who become ill. The HMO pays a fixed sum no matter how many services are provided. The providers, in contrast, earn no additional money yet spend a great deal of time and incur large office and hospital expenditures to care for people who are sick. (In the long term, HMOs do want to limit services in order to reduce provider pressure for higher capitation payments. And, as explained below, HMOs providing stop-loss coverage assume risk for high-cost cases.)

MODELS OF CAPITATION

> Dr. Fairbanks calls a meeting of all physicians in the IPA to share her newly acquired knowledge. She draws a diagram of the relationships between HMO, IPA, PCPs, specialists, and ancillary services (Figure 5–1). She decides to leave the complex HMO-physician-hospital relationship for the next meeting.
>
> Employers pay Apple a Day HMO $100 per month for each employee enrolled in the HMO. Apple a Day keeps $20 per member per month (pmpm) for administration and profits and contracts with several hospitals to care for its patients for $40 pmpm. The HMO pays the remaining $40 pmpm to two IPAs, including CapCap IPA, for professional and ancillary services.
>
> Of Apple a Day's enrollees, 80,000 have chosen CapCap IPA for physician services. Apple a Day sends CapCap IPA a monthly capitation check for $3.2 million—$40 for each enrollee. The IPA pays $10 pmpm to PCPs; Dr. Fairbanks, a general internist chosen by 1000 Apple a Day patients, receives a $10,000 monthly check from the IPA. The IPA keeps $4 pmpm for administration and places the remaining $26 pmpm in a referral risk pool. The referral risk pool is

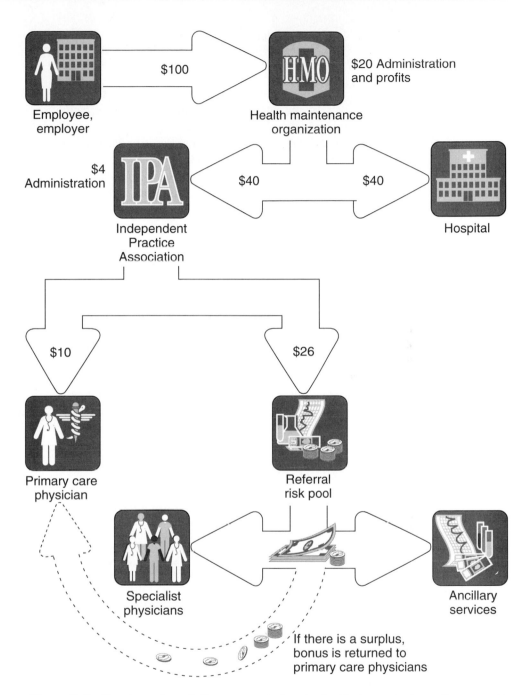

Figure 5–1. Structure of capitation payments in a typical independent practice association (IPA) arrangement. Dollar values indicate approximate amounts of typical "per member per month" payments.

used to pay for specialist care, laboratory and x-ray services, physical therapy, other ancillary services, and pharmacy services.

Capitation is a simple concept: payment of a lump sum per enrolled patient per month. However, in the current health care marketplace, capitation is anything but simple. Several models of capitation can be found, mirroring several models of HMOs (Gold et al, 1995). Dr. Fairbanks has described the IPA model (see Chapter 4), in which physicians in independent offices affiliate for purposes of contracting with managed care plans. Rather than paying each physician directly, an HMO makes capitated payments to the IPA as a whole for physician and related professional services. The IPA in turn pays each individual physician for each patient enrolled with that physician and assumes some responsibility for managing the costs and quality of care provided by participating physicians. Capitation can provide a remarkable cash flow to IPAs; a medium-sized IPA with 50,000 covered lives (enrolled patients are often called "covered lives") brings in $40 \times 50,000 = $2 million each month, or $24 million per year.

The IPA model is the most common capitation arrangement in the United States. Of the 547 HMOs in operation as of July 1, 1994, 59% used the IPA model. From 1989 through 1994, IPA-model HMOs grew somewhat faster than other HMO models (Interstudy, 1995b). Because so many physicians experience capitation through an IPA, this discussion of capitation will be from the IPA model. The general principles, however, apply to all capitation models. In essence, the IPA model involves a shift in the risk for physician and ancillary services from the HMO to the physician group. The HMO pays $40 pmpm to the IPA regardless of the quantity of services used.

CAPITATING PRIMARY CARE PHYSICIANS

Dr. Fairbanks concludes her presentation with a description of CapCap IPA's bonus system for PCPs. If PCPs are frugal about their diagnostic testing and specialty referrals, the referral risk pool will have money left at the end of the year, and the IPA will distribute a portion of this money to the PCPs as a bonus.

Dr. George Capwell explains why he likes the capitation system. He does not refer patients to specialists or for expensive diagnostic tests unless these referrals are clearly necessary. Dr. Capwell's partner, Dr. Reddink, has patients who wind up using far more specialty services. At the end of the year, CapCap IPA has $2 million remaining in the referral risk pool to distribute to its 80 PCPs. Although the average year-end bonus per PCP is $25,000, Dr. Capwell receives a bonus of $40,000, while Dr. Reddink receives a $6000 bonus. The IPA has in part used each physician's economic practice pattern to calculate how bonuses will be distributed to individual physicians.

Recall that risk refers to the potential to lose money, earn less money, or spend more time without additional payment. Capitation without the bonus feature places physicians at risk for their time. Capitation plus bonus, a far more common payment mode than capitation alone, places physicians at additional financial risk. How does the bonus payment represent financial risk?

In most IPA-type arrangements, the dollars paid by capitation to a PCP constitute a "base" payment. In Dr. Capwell's case previously, his base capitation earnings would be $10 per month per enrolled patient. Usually, the base payment rate is set below what a PCP has traditionally earned caring for the same types of patients. Dr. Capwell's yearly income from his base capitation payments would be less than what he would have earned caring for the same patients on a fee-for-service basis. However, most IPAs and HMOs set aside additional funds in various "risk pools." The most common form of risk pool consists of money available to pay for services provided by specialist physicians and for ancillary services such as laboratory and radiology procedures. A portion of the funds placed in these risk pools is usually referred to as dollars that are "withheld" because they are not included in the base capitation payment. If year-end specialty and ancillary costs are less than the amount set aside in the risk pool, PCPs receive the risk-pool surplus funds as additional compensation—often termed "bonus" payments. Under some managed care arrangements, the base capitation payments may be sufficient only to cover a physician's office overhead; the physician's take-home income may completely depend on the bonus payments he or she receives. In the marketplace of the mid-1990s, payers and HMOs were driving down capitation payments, thereby increasing the importance of bonus payments. The greater the degree to which earnings are determined by these risk-sharing arrangements, the more intense the pressure to restrict patient access to expensive specialty and diagnostic services (Woolhandler and Himmelstein, 1995).

A spectrum of methods exists for calculating physician bonus payments (Table 5–1). Each physician's referral costs may be tracked individually, with the end-of-year bonus determined by each physician's own cost to the IPA in specialty and ancillary referrals. Alternatively, IPAs may pay all physicians the same bonus pmpm according to how successfully the group as a whole has contained the use of specialty and ancillary services. This more collective approach means that all physicians in the

Table 5–1. Varieties of capitation payments.

Capitation without additional financial risk

Capitation with additional financial risk

    Withholds/bonuses distributed according to:

        A) Costs of referral and ancillary services
            Indexed to performance of individual physician or
            Indexed to performance of larger physician group
               or entire IPA
        B) Factors other than costs
            Quality of care, patient satisfaction
            Exclusivity of participation in IPA or HMO

Methods of Limiting or Adjusting Financial Risk

        A) "Carve-Outs"
            Based on:
               Type of service (eg, preventive care)
               Diagnoses or conditions (eg, AIDS)
               Referral specialty (eg, ophthalmology)
        B) Stop-loss insurance
        C) Risk-adjustment of capitation payments

IPA are penalized if their colleagues use many referral services. While the direct incentive to skimp on referrals is weaker, peer pressure to make fellow physicians practice a less costly style of medicine is stronger. Some IPAs use a method somewhere between these two extremes, blending both individual physician and overall IPA group performance into the formula for calculating bonus payments.

Factors other than how well physicians economize in their delivery of care may also be used to adjust compensation to individual physicians. Bonus payments from risk-pool residuals may be used to reward quality of care, with the payment adjusted upward for physicians who receive high marks on chart review and patient satisfaction surveys. HMOs and IPAs also prefer PCPs to care exclusively for their patients and to reject contracts with other HMOs or IPAs. Such exclusivity may be rewarded by giving them higher capitation payments than physicians who make nonexclusive arrangements with several HMOs or IPAs.

LIMITING FINANCIAL RISK

Primary Care Carve-Outs

> One of Dr. Fairbanks's former medical school classmates works in an IPA that pays PCPs only $8 capitation but pays extra fees for Pap smears, office EKGs, immunizations, minor office surgical procedures, and hospital visits. Dr. Fairbanks likes the idea because under her IPA, she has no financial incentive to be a conscientious physician and give all indicated immunizations, for which she receives no payment. In contrast with her former classmate, Dr. Fairbanks also receives no fee for hospital visits.

Certain methods have been developed to mitigate the financial risk associated with capitation payment. One method involves reintroducing fee-for-service payments for specified services. Such types of services provided but not covered within the capitation payment are called "carve-outs"; their reimbursement is "carved out" of the capitation payment and paid separately. CapCap IPA does not have primary care carve-outs; but for Dr. Fairbanks's classmate, Pap smears, immunizations, office EKGs, minor surgical procedures, and hospital visits are carved out and paid on a fee-for-service basis (Kongstvedt, 1989). Physicians can also attempt to remove high-cost diseases such as AIDS from their capitation agreements and receive reimbursement for patients with such diseases on a fee-for-service basis.

Stop-Loss Coverage

> One of Dr. Fairbanks's patients develops acute myelogenous leukemia. Because this patient requires hematology referrals, chemotherapy, treatment of leukopenic infections, and bone marrow transplantation, she will drastically elevate Dr. Fairbanks's average cost per patient per month. The amount of her bonus will take a steep dive. Dr. Fairbanks confides her discomfort to Mr. Jefferson, the IPA's executive director, who reassures her. "We have stop-loss insurance. If a patient incurs costs over $5000 during a year, the HMO picks up the tab above $5000."

Virtually every capitated physician or physician group is insured against high-cost patients through stop-loss coverage. The threshold of such coverage is the number of dollars in services one patient must incur during a year to trigger fee-for-service payments to physicians by the stop-loss carrier for additional services. The cost of stop-loss insurance is about $2 pmpm, roughly 20% of the primary care capitation payment. For stop-loss policies with a low threshold (for example, $5000 per patient), the cost is naturally more than for a high-threshold policy (eg, $25,000 per patient).

Commercial insurance companies sell stop-loss insurance, which is expected to become a multibillion dollar business. HMOs may offer stop-loss coverage for their physicians or physician groups; these HMOs reduce physician capitation payments to pay for the coverage. Large physician groups receiving a multimillion dollar capitation stream can self-insure for stop-loss protection.

RISK-ADJUSTED CAPITATION

> Dr. Reddink, who received only a small bonus because of high costs per patient per month, compared his list of patients with that of Dr. Capwell, whose costs were low. Dr. Reddink ended up seeing 18 AIDS patients; Dr. Capwell saw only 3. Dr. Reddink appealed the bonus payment, arguing that his costs were higher because his patients were, on the average, sicker.

As physicians and hospitals assume greater financial risk, they begin to experience the basic dynamic of insurance underwriting: Patients with costly illnesses are a financial liability, and patients in good health are a financial advantage. The intent of capitation is to encourage providers to make more efficient use of resources for a set bundle of services. However, just as insurance companies and HMOs have discovered an irresistible market logic in skimming off the healthiest subscribers, physicians such as Dr. Capwell and Dr. Reddink face a financial incentive to care for healthier patients. Concern about this socially undesirable risk-skimming incentive has given rise to attempts to "risk-adjust" reimbursement; that is, to pay a higher rate for higher-risk patients.

Fee-for-service payment has an intrinsic risk-adjustment factor. The sicker the patient, the more services provided and the greater the reimbursement. Risk adjustment has also been factored into the Medicare hospital diagnosis-related group (DRG) system, since more serious illnesses provide more payment to the hospital. DRG reimbursement is higher for a patient hospitalized for septic shock than for a patient admitted for elective cholecystectomy.

But risk selection is the Achilles' heel of capitation. If the same capitation rate applies to all patients, providers may be tempted to selectively enroll only healthier patients to minimize financial risk—a practice known by such gustatory terms as "cream skimming" or "cherry picking." Particularly for Medicare, physicians might well encourage their healthy patients to enroll in managed care plans while leaving their chronically ill patients in the fee-for-service system (Morgan et al, 1997). The crudest method for adjusting capitation payments is to set different rates by the age and sex of the patient; in general, persons in certain age–sex strata are more likely to use health services than individuals in other strata. For example, an HMO or an IPA may pay a monthly primary care capitation rate of $25 for a baby under 1 year, $5 for a teenager, $10 for a male age 45 to 64 years, $11.50 for a female age 45 to 64 years, and considerably more for people over 65 years. However, there is still enormous variation in health status and health care expenditures among individuals within specified age–sex groupings.

Why should one physician work harder than another without additional pay (or even with reduced pay resulting from lower bonuses) simply because he or she has sicker patients? Risk adjustment—setting capitation rates according to the health risk of the individual covered—poses a major challenge. Researchers have investigated measures for risk-adjusting capitation payments by more directly appraising an individual's state of health or risk of needing health care services. Unfortunately, these methods are often expensive to implement and have limited ability to explain the high degree of variation in health care costs across patients (Newhouse, 1994).

CAPITATING SPECIALISTS

To open a dialogue with the specialists on the hospital staff, Dr. Fairbanks meets with cardiologist Nancy Hartshorn. Dr. Hartshorn is worried. Many of the PCPs who provide her with referrals have joined CapCap IPA, which places them at risk for specialty consultations. She is no longer seeing patients with stable angina, atrial fibrillation, and congestive heart failure; the PCPs are caring for those problems without her help. The eight cardiologists on the hospital staff are competing for a smaller and smaller number of referrals. And the fees from the IPA seem to be dropping each year.

The next evening, Dr. Hartshorn goes to a lecture on specialty capitation; she cannot sleep that night thinking about it. She and three other cardiologists decide to approach CapCap IPA for a capitated contract that gives them the exclusive right to care for the IPA's cardiology patients. Three weeks later, the four-member cardiology group signs a contract to provide cardiology services, including angiograms and angioplasties, for $1 per patient per month. These payments are carved out of (subtracted from) the IPA's referral risk pool. Since the IPA has 80,000 enrollees, Dr. Hartshorn's cardiology group is guaranteed $80,000 per month, or $960,000 per year. The remaining four cardiologists at the hospital can no longer see CapCap IPA patients.

Several factors have combined to spur a new trend in managed care: specialty capitation. Specialists account for considerably more of the health care dollar than PCPs; eliminating specialists' fee-for-service incentive to provide more care has great potential to reduce health care costs for HMOs and employers. For PCPs whose bonuses go down as specialty referrals go up, specialty capitation limits the payout to specialists and reduces the pressure not to refer. For specialists, capitated contracts guarantee a flow of patients and money and may provide a major market advantage relative to colleagues/competitors who reject capitation payment.

Specialty capitation is another example of a capitation carve-out. As discussed above, a carve-out is money that is "carved out" of the pool of money available to compensate physicians and paid in a separate manner. Common specialty carve-outs are cardiology, oncology, orthopedics, and ophthalmology.

An essential feature of specialty capitation carve-outs is that they reduce risk (and also reduce potential profit) for PCPs. If PCPs refer to cardiologists at a low rate, costing less than $1 per patient per month on the average, then the cardiology capitation payment of $1 per patient per month will create a "loss" for the PCPs. If, on the other hand, PCPs refer many patients to cardiologists, the capitation contract will eliminate the risk of those referrals and will benefit the PCPs.

Under fee-for-service specialist reimbursement, PCPs and specialists are placed in conflict. PCPs tend to reduce referrals and to refer only the most difficult cases. Specialists have an incentive to perform as many services as possible. Specialty capitation alters this dynamic. Having capitated PCPs with capitated specialists creates the financial incentive for PCPs to send more patients to specialists; specialists, in contrast, benefit by performing few procedures and sending patients back to PCPs as soon as possible.

As with any capitated system, specialty capitation requires a clear delineation of which services are included in the capitation fee. For cardiologists, are invasive procedures included or not? If thallium treadmill tests are performed using a hospital nuclear scanner, is the facility cost of the scanner included in the capitation? Are electrophysiologic studies performed by an outside cardiologist at a tertiary care university hospital paid by the cardiology group out of the capitated fee, or does the HMO or IPA pay separately?

PHYSICIAN–HOSPITAL RELATIONS UNDER CAPITATION

The meetings go on and on. Jack Powers, administrator of the hospital, will not give in. Dr. Fairbanks, chief negotiator for CapCap IPA, continues to press for an agreement regarding the Apple a Day HMO contract held by the hospital and the IPA. The first bone of contention is the "split of the cap." Of the $80 pmpm paid out by the HMO, the hospital demands $50, leaving $30 for the physicians. The IPA feels that a $40/$40 split is a fair bargain.

The second major sticking point concerns the hospital risk pool. Capitation payments from Apple a Day to the hospital are placed in an account called a "risk pool." The risk pool pays the hospital a per diem of $1000 for each day an HMO enrollee spends in the hospital (in managed care–speak, the hospital "relieves" the risk pool of $1000). If money is left in the risk pool at year's end, that money is split between the physicians and the hospital. The hospital administrator wants any surplus to be split 50-50 between the hospital and the IPA. The IPA wants 75% of any surplus, arguing that the physicians, who work hard to reduce hospital days, should be rewarded for their efforts.

After several weeks of wrangling, a deal is cut. The hospital gets $42 of the $80 cap from the HMO, the IPA $38. The IPA gets 65% of the risk pool surplus, the hospital 35%. Several other issues are ironed out and a 2-year agreement is signed.

Capitation payment creates conflict. (Figure 5–2 shows a typical arrangement under managed care.) Under fee-for-service, payment to hospitals does not directly threaten payment to physicians. However, under capitation, the hospital, specialists, and PCPs are forced to fight one another over what proportion of the $80 pmpm payment each group gets. Skirmishes take place between PCPs and specialists over specialty fees or specialty capitation rates. But few battles are more heated than negotiations between physician groups and hospitals over the "split of the cap." For an IPA with 50,000 capitated "lives," a change in the split of the $80 pmpm from $40/$40 to $50 IPA/$30 hospital shifts $6 million per year from hospital to IPA. As the volume of hospital services drops, it is expected that the capitation split will evolve to favor physicians. Currently, many contracts contain a 50%/50% split; by the year 2000, physicians are projected to receive a larger share of the provider capitation dollar.

The hospital risk pool is also a contentious issue. A key statistic in managed care is the number of hospital days per 1000 enrollees per year. In 1993, the number of hospital days per 1000 enrollees under 65 years of age was 539. California physician groups with tight utilization review have reduced this number to 140. For Medicare,

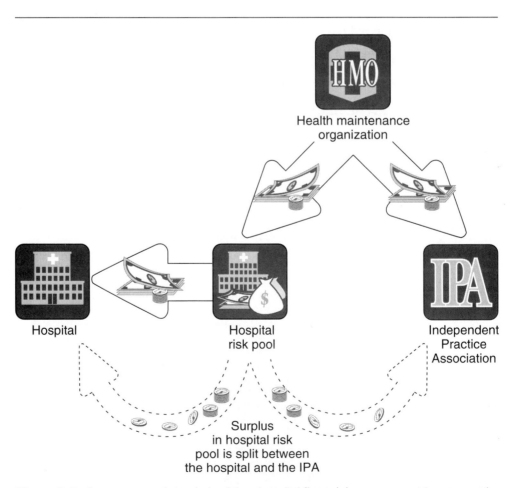

Figure 5–2. A common variety of physician–hospital financial arrangement in managed care.

patient hospital days per thousand average about 2000 nationally; some plans in California have reduced Medicare hospital days to below 900 (Robinson and Casalino, 1995). Under most arrangements, hospitals receive a per diem payment for each day an HMO patient spends in the hospital. The fewer the hospital days, the greater the hospital risk-pool surplus.

Hospitals tend to view these risk pools as their money. In negotiations with IPA physician groups, hospital representatives will argue that sufficient revenues must go to the hospital to maintain staffing, equipment, and overall infrastructure at a level that will support a high standard of care necessary for making the hospital and its associated physicians attractive to patients and HMOs. In reply, physicians tend to say, "Our efforts determine the number of hospital days, so we, not the hospital, should receive the risk-pool surplus." Many HMO contracts are structured such that physicians can only maintain their traditional level of income if they garner substantial bonuses from hospital risk pools. In some arrangements, the HMO and the physicians split the hospital risk-pool surplus, leaving the hospital out. In other cases, large physician groups receive the entire $80 capitation payment covering hospital, physician, and ancillary services; pay the hospital a per diem rate; and share the surplus with no one.

Hospital risk pools represent large amounts of money, especially for Medicare managed care patients whose capitation rates are far higher than those for enrollees under age 65 years. For 5000 Medicare enrollees, assuming a hospital capitation payment of $150 per month, the hospital risk pool would receive $9 million for a year. At a high hospitalization rate of 2000 days per thousand enrollees, with the hospital receiving a $1000 per diem payment for each day, the risk pool would owe the hospital $10 million, creating a $1 million deficit. The hospital-IPA contract would specify who is responsible for the deficit ("downside risk"); in most cases, it would be shared between the IPA and the hospital. In the case of a 50-physician IPA, $20,000 would be subtracted from the year-end bonus of each physician in the IPA.

If physicians keep their Medicare patient days to 1200 per thousand enrollees, the $9 million risk pool would owe the hospital $6 million in per diem payments for the year, thereby generating a profit of $3 million. If the risk-pool surplus is shared 50-50 between hospital and IPA, each physician in a 50-physician IPA would receive $30,000. If 75% of the risk pool goes to the IPA, each physician would receive $45,000. It is small wonder that negotiations over hospital risk pools are major events in the capitated medical marketplace.

THE PROMISE AND PERIL OF CAPITATION

Dr. Will Cope expected the worst when his group of a dozen pediatricians was thrust into the capitation environment. To his surprise, Dr. Cope has found some unanticipated benefits of capitation. He now receives a regularly updated list of all the patients enrolled in his practice. Previously, he was often frustrated by not knowing exactly which patients still considered him as their pediatrician. Reminders to families to bring their children in for their immunizations were often returned with notices that the families had moved away or changed their source of care. Dr. Cope can now track the patients for whom he remains responsible and monitor more accurately the patients who are behind on their checkups and immunizations. Dr. Cope's group also structured their bonus system to primarily reward quality of care, such as achieving high rates of immunization, rather than reduced services.

Dr. Gary Geld works as a PCP in a different practice. Dr. Geld is well aware that his IPA tracks the total costs incurred by his patients for diagnostic tests, specialty referrals, and hospital days. He also knows that his end-of-year bonus decreases as his total costs increase. Dr. Geld denies an emergency room visit to a patient with fever and vomiting; the patient becomes severely dehydrated and comes close to death. He also fails to admit a patient with unstable angina, resulting in the patient sustaining a serious myocardial infarct.

Capitation is neither entirely new nor uniquely American. Many of the benevolent and trade associations that introduced group insurance plans in Europe and the United States at the conclusion of the nineteenth century paid PCPs by capitation (Friedman, 1996). Capitation has been the principal mode of paying general practitioners for the past 50 years in the United Kingdom's National Health Service. Capitation has potential merits as a way to control costs by providing an alternative to the inflationary tendencies of fee-for-service payment. In addition, capitation has been advocated for its potential beneficial influence on the organization of care. Capitation payments require patients to register with a physician or group of physicians. As Dr. Cope found, the clearer enumeration of the population of patients in his practice offered advantages for monitoring appropriate use of services and planning for these patients' needs. Capitation also explicitly defines—in advance—the amount of money available to care for an enrolled population of patients, potentially providing a better framework for rational allocation of resources and innovation in developing more group-oriented and efficient modes of delivering services. For a large group of PCPs, the sheer size of the aggregated capitation payments provides clout and flexibility over how to best arrange ancillary and specialty services.

What is novel, however, about capitation in the United States is the degree to which it has become a high-risk, high-stakes proposition in the context of a fearsomely competitive, market-oriented health care system. Risk pools indexed to individual physician performance create the potential for massive swings in income, depending on a particular physician's "success" at minimizing hospitalizations, referrals, and diagnostic tests—or at avoiding high-risk patients. Acumen in negotiating "the split of the cap" can mean shifts of millions of dollars in revenue to the physician group. Rapid turnover of patients because of loss of insurance or involuntary change of health plan undermines the potential utility of capitation for planning for the needs of a population over time. The common practice of physicians belonging to multiple IPAs and contracting with several HMOs—each with their own referral and authorization requirements—has blunted the idea of an efficient, quality-oriented group practice culture. At this time, preoccupation with the fine print of HMO contracts and risk-pool bonus clauses has left much of the promise of capitation unrealized. The ethical issues generated by a payment system that rewards less care have been well summarized in a recent report of the AMA Council on Ethical and Judicial Affairs (1995). Public concern over the apparent denial of care to some HMO patients—allegedly linked with capitation-plus-bonus payment—has led to the introduction of over 1000 bills in state legislatures and Congress to regulate HMO practices (Bodenheimer, 1996).

Clancy and Brody (1995) have distinguished between "Jekyll and Hyde" forms of managed care. The Jekyll model, represented by some of the traditional nonprofit HMOs, encourages a primary care–oriented approach and population health perspective. This approach emphasizes creating a "culture of practice characterized by practitioners who equate good patient care with cost-effective care" and who strive for quality improvement. The Hyde model typifies those newer, commercially oriented HMOs that lack a cohesive practice culture and rely heavily on financial incentives to change physician practices, with success measured by the bottom line of return of profits to shareholders. Capitation, as a method of payment, may bring out either the Jekyll or the Hyde in physicians. While Dr. Jekyll responds to professional considerations and acts exclusively in the best interest of patients, Dr. Hyde is motivated entirely by economic self-interest. The capitation-plus-bonus payment mechanism attempts to control medical care costs by appealing to the economic concerns of physicians. This strategy "rests on the narrow model of homo economicus, which assumes that financial incentives alone shape human behavior." (Light and May, 1993).

The tension between the Jekyll and Hyde sides of physicians, between the homo medicus and the homo economicus, is accentuated by clinical uncertainty. In these situations, fee-for-service payment may tip the balance in favor of acting rather than waiting. In a similar circumstance, capitation-plus-bonus payment may encourage the physician to wait rather than to act. Capitation-plus-bonus reimbursement, by making a physician's livelihood dependent on the denial of services to patients, risks feeding the dollar-driven homo economicus at the expense of the professionally oriented homo medicus.

REFERENCES

AMA Council on Ethical and Judicial Affairs: Ethical issues in managed care. JAMA 1995;273:330.

Bodenheimer T: The HMO backlash: Righteous or reactionary? N Engl J Med 1996;335:1601.

Clancy CM, Brody H: Managed care: Jekyll or Hyde? JAMA 1995;273:338.

Friedman E: Capitation, integration, and managed care. JAMA 1996;275:957.

Gold MR et al: A national survey of the arrangements managed-care plans make with physicians. N Engl J Med 1995;333:1678.

Interstudy: Competitive Edge. Part II: Industry Report. Interstudy Publications; 1995a.

Interstudy: Competitive Edge. Part III: Regional Market Analysis. Interstudy Publications, 1995b.

Kongstvedt PR: The Managed Care Handbook. Aspen Publishers, 1989.

Light D, May A: Britain's Health System: From Welfare State to Managed Markets. Faulkner and Gray, 1993.

Morgan RO et al: The Medicare-HMO revolving door: The healthy go in and the sick go out. N Engl J Med 1997;337:169.

Newhouse JP: Patients at risk: Health reform and risk adjustment. Health Aff 1994;13(1):132.

Robinson JC, Casalino LP: The growth of medical groups paid through capitation in California. N Engl J Med 1995;333:1684.

Woolhandler S, Himmelstein DU: Extreme risk: The new corporate proposition for physicians. N Engl J Med 1995;333:1706.

How Health Care Is Organized—I   6

Frank Hope has walked with a limp since contracting polio in the 1940s. When he watches his daughter run after her young toddler, he feels a sense of gratitude that the era of vaccinations has protected his child and grandchild from such a disabling infection. He recalls the excitement that gripped the nation as the Salk polio vaccine was first tested and then adopted into widespread use. In Frank's mind, these types of scientific breakthroughs attest to the wonders of the United States health care system.

Frank's grandson attends a daycare program. Ruby, a 2-year-old girl in the program, was recently hospitalized for a severe case of measles complicated by pneumonia. She spent 2 weeks in a pediatric intensive care unit, including several days on a respirator. She had not received measles immunization, normally scheduled for 12–15 months of age. Ruby's mother works full time as a bus driver while raising three children. She has comprehensive private health insurance through her job, but finds it difficult to keep track of all her children's immunization schedules and to find a doctor's office that offers convenient appointment times. She takes her children to an evening-hours urgent care center when they have ear infections but never sees the same physician twice. She blames herself for Ruby's illness.

People in the United States rightfully take pride in the technologic accomplishments of their health care system. Innovations in biomedical science have almost eradicated scourges such as polio and measles and have allowed such marvels as organ transplantation, "knifeless" gamma ray surgery for brain tumors, and intensive care technology that saves the lives of children with measles complicated by pneumonia. Yet, for all its successes, the health care system also has its failures. In 1990, over 25,000 cases of measles were reported in the United States (CDC, 1990). Only two-thirds of preschool children have received the full schedule of immunizations. In some instances, scheduled immunizations are skipped because of inadequate insurance coverage. In other cases such as Ruby's, the failure is not related to financial barriers (Fielding et al, 1994) but rather reflects organizational problems, particularly in the delivery of primary care and preventive services.

The organizational task facing all health care systems, according to analyst Victor Rodwin (1984), is one of "assuring that the right patient receives the right service at the right time and in the right place." An additional criterion could be ". . . and by the right care giver." Ruby's missed vaccination is an example of this challenge. Who is responsible for planning and ensuring that every child receives the right service (vaccination) at the right time (on schedule for a vaccination series)? Can an urgent care center designed for episodic needs be held accountable for vaccinating all patients passing through its doors? Should parents be expected to make appointments for well-child visits at medical offices and clinics, or should public health nurses travel to day-care centers to provide vaccinations out in the community? What is the proper balance between intensive care units that provide life-saving services to critically ill patients and primary care services geared toward less dramatic medical and preventive needs?

The previous chapters have emphasized financial transactions in the health care system. In this chapter and the following one, the organization of the health care system will be the main focus. While considerable debate has dwelled on how to improve financial access to care, less emphasis has been given to the question, "access to what?" In this chapter, organizational systems will be viewed through a wide-angle lens, with emphasis on such broad concepts as the relationship between primary, secondary, and tertiary levels of care, and the influence of the biomedical paradigm and medical professionalism in shaping United States health care delivery. In Chapter 7, a zoom lens will be used to focus on specific organizational models that have appeared (often only to disappear) in this country over the past century.

MODELS OF ORGANIZING CARE

Primary, Secondary, & Tertiary Care   One concept is essential in understanding the "topography" of any health care system: the organization of care into primary, secondary, and tertiary levels. In the Lord Dawson Report, an influential British study written in 1920, the author (1975) proposed that each of the three levels of care should correspond with certain unique patient needs.

(1) Primary care involves common health problems (eg, sore throats, sprained ankles, hypertension) and preventive measures (eg, vaccinations) that account for 80–90% of visits to a physician or other care giver.

(2) Secondary care involves problems that require more specialized clinical expertise such as hospital care for a patient with acute renal failure.

(3) Tertiary care, which lies at the apex of the organizational pyramid, involves the management of rare and complex disorders such as pituitary tumors and congenital malformations.

Two contrasting approaches can be used to organize a health care system around these levels of care: (1) the carefully structured Dawson model of regionalized health care, and (2) a more free-flowing model.

(1) One approach uses the Dawson model as a scaffold for a highly structured system. This model is based on the concept of regionalization: the organization and coordination of all health resources and services within a defined area (Bodenheimer, 1969). In a regionalized system, different types of personnel and facilities are assigned to distinct tiers in the primary, secondary, and tertiary levels, and the flow of patients across levels occurs in an orderly, regulated fashion. This model emphasizes the primary care base.

(2) An alternative model allows for more fluid roles for care givers, and more free-flowing movement of patients, across all levels of care. This model tends to place a higher value on services at the tertiary care apex than at the primary care base.

Although most health care systems embody elements of both models, some gravitate closer to one polarity or the other. The British National Health Service (NHS), and more recently some health maintenance organizations (HMOs) in the United States, resemble the regionalized approach, while United States health care as a whole approximates the more dispersed format.

The Regionalized Model: The Traditional British National Health Service

> Basil, a 60-year-old man living in a London suburb, is registered with Dr. Prime, a general practitioner in his neighborhood. Basil goes to Dr. Prime for most of his health problems, including hay fever, back spasms, and hypertension. One day, he experiences numbness and weakness in his face and arm. By the time Dr. Prime examines him later that day, the symptoms have resolved. Suspecting that Basil has had a transient ischemic attack, Dr. Prime prescribes aspirin and refers him to the neurologist at the local hospital, where a carotid artery sonogram reveals high-grade carotid stenosis. Dr. Prime and the neurologist agree that Basil should make an appointment at a London teaching hospital with a vascular surgeon specializing in head and neck surgery. The surgeon recommends that Basil undergo carotid endarterectomy on an elective basis to prevent a major stroke. Basil returns to Dr. Prime to discuss this recommendation and inquires whether the operation could be performed at a local hospital closer to home. Dr. Prime informs him that only a handful of London hospitals are equipped to perform this type of specialized operation. Basil schedules his operation in London and several months later has an uncomplicated carotid endarterectomy. Following the operation, he returns to Dr. Prime for his ongoing care.

The British NHS has traditionally typified a relatively regimented primary-secondary-tertiary care structure (Figure 6–1).

(1) For physician services, the primary care level is virtually the exclusive domain of general practitioners (commonly referred to as GPs), who practice in small- to medium-sized groups and whose main responsibility is ambulatory care. Two-thirds of all physicians in the United Kingdom are GPs (Grumbach and Fry, 1993).

(2) The secondary tier of care is occupied by physicians in such specialties as internal medicine, pediatrics, neurology, psychiatry, obstetrics and gynecology, and general surgery. These physicians are located at hospital-based clinics and serve as consultants for outpatient referrals from GPs, in turn routing most patients back to GPs for ongoing care needs. Secondary-level physicians also provide care to hospitalized patients.

(3) Tertiary care subspecialists such as cardiac surgeons, immunologists, and pediatric hematologists are located at a few tertiary care medical centers.

Hospital planning follows the same regionalized logic as physician services. District hospitals are local facilities equipped for basic inpatient services. Regional tertiary care medical centers handle highly specialized inpatient care needs.

Planning of physician and hospital resources within the NHS occurs with a population focus. GP groups provide care to a base population of 5000–50,000 persons, depending on the number of GPs in the practice. District hospitals have a catchment area population of 50,000–500,000, while tertiary care hospitals serve as referral centers for a population of 500,000 to 5 million (Fry, 1980).

Patient flow moves in a stepwise fashion across the different tiers. Except in emergency situations, all patients are first seen by a GP, who may then steer patients toward more specialized levels of care through a formal process of referral. Patients may not directly refer themselves to a specialist.

While nonphysician health professionals such as nurses play an integral role in staffing hospitals at the secondary and tertiary care levels, especially noteworthy is the NHS's multidisciplinary approach to primary care. GPs work in close collaboration with practice nurses (similar to nurse practitioners in the United States), home health visitors, public health nurses, and midwives (who attend most deliveries in the United Kingdom). Such teamwork, along with accountability for a defined population of enrolled patients and universal health care coverage, helps to avert such problems as missed childhood vaccinations. Public health nurses visit all homes in the first weeks after a birth to provide education and assist with scheduling of initial GP appointments. A national vaccination tracking system notifies parents about each scheduled vaccination and alerts GPs and public health nurses if a child has not appeared at the appointed time. As a result, over 85% of British preschool children receive a full series of immunizations. (The British NHS is discussed at greater length in Chapter 14.)

A number of other nations, ranging from industrialized countries in Scandinavia to developing nations in Latin America, have adopted a similar approach to organizing health services. In developing nations, the primary care tier relies more on community health educators and other types of public health personnel than on physicians.

The Dispersed Model: Traditional United States Health Care Organization

> Polly Seymour, a 55-year-old woman with private health insurance who lives in the United States, sees several different physicians for a variety of problems: a dermatologist for eczema, a gastroenterologist for recurrent heartburn, and an orthopedist for tendinitis in her shoulder. She may ask her gastroenterologist to treat a few general medical problems, such as borderline diabetes. On occasion, she has gone to the nearby hospital emergency room for treatment of urinary tract infections. One day, Polly feels a lump in her breast and consults a gynecologist. She is referred to a surgeon for biopsy, which indicates cancer. After discussing treatment options with Polly, the surgeon performs a lumpectomy and refers her to an oncologist and radiation therapy specialist for further therapy. She receives all of these treatments at a local hospital a short distance from her home.

The United States health care system has had a far less structured approach to levels of care than the British NHS. In contrast with the stepwise flow of patient referrals in the United Kingdom, insured patients in the United States such as Polly Seymour have traditionally been able to refer themselves and enter the system directly at any level. Rather than having a designated primary care physician (PCP) to initially evaluate all of their problems, patients in the United States have become accustomed to taking their symptoms directly to the specialist of their choosing.

Physicians in the United States have less clearly defined roles than physicians in systems such as the NHS. Primary care, rather than being a unique ecologic niche for GPs and nonphysician primary providers, has become integrated into the practices of many specialist physicians. This diffuse approach to primary care was partly born out of necessity, as only 13% of physicians in the United States are general or family practitioners. The relative decline in the numbers of these practitioners has been a steady trend since 1940, when three-fourths of physicians were GPs (Starr, 1982).

One unique aspect of the United States approach to primary care has been to broaden the role of internists and pediatricians. Whereas general internists and general pediatricians in the United Kingdom and most European nations serve principally as referral physicians in the secondary tier, their United States counterparts share in providing primary care. Moreover, the overlapping roles among "generalists" in the United States (GPs, family physicians, general internists, and general pediatricians) are not limited to the outpatient sector. GPs and family physicians in the United States have taken on a number of secondary care functions by providing substantial amounts of inpatient care. Only recently have some settings in the United States adopted the European model that removes inpatient care from the domain of PCPs and assigns this work to "hospitalists"—physicians who exclusively practice within the hospital (Wachter and Goldman, 1996). Under managed care, this trend is expected to grow.

Including general internists and general pediatricians, the total supply of generalists amounts to about one-third of all physicians in the United States, a number well below the 50% or more found in Canada and many European nations (Starfield, 1992). To fill in the primary care gap, some physicians at the tertiary care level in the United States have also acted as PCPs for many of their patients. Studies in the 1970s indicated that nearly 20% of persons in the United States relied on a nongeneralist physician for their principal care (Aiken et al, 1979).

United States hospitals also are not constrained by rigid secondary and tertiary care boundaries. Instead of a pyramidal system featuring a large number of general community hospitals at the base and a limited number of tertiary care referral centers at the apex, the United States features a collection of autonomous hospitals, each aspiring to offer the latest in specialized care. In most urban areas, for example, several hospitals perform open heart surgery, organ transplants, radiation therapy, and high-risk obstetric procedures. The resulting structure resembles a diamond more than a pyramid, with a small number of hospitals (mostly rural) that lack specialized units at the base, a small number of elite university medical centers providing "quaternary" superspecialized referral services at the apex, and the bulk of hospitals providing a wide range of secondary and tertiary services in the middle (Freymann, 1977). (Chapter 7 discusses alternative models in the United States, such as community health centers and prepaid group practice HMOs that deviate from this "traditional" organizational form.)

Which Model Is Right? Critics of the United States health care system find fault with its "top-heavy" specialist and tertiary care orientation and lack of organizational coherence. Analyses of health care in the United States over the past half century abound with such descriptions as "the nonsystem of care," "fragmentation, chaos, and disarray," "a collection of bits and pieces," and "uncontrolled growth and pluralism verging on anarchy" (Somers, 1972). The high cost of health care has been attributed in part to this organizational disarray. Quality of care may suffer, also. For example, when many hospitals each perform small numbers of surgical procedures such as coronary artery bypass grafts, mortality rates are higher than when such procedures are regionalized in a few higher-volume centers (Grumbach et al, 1995).

Defenders of the dispersed model reply that pluralism is a virtue, promoting flexibility and convenience in the availability of facilities and personnel. In this view, the emphasis on specialization and technology is compatible with values and expectations in the United States, with patients placing a high premium on direct access to specialists and tertiary care services, and on autonomy in selecting care givers of their choosing for a particular health care need. A New York Times reporter recently observed that

> . . . nostalgia for Marcus Welby competes with the Mayo Clinic syndrome. . . . [Americans] may love their family doctor, but the phrase "the best in his field" has a powerful allure. (Toner R: The family doctor is rarely in. New York Times, Feb 6, 1994.)

Similarly, the desire for the latest in hospital technology located a convenient distance from home competes with plans to regionalize tertiary care services at a limited number of hospitals.

Balancing the Different Levels of Care

> Dr. Billie Ruben completed her residency training in internal medicine at a major university medical center. Like most of her fellow residents, she went on to pursue subspecialty training—in her case, gastroenterology. Dr. Ruben chose this career after caring for a young woman who developed irreversible liver failure following toxic shock syndrome. After a nerve-racking touch-and-go effort to secure a donor liver, transplantation was performed, and the patient made a complete recovery.

> Upon completion of her training, Dr. Ruben joined a growing subspecialty practice at Atlantic Heights Hospital, a successful private hospital in the city. Even though the metropolitan area of 2 million people already has two liver transplant units, Atlantic Heights has just opened a third such unit, feeling that its reputation for excellence depends on delivering tertiary care services at the cutting edge of biomedical innovation. In her first 6 months at the hospital, Dr. Ruben participates in the care of only two patients requiring liver transplantation. Most of her patients seek care for chronic, often ill-defined abdominal pain and digestive problems. As Dr. Ruben begins seeing these patients on a regular basis, she starts to give preventive care and treat nongastrointestinal problems such as hypertension and diabetes. At times, she wishes she had experienced more general medicine during her training.

Advocates of a stronger role for primary care in the United States believe that it is too important to be considered an afterthought in health planning. In this view, overemphasis on the tertiary care apex of the pyramid creates a system in which health care resources are not well matched to the prevalence and incidence of health problems in a community. In an article entitled "The Ecology of Medical Care," published over 3 decades ago, Kerr White recorded the monthly prevalence of illness for a general population of 1000 adults (White et al, 1961). In this group, 750 experienced one or more illnesses or injuries during the month. Of these patients, 250 visited a physician at least once during the month, nine were admitted to a hospital, and only one was referred to a university medical center. Dr. White voiced concern that the training of health care professionals at tertiary care–oriented academic medical centers gave trainees like Dr. Billie Ruben an unrepresentative view of the health care needs of the community:

> Serious questions can be raised about the nature of the average medical student's experience, and perhaps that of some of his clinical teachers, with the substantive problems of health and disease in the community. In general, this experience must be both limited and unusually biased if, in a month, only 0.0013 of the "sick" adults . . . or 0.004 of the patients . . . in a community are referred to university medical centers. . . . Medical, nursing, and other students of the health professions cannot fail to receive unrealistic impressions of medicine's task in contemporary Western society. . . . (White KL, Williams F, Greenberg BG: The ecology of medical care. N Engl J Med 1961;265:885.)

An English GP, John Fry (1980), conducted a related study of the ecology of care, in which he systematically recorded the types of health problems that brought patients to his office in the 1970s. Because of the GP's function as gatekeeper under the NHS, Dr. Fry's investigation provides a close approximation of the full incidence and prevalence of diseases requiring medical attention among his population of registered patients (Table 6–1). The dominant "pathology" in this unselected population consisted of minor ailments (many of which would have improved without treatment), chronic conditions such as hypertension and arthritis, and gradations of mental illness. The incidence of new cancers was relatively rare, and only a handful of patients manifested complex syndromes such as multiple sclerosis. Dr. Fry's study confirms the adage that "common disorders commonly occur and rare ones rarely happen."

Although the analyses of Kerr White and John Fry suggest that most health needs can be met at the primary care level, this observation should not imply that most health care resources should be devoted to primary care. The minority of patients with severe or complicated conditions requiring secondary or tertiary care will command a much larger share of health care resources per capita than the majority of people with less dramatic health care needs. Treating a patient with liver failure costs a great deal more than treating a patient for a sore throat. Even in the United Kingdom, where the 65% of physicians who are GPs provide 60% of all ambulatory care, expenditures on their services account for less than 10% of the overall NHS budget, whereas the cost of inpatient and outpatient hospital care at the secondary and tertiary levels consumes nearly two-thirds of the budget (Sidel and Sidel, 1983). Thus, the pyramidal shape shown in Figure 6–1 better represents the distribution of health

Table 6–1. Persons per year seeking care in a general practitioner practice with a registered population of 2500, according to problem.[1]

		Persons Per Year Seeking Care
Minor Illness		
General disorders		
Upper respiratory infections		600
Skin disorders		325
Emotional problems		300
Gastrointestinal disorders		300
Accidents		200
Specific disorders		
Acute tonsillitis		100
Acute otitis media		75
Acute urinary infections		50
"Acute back" syndrome		50
Migraine headache		25
Hay fever		25
Preventive care needs		
(eg, immunization, checkup, prenatal care)		300
Major illness		
Pneumonia		20
Severe depression		10
Suicide attempt	3	
Suicide	1 in 4 years	
Acute myocardial infarction		8
Acute appendicitis		5
Acute strokes		5
New cancers		5
Lung	2 per year	
Breast	1 per year	
Large bowel	2 every 3 years	
Stomach	1 every 2 years	
Prostate	1 every 2 years	
Cervix	1 every 4 years	
Brain	1 every 10 years	
Lymphoma	1 every 15 years	
Thyroid	1 every 20 years	
Chronic illness		
Chronic arthritis		100
Chronic psychiatric problems		60
High blood pressure		50
Obesity		40
Chronic bronchitis		35
Chronic heart failure		30
Cancers (new and old)		30
Asthma		25
Peptic ulcers		20
Coronary artery disease		20
Cerebrovascular disease		15
Epilepsy		10
Diabetes		10
Thyroid disease		7
Parkinsonism		3
Multiple sclerosis		1
Chronic renal disease		less than 1

[1] Adapted and reproduced, with permission, from Fry J: Primary care. In: Primary Care. Fry J (editor). William Heinemann, 1980.

care problems in a community than the apportionment of health care expenditures. While almost all industrialized nations devote a dominant share of health care resources to secondary and tertiary care, the ecologic view reminds us that most people have health care needs at the primary care level.

Defining Practitioner Roles No health care system considers it appropriate for family physicians to perform cardiac catheterizations, yet in the United States, primary care is often considered to be within the reasonable scope of practice for cardiologists. Because primary care concentrates on "common problems that are common," there is a tendency to consider it routine and not requiring special expertise. This notion is increasingly being challenged. Barbara Starfield (1992) is a leading proponent of the need to train generalist physicians (ie, family physicians, general internists, and GPs) specifically to fill the primary care niche. In her view:

> . . . the goals of primary care are better served by practitioners trained and organized to provide primary care than by practitioners trained to focus on particular illnesses, organ systems, or pathogenetic mechanisms. (Starfield B: Primary Care. Oxford Univ Press, 1992.)

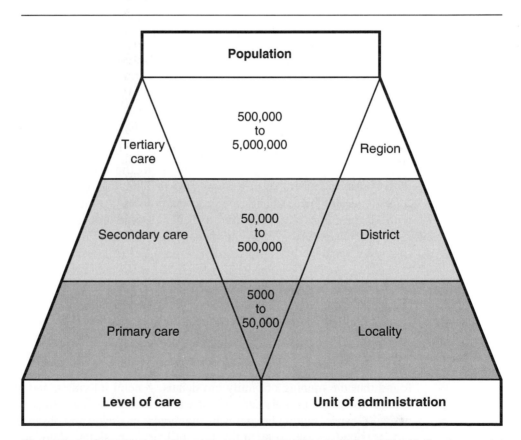

Figure 6–1. Organization of services under the traditional National Health Service model in the United Kingdom. Care is organized into distinct levels corresponding to specific functions, roles, administrative units, and population bases.

Just as an invasive cardiologist must master the skills needed to perform coronary angioplasty, special competencies are required of primary care practitioners. Dr. Starfield has formulated the key tasks of primary care as follows: (1) first contact care, (2) longitudinality, (3) comprehensiveness, and (4) coordination.

> Dr. O. Titus Wells has cared for all six of Bruce and Wendy Smith's children. As a family physician whose practice includes obstetrics, Dr. Wells attended the births of all but one of the children. The Smith's 18-month-old daughter, Ginny, has had many ear infections. Even though this is a common problem, Dr. Wells finds that it presents a real medical challenge. Sometimes, examination of Ginny's ears indicates a raging infection and, at other times, the presence of middle ear fluid, which may or may not represent a bona fide bacterial infection. He tries to reserve antibiotics for clear-cut cases of bacterial otitis. He feels it is important that he be the one to examine Ginny's ears because her eardrums never look entirely normal and he knows what degree of change is suspicious for a genuinely new infection.
>
> When Ginny is 2 years old, Dr. Wells recommends to the Smiths that she see an otolaryngologist and audiologist to check for hearing loss and language impairment. The audiograms show modest diminution of hearing in one ear. The otolaryngologist informs the Smiths that ear tubes are an option. At Ginny's return visit with Dr. Wells, he discusses the pros and cons of tube placement with the Smiths. He also uses the visit as an opportunity to encourage Mrs. Smith to quit smoking, mentioning that research has shown that exposure to tobacco smoke may predispose children to ear infections.

Dr. Wells's care of the Smith family illustrates the essential features of primary care. He is the first-contact physician performing the initial evaluation when Ginny or other family members develop symptoms of illness. Longitudinality (or continuity) refers to sustaining a patient–care giver relationship over time. Dr. Wells's familiarity with Ginny's condition helps him to better discern an acute infection. Comprehensiveness consists of the ability to manage a wide range of health care needs, in contrast with specialty care, which focuses on a particular organ system or procedural service. Dr. Wells's comprehensive family-oriented care makes him aware that Mrs. Smith's smoking cessation program is an important part of his treatment plan for Ginny. Coordination builds upon longitudinality. Through referral and follow-up, the primary care provider integrates services delivered by other care givers.

The dispersed model of care in the United States has given rise to debate about which types of physicians are best equipped to perform these primary care functions. In a review of specialty training programs in the United States, Rivo et al (1994) found that the training of family physicians, general internists, and general pediatricians emphasized primary care competencies such as comprehensiveness and coordination of care. Training programs in emergency medicine and obstetrics and gynecology provided less preparation for these primary care skills. Many nurse practitioners and physician assistants in the United States also receive training in these primary care competencies.

Several studies have found that the elements of good primary care contribute to higher patient satisfaction and better patient outcomes (Starfield, 1992). For example, increased continuity is associated with greater use of preventive services (Benson et al, 1984), higher compliance with appointment keeping and use of medications (Charney et al, 1967), better pregnancy outcomes (Shear et al, 1983), reductions in hospitalizations (Wasson et al, 1984), and declines in overall costs (Weiss and Blustein, 1996). There is evidence that having a regular source of care results in better control of hypertension and less reliance on emergency department services (Shea et al, 1992). Persons whose care meets a primary care–oriented model have better perceived access to care and are more likely to receive recommended preventive services (Bindman et al, 1995; Stewart et al, 1997). Additional research indicates that primary care features such as continuity and coordination are more likely to be present when care is provided by generalists rather than specialists (Starfield, 1992).

An unresolved question remains about the quality of care that may be provided by primary care–oriented generalist physicians as opposed to specialists oriented toward expertise in specific areas of medicine and surgery. Direct access by patients to different specialists might result in a less integrated model of care but might, on the other hand, allow access to physicians with the most extensive training and experience at managing individual conditions within each organ-based specialty area. Many studies have found that generalists and specialists provide a comparable quality for a variety of conditions such as diabetes, hypertension, low back pain, and childbirth (Greenfield et al, 1995; Carey et al, 1995; Hueston et al, 1995). Specialists may in some instances perform better than generalists when managing conditions within their particular specialty domain, for example, cardiologists treating patients with acute myocardial infarction (Jollis et al, 1996). On the other hand, specialists who devote a substantial amount of their practice to primary care or nonreferral cases may not be able to maintain as much expertise in their specialty area as those who concentrate more fully on secondary and tertiary care problems (Menken, 1988).

In terms of costs, research supports the view that generalist physicians practice a less resource-intensive style of medicine than specialists and therefore may represent a more economical approach to the provision of primary care (Starfield, 1992; Franks et al, 1993; Carey et al, 1995). The most rigorously conducted cost-comparison study found that even after controlling for potential differences in severity of illness, patients with a general internist or family physician as a regular physician used fewer resources than similar patients with a specialist as a regular physician (Greenfield et al, 1992). Other studies have shown that health care costs are higher in regions with higher ratios of specialist-to-generalist physicians (Starfield, 1992; Welch et al, 1993). Studies of patients with low-risk pregnancies have found that certified nurse midwives provided a less interventionist and costly style of care than obstetricians, resulting in one-third fewer cesarean sections (Rosenblatt et al, 1997).

Gatekeeping & Structured Patient Flow

> Polly Seymour, described earlier in the chapter, feels terrible. Every time she eats she feels nauseated, and frequently she vomits. She has lost 8 pounds, and her oncologist is worried that her breast cancer has spread. She undergoes blood tests, an abdominal CT scan, and a bone scan, all of which are normal. She returns to her gastroenterologist,

who tells her to stop the ibuprofen she has been taking for tendinitis. Her problem persists, and the gastroenterologist performs an endoscopy, which shows mild gastric irritation. A month has passed, $3000 has been spent, and Polly continues to vomit.

Polly's friend Martha recommends a nurse practitioner who has been caring for Martha for many years and who, in Martha's view, seems to spend more time talking with patients than do many physicians. Polly makes an appointment with the nurse practitioner, Sara Steward. Ms. Steward takes a complete history, which reveals that Polly is taking tamoxifen for her breast cancer and that she began to take aspirin after stopping the ibuprofen. Ms. Steward explains that either of these medications can cause vomiting and suggests that they be stopped for a week. Polly returns in a week, her nausea and vomiting resolved. Ms. Steward then consults with Polly's oncologist, and together they decide to restart the tamoxifen but not the aspirin. Polly becomes nauseated again, but eventually begins to feel well and gains weight while taking a reduced dose of tamoxifen. In the future, Ms. Steward handles Polly's medical problems, referring her to specialty physicians when needed, and making sure that the advice of one consultant does not interfere with the therapy of another specialist.

A concept that incorporates many of the elements of primary care is that of the primary care provider as gatekeeper. Gatekeeping has taken on pejorative connotations in the era of managed care, where some types of financial arrangements with PCPs may provide incentives for them to "shut the gate" in order to limit specialist referrals, diagnostic tests, and other services (see Chapters 4 and 5). Stories such as Polly's may restore some of the gatekeeper's historical luster, which has been lost as a result of managed care's conversion of gatekeepers into gateshutters. Peter Franks and colleagues (1992) have written a review describing gatekeeping as "a core function of primary care," defined as "the process of matching patients' needs and preferences with judicious use of medical services." The health care provider as gatekeeper is

> . . . an advocate who can protect patients from the possible adverse effects of unnecessary care, and . . . a critical decision maker who can ensure the appropriate use of health care services. (Franks P, Clancy CM, Nutting PA: Gatekeeping revisited: Protecting patients from overtreatment. N Engl J Med 1992;327:424.)

This view of the gatekeeper role corresponds with the main organizational challenge in the delivery of care: assuring that each patient gets "the right service at the right time and in the right place." Dr. Wells and Ms. Steward both act as gatekeepers in serving as health care provider of first contact, deciding when a specialty consultation is appropriate, and coordinating medical and preventive care. A Canadian study of gatekeeping found that children undergoing tonsillectomy were more likely to have the operation performed for appropriate indications when they were referred to the otolaryngologist by a pediatrician than when care was directly sought from the otolaryngologist (Roos, 1979). This suggests that the gatekeeper can play a positive role in "ensuring appropriate use of health care services."

Accountability for Health Care

> Through the HMO she works for, 2000 people have signed up with Dr. Lisa Service. One day, over a couple of ginger ales, Dr. Service makes a bet with her colleague, Dr. Henry Caire, that she can make her 2000 patients healthier than the patients enrolled with Dr. Caire. They will meet in a year and compare statistics. Dr. Service turns on her computer and finds that she has seen 1200 of her enrollees in the past year and has not seen 800. The computer also tells her who has had Pap smears, mammograms, blood pressure checkups, well-baby care, and immunizations; when they had them; and who was not receiving proper preventive services. She arranges that each month, her receptionist will contact any of the 2000 patients due for a preventive service, hypertensives due for blood pressure checkups, and diabetics due for blood sugar evaluations. Dr. Caire, in contrast, simply provides high-quality medical care to those patients who come to see him. At the end of the year, the two doctors ask a nurse specialized in quality improvement to audit their charts. Dr. Service wins the bet.

In the dispersed model of medical care, with several specialists each concerned with one organ system of the body, accountability for the care of the whole patient may be lacking, even if each specialist gives the highest quality of care. The idea of gatekeeper as patient advocate may advance the ideal of accountability by giving one care giver responsibility for providing or coordinating a person's overall care. Yet even in the gatekeeper model, much of the responsibility for receipt of service is placed on the individual patient. While physicians and other care givers have an obligation to provide the highest-quality services to patients seeking care, this obligation does not usually extend to identifying and targeting services for patients who do not initiate contact with the medical system.

Systems such as the British NHS consider accountability in primary care to extend beyond individual patient encounters to encompass the wider population. For example, as noted above, GPs are expected to achieve targeted rates of vaccination among all children enrolled in the practice, and the medical care and public health systems collaborate in tracking and performing outreach for immunizations.

A number of analysts have called on the United States to adopt more of such a population-oriented model of primary care—the model used by Dr. Service to win her bet. Advocates of this approach have used the term *community-oriented primary care* to refer to a model that incorporates efforts to systematically define a target population, determine its health needs, and develop community-based interventions to address these needs (Nutting, 1990). Attempts to practice community-oriented primary care in the United States have often been frustrated by difficulties in defining a relevant population in the fee-for-service, multipayer system with ill-defined gatekeeper responsibilities. In addition, the historically rigid boundaries between public health activities and private medical practice have contributed to the view that population health concerns fall under the purview of public health departments. Just as automobile mechanics are expected to competently work on cars brought in for servicing but are not held accountable for the failure of car owners to bring their cars in for tune-ups, some consider it unreasonable to expect physicians to be responsible for the state of health of a community rather than of individual patients seeking services.

The conceptualization of primary care continues to undergo redefinition as health care planners grapple with the challenges of organizing systems responsive to the public's needs. The Institute of Medicine has recently promulgated a revised definition of primary care: "Primary care is the provision of integrated, accessible health care services by clinicians who are accountable for addressing a large majority of personal health care needs, developing sustained partnerships with patients, and practicing in the context of family and community" (Institute of Medicine, 1996).

FORCES DRIVING THE ORGANIZATION OF HEALTH CARE IN THE UNITED STATES

The Biomedical Model   The dispersed mode of health care delivery in the United States for the past several decades was shaped by several forces. One influential factor was the preeminence of the biomedical model among medical educators and young physicians throughout the twentieth century. The combination of stricter state licensing laws and an influential national study, the Flexner report of 1906, led to consolidation of medical training in academically oriented medical schools (Starr, 1982). These academic centers embraced the biomedical paradigm that was the legacy of such renowned nineteenth century European microbiologists as Pasteur and Koch. Departing from the empiricism and mysticism that characterized most healing practices prior to the twentieth century, the biomedical model fed an optimism that the union of technologic innovation and expertise in basic science would produce cures for most human afflictions. The antimicrobial model engendered the faith that every illness has a discrete, ultimately knowable cause and that "magic bullets" can be crafted to eradicate these sources of disease. Physicians were trained to master pathophysiologic changes within a particular organ system, leading to the development of specialization (Luce and Byyny, 1979).

The scientific biomedical paradigm became preeminent not only among physicians and other health professionals but also among the general population in the United States. The often dramatic accomplishments of modern medicine were bolstered by broader historical events. The Manhattan Project's success in designing an atomic bomb convinced the nation after World War II of the value of basic science and research. In the 1950s and 1960s, the launching of Sputnik by the Soviet Union and the landing of the first man on the moon by the United States captured the public imagination. In 1941, federal spending for medical research was $3 million, but by 1951, it had jumped to $75 million. In 1955, Congress established the National Institutes of Health, with a budget of $81 million, and its appropriations rose 500% over the next 5 years (Starr, 1982).

Advocates of a larger role for generalism in United States health care have not so much rejected the concepts of scientific medicine and professional specialism as they have attempted to broaden the interpretation of these terms. They have called for a more integrated scientific approach to understanding health and illness that incorporates information about the individual's psychosocial experiences and family, cultural, and environmental context as well as physiologic and anatomic constitution (Engel, 1977). The attempt to more rigorously define the scientific and clinical basis of generalism contributed to the emergence of family medicine in the 1970s as a specialty discipline in its own right, and the 1-year general practice internship was re-placed by a 3-year residency program and specialty board certification.

Financial Incentives   A second and related factor influencing the structure of health care was the financial incentive for physician specialization and hospital ex-pansion, which played out in a number of ways.

(1) Insurance benefits first offered by Blue Cross covered hospital costs but not physician visits and other outpatient services.

(2) As physician services came to be covered later under Blue Shield and other plans, a growing differential in reimbursement between generalist and specialist physicians developed. New technologic and other procedures often required consid-erable physician time when first introduced, and higher fees were justified for these procedures. But as the procedures became routine, fees remained high while the time and effort required to perform them declined (Starr, 1982); this resulted in an increas-ing disparity in income between PCPs and specialists (Gonzalez, 1997). The current magnitude of these disparities is shown in Table 6–2.

(3) Federal involvement in health care financing further fueled the expansion of hos-pital care and specialization. One of the first major federal government investments in health care was the Hill-Burton Hospital Construction Act of 1946, which allocated nearly $4 billion between 1946 and 1971 for expansion of hospital capacity rather than development of ambulatory services (Starr, 1982). The subsequent enactment of Medicare and Medicaid in 1965 perpetuated the private insurance tradition of higher reimbursement for procedurally oriented specialists than for generalists. Medicare

Table 6–2. Physician net income in the United States (1996).[1]

	Mean	Median
All physicians	$195,500	$160,000
Specialty		
General or family practice	131,200	124,000
Internal medicine	185,700	150,000
General internal medicine	159,500	138,000
Cardiovascular diseases	292,000	210,000
Surgery	269,000	225,000
General surgery	244,400	203,000
Otolaryngology	232,300	206,000
Orthopedic surgery	323,200	250,000
Ophthalmology	240,800	194,000
Urologic surgery	243,400	220,000
Pediatrics	140,500	129,000
Obstetrics and gynecology	244,300	200,000
Radiology	244,400	230,000
Psychiatry	137,200	124,000
Anesthesiology	215,100	203,000
Pathology	209,400	185,000
Emergency medicine	184,400	170,000

[1] Reproduced, with permission, from Gonzalez M: Physician Marketplace Statistics. American Medical Association, 1997.

further encouraged specialization through its policy of extra payments to hospitals to cover costs associated with residency training. Furthermore, Medicare teaching payments were linked to the hospital's level of inpatient, but not outpatient, service, adding yet another bias against community-based primary care training.

The growth of hospitals and medical specialization were intertwined. Hospitals are by definition sites of secondary and tertiary care, with the exception of hospital-based primary care clinics. As medical practice became more specialized and dependent on technology, the site of care increasingly shifted from the patient's home or physician's office to the hospital.

The emphasis on acute hospital care had an effect on the nursing profession comparable to the effect that hospitals had in promoting specialization among physicians. World War I was a watershed period in the transition of nursing from a community-based to a hospital-based orientation. During the war, United States military hospitals overseas were much heralded for their success in treating acute war injuries. At the war's conclusion, the nation rallied behind a policy of boosting the civilian hospital sector. According to Rosemary Stevens (1989):

> Before the war public-health nursing was the elite area; nurses had been instrumental in the campaigns against tuberculosis and for infant welfare. . . . In contrast, the war emphasized the supremacy and glamour of hospitals . . . nurses, like physicians, were trained—and ready—to perform in an increasingly specialized, acute-care medical environment rather than to expand their interests in social medicine and public health. (Stevens R: In Sickness and in Wealth: American Hospitals in the Twentieth Century. Basic Books, 1989.)

Professionalism   The final, and in many ways most critical, factor accounting for the organizational evolution of United States health care delivery was the nature of control over health planning. The United States is unique in its relative laxity of public regulation of health care resources. In most industrialized nations, governments wield considerable control over health planning through measures such as regulation of hospital capacity and technology, allocation of the number of residency training positions in generalist and specialist fields, and coordination of public health with primary, secondary, and tertiary medical care services. In the United States, the government has provided much of the financing for health care but without an attendant degree of administrative control. The Hill-Burton program, for example, did not make grants for hospital construction contingent upon any rigorous community-wide plan for regionalized hospital services. Federal funding for expansion of the physician work force did not stipulate any particular distribution of training positions according to specialty. Government ventures into health planning, such as transient establishment of regional health planning agencies in the 1970s, often had few regulatory "teeth" and exerted little control over the organization of services.

With government controls kept largely at bay, the professional "sovereignty" of physicians emerged as the preeminent authority in health care (Starr, 1982). According to sociologists, an occupation takes on the mantle of a profession when it achieves several key characteristics. First, members of a profession have considerable control over their own work. This control consists of autonomy in daily occupational tasks and working conditions, as well as control over occupational standards and entry through processes such as licensing. In addition, the high level of "professional dominance" achieved by physicians is explained by the power of physicians to "control the work of others in one's domain," such as nurses, medical technicians, and other health care workers (Friedson, 1970; Light and Levine, 1988). Societies grant occupations these professional prerogatives because of the special knowledge and skill required of members of the profession and the expectation that this knowledge and skill will be applied beneficially. Professionalism thus involves a social contract; in return for the privilege of autonomy, physicians bear the responsibility for acting as the patient's agent, and the profession must regulate itself to preserve the public trust.

Their professional status vested physicians with special authority to guide the development of the United States health care system. As described in Chapter 2, third-party payment for physician services was established with physician control of the initial Blue Shield insurance plans. Physician judgment about the need for technology and greater inpatient capacity drove the expansion of hospital facilities.

What was the nature of the profession that so heavily influenced the development of the United States health care organization? It was a profession that, because of the primacy of the biomedical paradigm and the nature of financial incentives, was weighted toward hospital and specialty care. Small wonder that United States health care has emphasized its tertiary care apex over its primary care base.

CONCLUSION

> Jeff leaves a town forum at the local medical center feeling confused. It featured two speakers, one of whom criticized the medical center as being out of touch with the community's needs, and the other of whom defended the center's contributions to society. Jeff found the first speaker very convincing about the need to pay more attention to primary care, prevention, and public health. He had never had a regular primary care doctor, and the idea of having a family physician appealed to him. He was equally impressed by the second speaker, whose account of how research at the medical center had led to life-saving treatment of children with a hereditary blood disorder was very moving and whose description of the hospital's plan for a new imaging center was spellbinding. Jeff felt that if he ever became seriously ill, he would certainly want all the specialized services the medical center had to offer.

The professional model and the biomedical paradigm are responsible for many of the attractive characteristics of the United States health care system. The biomedical model has instilled respect for the scientific method and has helped to curtail medical quackery. Professionalism has directed physicians to serve as agents acting in their patients' best interests and has made the practice of medicine more than just another business. Expansion of hospital facilities has meant that people with health insurance have had convenient access to tertiary care services and new technology. Patients have been able to take advantage of the expertise and availability of a wide variety of specialists. In many circumstances, the system is well organized to deliver the "right care." For a patient in cardiogenic shock, the right place to be is in an intensive care unit; for a patient with a detached retina, an ophthalmologist's office is the right place to be.

There is widespread concern, however, that despite the benefits of biomedical science and medical professionalism, the United States health care system is precariously off balance. A model of excellence focused on specialization, technology, and curative medicine has led to relative inattention to basic primary care services, including such needs as disease prevention and supportive care for patients with chronic and incurable ailments. The value placed on individualism and autonomy for health care professionals and institutions has contributed to a pluralistic delivery system in which care is often fragmented and lacking in coordination. A system that prizes specialists who focus on organ systems and researchers who concentrate on splitting genes has bred apprehension that health care has somehow lost sight of the whole person and the whole community. The net result is a system structured to perform miraculous feats for individuals who are ill but at great expense and often without satisfactorily attending to the full spectrum of health care needs of the entire population.

The sovereignty of the medical profession and its role in commanding the "dispersed" course of health policy in the United States has only recently been seriously challenged. Although physicians in the United States have long perceived government as the main threat to their professional autonomy and authority, the force that has begun to erode professional dominance has not been government but the large private managed care corporations that are forcefully asserting their influence in the emerging competitive market. These newly changing roles and power relationships are discussed in greater detail in Chapter 16.

REFERENCES

Aiken LH et al: The contribution of specialists to the delivery of primary care. N Engl J Med 1979;300:1363.

Benson P et al: Preventive care and overall use of services: Are they related? Am J Dis Child 1984;138:74.

Bindman AB et al: Primary care and receipt of preventive services. J Gen Intern Med 1996;11:269.

Bodenheimer TS: Regional medical programs: No road to regionalization. Med Care Rev 1969;26:1125.

Carey TS et al: The outcomes and cost of care for acute low back pain among patients seen by primary care practitioners, chiropractors, and orthopedic surgeons. N Engl J Med 1995;333:913.

Centers for Disease Control: Cases of specified notifiable diseases, United States, weeks ending June 30, 1990, and July 1, 1989. MMWR 1990;39:448.

Charney E et al: How well do patients take oral penicillin? A collaborative study in private practice. Pediatrics 1967;40:188.

Dawson W: Interim report on the future provision of medical and allied services. In: The Regionalization of Personal Health Services. Saward EW (editor). Prodist, 1975.

Engel GL: The need for a new medical model: A challenge for biomedicine. Science 1977;196:129.

Fielding JE, Cumberland WG, Pettitt L: Immunization status of children of employees in a large corporation. JAMA 1994;271:525.

Franks P, Clancy CM, Nutting PA: Gatekeeping revisited: Protecting patients from overtreatment. N Engl J Med 1992;327:424.

Franks P, Nutting PA, Clancy CM: Health care reform, primary care, and the need for research. JAMA 1993;270:1449.

Freymann JG: The American Health Care System: Its Genesis and Trajectory. Krieger, 1977.

Friedson E: Professional Dominance: The Social Structure of Medicine. Atherton, 1970.

Fry J: Primary care. In: Primary Care. Fry J (editor). William Heinemann, 1980.

Gonzalez M: Physician Marketplace Statistics. American Medical Association, 1997.

Greenfield S et al: Outcomes of patients with hypertension and non-insulin dependent diabetes mellitus treated by different systems and specialties. JAMA 1995;274:1436.

Greenfield S et al: Variations in resource utilization among medical specialties and systems of care. JAMA 1992;267:1624.

Grumbach K, Fry J: Managing primary care in the United States and in the United Kingdom. N Engl J Med 1993;328:940.

Grumbach K et al: Regionalization of cardiac surgery in the United States and Canada: Geographic access, choice, and outcomes. JAMA 1995;274:1282.

Hueston et al: Practice variation between family physicians and obstetricians in the management of low-risk pregnancies. J Fam Pract 1995;40:345.

Institute of Medicine: Primary Care: America's Health in a New Era. National Academy Press, 1996.

Jollis JG et al: Outcome of acute myocardial infarction according to the specialty of the admitting physician. N Engl J Med 1996;335:1880.

Light D, Levine S: The changing character of the medical profession: A theoretical overview. Milbank Mem Fund Q 1988;66:10.

Luce JM, Byyny RL: The evolution of medical specialism. Perspect Biol Med 1979;22:377.

Menken M: Generalism and specialism revisited: The case of neurology. Health Aff 1988;7(5):115.

Nutting PA (editor): Community Oriented Primary Care: From Principle to Practice. Univ New Mexico Press, 1990.

Rivo ML et al: Defining the generalist physician's training. JAMA 1994;271:1499.

Rodwin VG: The Health Planning Predicament. Univ California Press, 1984.

Roos N: Who should do the surgery? Tonsillectomy-adenoidectomy in one Canadian province. Inquiry 1979;16:73.

Rosenblatt R et al: Interspecialty differences in the obstetric care of low-risk women. Am J Public Health 1997;87:344.

Shea S et al: Predisposing factors for severe, uncontrolled hypertension in an inner-city minority population. N Engl J Med 1992;327:776.

Shear CL et al: Provider continuity and quality of medical care: A retrospective analysis of prenatal and perinatal outcome. Med Care 1983;21:1204.

Sidel V, Sidel R: A Healthy State. Pantheon Books, 1983.

Somers AR: Who's in charge here? Alice searches for a king in Mediland. N Engl J Med 1972;287:849.

Starfield B: Primary Care. Oxford Univ Press, 1992.

Starr P: The social transformation of American medicine. Basic Books, 1982.

Stevens R: In Sickness and in Wealth: American Hospitals in the Twentieth Century. Basic Books, 1989.

Stewart AL et al: Primary care and patient perceptions of access to care. J Fam Pract 1997;44:177.

Toner R: The family doctor is rarely in. New York Times, Feb 6, 1994.

Wachter RM, Goldman L: The emerging role of "hospitalists" in the American health care system. N Engl J Med 1996;335:514.

Wasson JH et al: Continuity of outpatient medical care in elderly men: A randomized trial. JAMA 1984;252:2413.

Weiss LJ, Blustein J: Faithful patients: The effect of long-term physician-patient relationships on the costs and use of health care by older Americans. Am J Public Health 1996;86:1742.

Welch WP et al: Geographic variation in expenditures for physicians' services in the United States. N Engl J Med 1993;328:621.

White KL, Williams F, Greenberg BG: The ecology of medical care. N Engl J Med 1961;265:885.

How Health Care Is Organized—II

7

The last chapter explored some general principles of health care organization, including levels of care, regionalization, physician and other practitioner roles, and patient flow through the system. The regionalized model of organizing care was contrasted with the dispersed model. This chapter looks more closely at actual structures of medical practice.

The traditional dispersed model of United States medical practice has often been referred to as a "cottage industry" of independent private physicians working as solo practitioners or in small groups. A number of alternative organizational forms have existed in the United States, ranging from community health centers to prepaid group practices. The traditional model is giving way to a system of larger practice organizations and networks structured along a more "corporate" model of health care delivery.

THE TRADITIONAL STRUCTURE OF MEDICAL CARE

Physicians & Hospitals

> Dr. Harvey Commoner finished his residency in general surgery in 1956. For the next 30 years, he and another surgeon practiced medicine together in a middle class suburb near St. Peter's Hospital, a nonprofit church-affiliated institution. Dr. Commoner received most of his cases from general practitioners (GPs) and internists also on the St. Peter's medical staff. By 1965, the number of surgeons operating at St. Peter's had grown. Because Dr. Commoner was not getting enough cases, he and his partner joined the medical staffs of Top Dollar Hospital, a for-profit facility 3 miles away, and University Hospital downtown. On an average morning, Dr. Commoner drove to all three hospitals to perform operations or to do postoperative rounds on his patients. The afternoon was spent seeing patients in his office. He was on call every other night and weekend.

> Dr. Commoner was active on the St. Peter's medical staff executive committee, where he frequently proposed that the hospital purchase new radiology and operating room equipment needed to keep up with advances in surgery. Because the hospital received hundreds of thousands of dollars each year for providing care to Dr. Commoner's patients, and because Dr. Commoner had the option of admitting his patients to Top Dollar or University, the St. Peter's administration usually purchased the items that Dr. Commoner recommended. The Top Dollar Hospital administrator did likewise.

During the period when Dr. Commoner was practicing, most medical care was delivered by fee-for-service private physicians in solo or small group practices. Most hospitals were private nonprofit institutions, sometimes affiliated with a church, occasionally with a medical school, often run by an independent board of trustees composed of prominent people in the community. Most physicians in traditional fee-for-service practice were not employees of any hospital, but joined one or several hospital medical staffs, thereby gaining the privilege of admitting patients to the hospital and at times acquiring the responsibility to assist the hospital through work on medical staff committees or by caring for emergency room patients who have no physician.

For many years, the physicians were the dominant power in the hospital, because physicians admit the patients—and hospitals without patients have no income. Because physicians were free to admit their patients to more than one hospital, the implicit threat to take their patients elsewhere gave them influence. Recently, as hospitals have begun to build a patient base through health maintenance organization (HMO) contracts rather than through physician loyalty, hospital administrators have gained in authority, but they must always perform a balancing act to satisfy both the business and the medical sides of the hospital (Stevens, 1989).

Under traditional fee-for-service medicine, physicians used informal referral networks, often involving other physicians on the same hospital medical staff. In metropolitan areas with a high ratio of physician specialists to population, referrals could become a critical economic issue. Most surgeons obtained their cases by referral from primary care physicians (PCPs) or medical specialists; surgeons like Dr. Commoner who were not readily available when called, soon found their case load drying up.

THE SEEDS OF NEW MEDICAL CARE STRUCTURES

The dispersed structure of independent, fee-for-service private practice was not always the dominant model in the United States. When modern medical care took root in the first half of the twentieth century, a variety of structures blossomed. Among these were contract doctors, multispecialty group practices, community health centers, and prepaid group practices. Some of these flourished but then wilted, while others became the seeds from which germinated the future health care system of the twenty-first century.

Contract Doctors

> Dr. Jerome Trainer was a surgeon employed by the Union Pacific Railroad in the 1890s to care for railroad workers injured on the job. His work occasionally brought him to Colorado, where he would visit with his old friend Dr. Thomas Silver, who worked for a mining company in the mountainous regions of the state. Both physicians received a salary paid out of mandatory deductions from the paychecks of their companies' workers.

Company-run medical care with salaried physicians was usually confined to remote areas of the country where private physicians were unlikely to live, and thus was limited to such industries as railroads, mining, and logging.

> Dr. Aaron Bernstein worked as a general practitioner in New York City in the early 1900s. He had a contract to pro-

> vide services to members of the Jewish Benevolent Society
> health insurance fund, receiving payment on a capitated ba-
> sis for each fund member in his practice.

Many benevolent societies at the turn of the twentieth century sought a more direct
role in delivering services than was typical under traditional insurance arrangements
with independent practitioners. Funds arranged contracts with particular physicians
to serve plan members, often under salaried or capitated payment (Abel-Smith, 1988;
Starr, 1982).

By the 1930s, the "contract doctor" form of health care organization was nearly ex-
tinct in the United States, largely due to fierce political opposition from the medical
profession. Competition among physicians for contracts was threatening to drive
down physician fees, jeopardizing the economic interests of physicians in independent private practice as well as those bargaining for contracts. The contract doctor
model, however, was not entirely extinguished in the United States. As discussed below, company-sponsored medical care in a remote area in Washington State in 1938
became the progenitor of Kaiser-Permanente and the modern HMO, the most substantial alternative to traditional fee-for-service practice. Before discussing this
legacy of the contract doctor model of care, however, some additional models deserve
mention.

Multispecialty Group Practice

> In 1905, Dr. Geraldine Giemsa joined the department of
> pathology at the Mayo Clinic. The clinic, led by the broth-
> ers William and Charles Mayo, was becoming a nationally
> renowned referral center for surgery and was recruiting
> pathologists, microbiologists, and other specialized diag-
> nosticians to support the work of the clinic's group of sur-
> geons. Dr. Giemsa received a salary and became an em-
> ployee of the group practice. With time, she became a
> senior partner and part owner of the Mayo Clinic.

Together with their father, the Mayo brothers, who were general practitioners
skilled at surgical techniques, formed a group practice in the small town of
Rochester, Minnesota, in the 1890s. As the brothers' reputation for clinical excellence grew, the practice added several surgeons and physicians in laboratory-oriented
specialties. By 1929, the Mayo Clinic had over 375 physicians and 900 support staff
(Starr, 1982). Although the clinic paid its physician staff by salary, the clinic itself
billed patients, and later third-party insurance plans, on a fee-for-service basis. Unlike the contract doctor model, the Mayo Clinic did not merge the financing and delivery of care into a single organizational structure. Physicians worked in a group setting that preserved private practice's traditional independence from the payers of
care.

The Mayo Clinic was the inspiration for other group practices that developed in
the United States, such as the Menninger Clinic in Topeka, Kansas, and the Palo
Alto Clinic in California. These clinics were owned and administered by physicians
and featured physicians working in various specialties—hence, the common use of
the term "multispecialty group practice" to describe this organizational model. As in
the case of the Mayo Clinic, these multispecialty group practices were innovative

in the manner in which they brought large numbers of physicians together under one roof to deliver care.

By formally integrating specialists in a single clinic structure, group practice attempted to promote a collaborative style of care. Lacking a strong role for the PCP as coordinator of services, the specialty-oriented group practice model attempted to use the structure of the practice organization itself as a means of creating an environment for coordinated care among specialist physicians. Enhancement of quality of care was also expected from the greater opportunity for formal and informal peer review and continuing education when colleagues worked together and shared responsibility for the care of patients. Critics of group practice warned that large practice structures would jeopardize the intimate patient-physician relationship possible in a solo or small group setting. Large groups would subject patients to an impersonal style of care with no single physician clearly accountable for the patient's welfare. The physician's clinical and financial autonomy would also be compromised by large group practice (Silver, 1963).

In 1932, the blue ribbon Committee on the Costs of Medical Care recommended that the delivery of care be organized around large group practices (Starr, 1982; Silver, 1963). The eight physicians in private practice who were members of the committee dissented from the recommendations, roundly criticizing the sections on group practice. An editorial in the *Journal of the American Medical Association* was even more scathing in its attack on the committee's majority report:

> The physicians of this country must not be misled by utopian fantasies of a form of medical practice which would equalize all physicians by placing them in groups under one administration. The public will find to its cost, as it has elsewhere, that such schemes do not answer that hidden desire in each human breast for human kindliness, human forbearance and human understanding. It is better for the American people that most of their illnesses be treated by their own doctors rather than by industries, corporations or clinics. (The Committee on the Costs of Medical Care. [Editorial.] JAMA, 1932;99:1950.)

Several multispecialty group practices flourished during the period between the world wars, and to this day remain among the most highly regarded systems of care in the United States. Yet multispecialty group practice did not become the dominant organizational structure envisioned by the Committee on the Costs of Medical Care. In part, resistance to this model by professional societies blunted the potential for growth. In addition, as hospitals assumed a central role in medical care, group practice lost some of its unique attractions. Hospitals could provide the ancillary services physicians needed for the increasingly specialized and technology-dependent work of medicine. Hospitals also served as an organizational focus for the informal referral networks that developed among private physicians in independent practice.

Community Health Centers

> The year is 1915 and a rural community in Iowa has just hired Rose LeCroix as director of the newly formed public health nursing agency. Local clergy, teachers, business owners, Red Cross administrators, and physicians have

come together to develop a regional plan for improving the
health of the population. The focal point is to be the public
health nursing agency. Ms. LeCroix's first tasks are to develop a team of health workers to evaluate all children in
the region for nutritional status, symptoms of tuberculosis,
and housing conditions.

One of the most far-reaching alternatives to fee-for-service medical practice is the
community health center, one of whose goals is to practice community-oriented primary care (see Chapter 6), taking responsibility for the health status of the entire
community served by the health center. One example of such an institution was the
Greater Community Association at Creston, Iowa. The association brought together
civic, religious, education, and health care groups in a coordinated system centered
on the community hospital serving a six-county area with 100,000 residents. The
plan placed its greatest emphasis on preventive care and public health measures administered by public health nurses. In describing the association, A.E. Kepford
(1919) wrote:

> The motto of the Greater Community Association is "Ser-
> vice." Among the principles of the hospital management are
> the precept that it shall be a long way from the threshold of
> the hospital to the operating room . . . We have a hospital
> which makes no attempt to pattern after the great city insti-
> tutions, but is organized to meet the needs of a rural neigh-
> borhood. The Greater Community Association has been
> taught to regard the hospital as a repair shop, necessary
> only where preventive medicine has failed. (Kepford AE:
> The Greater Community Association at Creston, Iowa. Mod
> Hosp 1919;12:342.)

The Creston, Iowa, experiment was attempting to reconcile an unfortunate "divorce" between public health and medical care. Public health centers working to improve the health status of defined communities have seldom offered medical care for
illness, usually because of opposition from organized medicine fearing competition
with fee-for-service practice (Geiger, 1984). Medical care facilities have focused on
the care of sick individuals and have not seen themselves as responsible for the health
of the overall community. The Committee on the Costs of Medical Care recommended in 1932 that curative medicine and public health be joined in local centers
serving defined populations, but organized medicine rejected this concept.

> In 1928, Sherry Kidd joined the Frontier Nursing Service in
> Appalachia as a nurse midwife. For $5 per year, families
> could enroll in the service and receive pregnancy-related
> care. Sherry was responsible for all enrolled families in a
> region within a 100-mile diameter. She referred patients
> with complications to an obstetrician in Lexington, Ken-
> tucky, who was the service's physician consultant.

The Frontier Nursing Service was established by Mary Breckinridge, an English-
trained midwife, in 1925 (Dye, 1983). Breckinridge designed the service to meet the
needs of a poor rural area in Kentucky that lacked basic medical and obstetric care
and suffered from high rates of maternal and infant mortality. The Frontier Nursing
Service shared many of the features of the Creston, Iowa, model: regionalized ser-

vices planned on a geographic basis to serve rural populations, with an emphasis on primary care and health education. Like the Creston system, the service relied on nurses to provide primary care, with physicians reserved for secondary medical services on a referral basis.

These rural programs had their urban counterparts in health centers that focused on maternal and child health services during the early 1900s (Rothman, 1978; Stoeckle and Candib, 1969). The clinics primarily served populations in low-income districts in large cities and were often involved with large immigrant populations. As in the rural systems, public health nurses played a central role in an organizational model geared toward health education, nutrition, and sanitation. Both the urban and rural models of community health centers waned during the middle years of this century. Public health nursing declined in prestige as hospitals became the center of activity for nursing education and practice (Stevens, 1989). A team model of nurses working in collaboration with physicians withered under a system of hierarchical professional roles.

The community health center model was revived in the 1960s as part of the Great Society reforms. In 1965, the federal Office of Economic Opportunity, the agency created to implement the "War on Poverty," initiated its program of neighborhood health centers with several goals, including the combining of comprehensive medical care and public health to improve the health status of defined low-income communities, the building of multidisciplinary teams to provide health services, and participation in the governance of the health centers by community members.

> Dr. Franklin Jefferson was professor of hematology at a prestigious medical school. His distinguished career was based on laboratory research, teaching, and subspecialty medical practice, with a focus on sickle cell anemia. Dr. Jefferson felt that his work was serving his community but that he would like to do more. In 1965, with the advent of the federal neighborhood health center program, he left his laboratory in the hands of a well-trained assistant and began to talk with community leaders in the poor neighborhood that surrounded the medical school. After a year, the trust developed between Dr. Jefferson and members of the neighborhood bore fruit in a decision to approach the medical school dean about a joint medical school–community application for funds to create a neighborhood health center. Two years later, the center opened its doors, with Dr. Jefferson as its first medical director.

By the early 1980s, 800 neighborhood health centers were serving 4.2 million people. Some were run by hospitals, medical schools, or local public health departments, and many were controlled by community groups, often with boards elected by the neighborhood or by the patients enrolled in the health center. Many of the centers trained community members as outreach workers, who became members of health care teams that included public health nurses, physicians, mental health workers, and health educators. Some of the health centers made a serious attempt to meld clinical services with public health activities in programs of community-oriented primary care. For example, the rural health center in Mound Bayou, Mississippi, helped to organize a cooperative farm to improve nutrition in the county, dig wells to supply safe drinking water, and train community residents to become health professionals.

The neighborhood health centers made important contributions. By improving the care of low-income ambulatory patients, the centers were able to reduce hospitalization and emergency department visits by their patients. Neighborhood health centers also had some success in improving community health status, particularly by reducing infant and neonatal mortality rates among African-Americans (Geiger, 1984).

Despite these successes, during the 1980s neighborhood health centers fell out of favor politically, and funding was deemphasized by the federal government. Consequently, health centers were forced to generate income through billing of patients and insurers (chiefly Medicare and Medicaid). Yet the energy and commitment of health care organizers around the nation transformed hundreds of community health centers (neighborhood health centers, rural migrant worker clinics, homeless clinics, and clinics for immigrant populations) into fiscally viable "safety net" organizations (Schauffler and Wolin, 1996). In 1996, 900 community health centers at 3000 sites were serving 10 million people, many of them without health insurance.

Prepaid Group Practice & HMOs   Historically, one alternative to small office-based fee-for-service practice became the major challenge to that traditional model: prepaid group practice. Company hired doctors play a minimal role in contemporary health care, and community health centers are important institutions only in a limited number of communities. Prepaid group practice, in contrast, became one of the models upon which the modern HMO is based.

In 1929, the Ross-Loos Clinic began to provide medical services for employees of the Los Angeles Department of Water and Power on a prepaid basis. By 1935, the clinic had enrolled 37,000 employees and their dependents, who each paid $2 per month for a specified list of services. Also in 1929, an idealistic physician, Dr. Michael Shadid, organized a medical cooperative in Elk City, Oklahoma, based on four principles: group practice, prepayment, preventive medicine, and control by the patients who were members of the cooperative. In the late forties, over a hundred rural health cooperatives were founded, many in Texas, but they tended to fade away, partly from the stiff opposition of organized medicine. In the 1950s, another version of the consumer-managed prepaid group practice sprang up in Appalachia, where the United Mine Workers established union-run group practice clinics, each receiving a budget from the union-controlled, coal industry-financed medical care fund. Meanwhile, the Group Health Association of Washington, D.C., had been organized in 1937 as a prepaid group practice whose board was elected by the cooperative's membership. A few years later in Seattle, Group Health Cooperative of Puget Sound acquired its own hospital, began to grow, and by the mid 1970s had 200,000 subscribers, a fifth of the Seattle-area population. In 1947, the Health Insurance Plan (HIP) of New York opened its doors, operating 22 group practices; within 10 years, HIP's enrollment approached 500,000 (Starr, 1982).

The most successful of the prepaid group practices that emerged in the 1930s and 1940s was the Kaiser Health Plan. In 1938, a surgeon named Sidney Garfield began providing prepaid medical services for industrialist Henry J. Kaiser's employees working at the Grand Coulee Dam in Washington State. Rather than receiving a salary from Kaiser, Garfield was prepaid a fixed sum per employee, a precursor to modern capitation payment. Kaiser transported this concept to 200,000 workers in his shipyards and steel mills on the West Coast during World War II (Starr, 1982; Garfield, 1970). In this way, company-sponsored medical care in a remote area gave birth to today's largest alternative to fee-for-service practice. Starting in the contract doctor tradition, Kaiser opened its doors to the general public after World War II. By 1997, Kaiser had facilities in many United States cities and had enrolled over 8 million people.

The contemporary systems that grew out of the Kaiser and consumer cooperative models share several important features. Rather than preserving a separation between insurance plans and the providers of care, these models attempt to meld the financing and delivery of care into a single organizational structure. Paying a premium for health insurance coverage in this approach does not just mean that a third-party payer will reimburse some or all of the costs of care delivered by independent practitioners. Rather, the premium serves to directly purchase, in advance, health services from a particular system of care. This is the notion of "prepaid" care that is one component of the prepaid group practice model. (As discussed in Chapter 2, the Baylor Hospital plan in the 1930s was a parallel attempt to develop a model of prepaid hospital care.) The second component is care delivered by a large group of practitioners working under a common administrative structure—the "group practice" aspect of prepaid group practice.

Systems such as Kaiser and Group Health Cooperative of Puget Sound were commonly referred to as prepaid group practices until the 1970s, when terminology underwent a transformation as part of a political effort to sell the public and Congress on this model of care as a centerpiece of health care reform under the Nixon administration. Paul Ellwood, a Minnesota physician and advisor to the Nixon administration, suggested that prepaid group practices be referred to as "health maintenance organizations" (Ellwood et al, 1971; Starr, 1982). This change in name was intended in part to break from the political legacy of the prepaid group practice movement, a legacy colored with populist tones from the cooperative plans and tainted by organized medicine's common criticism of prepaid group practice as a socialist threat. The term *health maintenance* was also designed to suggest that these systems would place more emphasis on preventive care than had the traditional medical model. Although HMOs were initially synonymous with prepaid group practice, by the 1980s several varieties of HMO plans emerged that departed from the prepaid group practice organizational form. We describe the Kaiser model to more fully illustrate the first-generation HMO model, and then proceed to discuss the second-generation HMOs known as independent practice association (IPA) HMOs.

FIRST-GENERATION HMOs AND VERTICAL INTEGRATION: THE KAISER–PERMANENTE MEDICAL CARE PROGRAM

Mario Fuentes was a professor at the University of California. He and his family belonged to the Kaiser Health Plan, and the university paid his family's premium. Professor Fuentes had once fractured his clavicle, for which he went to the urgent care clinic at Kaiser Hospital in Oakland; otherwise, he had not used Kaiser's facilities. Mrs. Fuentes suffered from rheumatoid arthritis; her regular physician was a salaried rheumatologist at the Permanente Medical Clinic, the group practice in which Kaiser physicians work. One of the Fuentes' sons, Juanito, had been in an automobile accident a year earlier near a town 90 miles away from home. He had been taken to a local emergency room and released; Kaiser had paid the bill because no Kaiser facility was available in the town. Three days after returning home, Juanito developed a severe headache and became drowsy; he was taken to the urgent care clinic, received a CT scan, and was found to have a subdural hematoma. He was immediately transported to Kaiser's regional neurosurgery center in Redwood City, California, where he underwent surgery to evacuate the hematoma.

Dr. Roberta Short had mixed feelings about working at Kaiser. She liked the hours, the salary, and the paucity of administrative tasks. She particularly liked working in the same building with other general internists and specialists, providing the opportunity for frequent discussions on diagnostic and therapeutic problems. She was not happy, though, about the regimented schedule. Every hour seemed to comprise either two short visits (of 10 minutes each) combined with two long visits (of 20 minutes each), or four "shorts" and one "long." Such a pace seemed to leave little time to talk to the patients or to make important phone calls to patients or specialists. It was tough for Dr. Short's patients to get appointments with her, and it was even harder to arrange prompt appointments with specialists, who were as busy as she was. Moreover, the rules for ordering MRIs and other expensive tests were strict, though by and large reasonable. Overall, Dr. Short felt that the Kaiser system worked well but needed more physicians per enrolled patient.

The Kaiser–Permanente Medical Care Program is the largest of the nation's prepaid group practice HMOs, consisting of three interlocking administrative units:

(1) The Kaiser Foundation Health Plan, which performs the functions of health insurer, such as administering enrollment and other aspects of the financing of care;

(2) The Kaiser Foundation Hospitals Corporation, which owns and administers Kaiser hospitals (the same individuals sit on the boards of directors for the Health Plan and the Hospitals corporation); and

(3) The Permanente Medical Group, the physician organization that administers the group practice and provides medical services to Kaiser plan members under a capitated contract with the Kaiser plan (Luft, 1987).

The organizational model typified in the Kaiser–Permanente HMO has come to be known as "vertical integration." Vertical integration refers to consolidating under one organizational roof and common ownership all levels of care, from primary to tertiary care, and the facilities and staff necessary to provide this full spectrum of care (Figure 7–1). Although structures differ somewhat across Kaiser's 12 regional health plans, most Kaiser–Permanente regional units own their hospitals and clinics, hire the nurses and other personnel staffing these facilities, and contract with a single large group practice (the Permanente Medical Group) to exclusively serve patients covered by the Kaiser health plan.

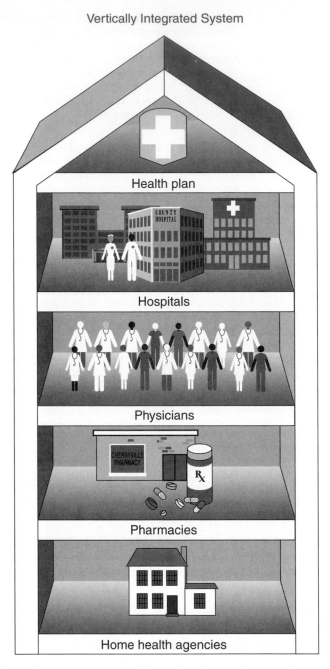

Vertically Integrated System

Health plan

Hospitals

Physicians

Pharmacies

Home health agencies

Figure 7–1. Vertical integration consolidates health services under one organizational roof.

The Kaiser form of HMO differs from traditional fee-for-service models in how it pays physicians (salary) and hospitals (global budget). It also differs in how health services are organized. Most obvious is the prepaid group practice structure that contrasts with the traditional United States style of solo, independent private practice. In addition, Kaiser has typically regionalized tertiary care services at a select number of specialized centers. For example, Northern California Kaiser has centralized all neurosurgical care at a single hospital; patients with spinal cord injuries, brain tumors, and other neurosurgical conditions are referred to this center from other Northern California Kaiser hospitals. The distribution of specialties within the physician staff in the Permanente Medical Group is about half generalists and half specialists. Some regions have also integrated nonphysicians such as nurse practitioners and physician assistants into the primary care team.

Many observers consider this ability to coherently plan and regionalize services to be a major strength of vertically integrated systems (Figure 7–1). Unlike a public District Health Authority in the United Kingdom, an HMO such as Kaiser–Permanente is not responsible for the entire population of a region, but these private, vertically integrated systems in the United States do assume responsibility for organizing and delivering services to a population of plan enrollees. The prepaid nature of enrollment in the Kaiser plan, in theory, permits Kaiser to orient its care more toward a population health model. Although the opportunity to evaluate a defined population of enrollees has spurred considerable epidemiologic research activity within the Kaiser system, the HMO has not been particularly innovative in applying these methods to the practice of community-oriented primary care.

SECOND-GENERATION HMOs AND "VIRTUAL INTEGRATION": INDEPENDENT PRACTICE ASSOCIATIONS

> The phone rang at 3:15 AM. It was the emergency department. "We have a Good Health IPA patient named Buster with a severe leg injury. Can you authorize the visit?" Dr. Monica Byrne was hot under the collar. It happened every night she was on call. Stupid requests from the emergency room asking permission to see a patient who obviously needed to be seen. At 3:45 AM the emergency room called again. "Buster has a displaced tibia fracture. Which orthopedist do you want?" "I don't know," seethed Dr. Byrne, "it depends who's on the Good Health referral list. I don't sleep with the list under my pillow. Get anyone. We'll sort it out in the morning."
>
> Dr. Byrne's troubles were not over. Buster called at 6 AM "The orthopedist I saw last night isn't on my Good Health list. What should I do?" The office manager of Dr. Byrne's primary care practice spent two hours that morning getting approval from Good Health IPA for the non-IPA orthopedic emergency room consultation, calling four Good Health orthopedists before finding one who would see Buster that day, and getting on the phone to Good Health and Buster 7 more times for the proper urgent authorizations and patient instructions. As Dr. Byrne said to her seven-year-old at dinner that night, "A child could figure out a better system than this."

In 1954, the medical society in San Joaquin County, California, fretted about the possibility of Kaiser moving into the county. Private fee-for-service patients might go to the lower cost Kaiser, and physicians' incomes would fall. An idea was born: To compete with Kaiser, the San Joaquin Foundation for Medical Care was set up to contract with employers for a monthly payment per enrollee; the foundation would then pay the physicians on a discounted fee-for-service basis and conduct utilization review to discourage overtreatment (Starr, 1982). The plan hoped to reduce the costs to employers, who would choose the foundation rather than Kaiser. The San Joaquin Foundation for Medical Care was the first IPA.

When the Health Maintenance Organization Act of 1973 was enacted into law as the outcome of President Nixon's health care reform strategy, IPA-model HMOs were included along with prepaid group practice as legitimate HMOs. The HMO law stimulated HMO development by requiring large and medium-sized businesses that provided health insurance to their employees to offer at least one federally qualified HMO as an alternative to traditional fee-for-service insurance if such an HMO existed in the vicinity (Starr, 1982). IPA-model HMOs were far easier to organize than prepaid group practices; a county or state medical society, a hospital, or an insurance company could simply recruit the office-based fee-for-service physicians practicing in the community into an IPA, and thereby create the basis for an HMO. The physicians could continue to see their non-IPA patients as well. The inclusion of the IPA form of HMO in the 1973 legislation ensured that the HMO movement would emphasize changes in physician and hospital reimbursement, but would not produce rapid alterations in the traditional mode of delivering medical care.

Some of the initial IPA-model HMOs were organized on the "two-tier" payment model described in Chapter 4. Under this model, an HMO contracts with many individual physicians to care for HMO enrollees. Many IPA-model HMOs have evolved into models that use a "three-tier" payment structure whereby the HMO does not contract directly with individual physicians but rather with a large group of physicians. These groups may take several forms. One form, the IPA, refers to a network of physicians that agree to participate in an association for purposes of contracting with HMOs and other managed care plans. Physicians maintain ownership of their practices and administer their own offices. The IPA serves as a vehicle for negotiating and administering HMO contracts. The IPA also accepts the capitation payment from HMOs and distributes these revenues to the physicians participating in the IPA. The IPA maintains its internal network of primary care and specialist physicians irrespective of the patient's HMO plan.

Unlike the "monogamous" arrangement between Kaiser and the Permanente Medical Group, physicians can establish contractual relationships with numerous HMOs and IPAs. The result of this more open HMO–physician relationship is a series of physician panels in the same community that overlap partially, but not completely, for patients covered by different HMOs.

IPAs initially did little more than act as brokers between physicians and HMOs, replacing the need for physicians to negotiate contracts on an individual basis. As these IPAs have assumed a larger portion of financial risk for care (see Chapters 4 and 5), they have developed a more active role in authorizing utilization of services, assessing quality of care, and deciding which physicians may participate in the IPA. Some observers believe that IPAs may become "group practices without walls," promoting the positive features of physician-directed group practice while allowing physicians to maintain independence in the ownership and administration of their individual practice (Robinson and Casalino, 1996; Shenkin, 1995). Critics contend that the loose structure of IPAs will inevitably undermine the goal of achieving a more cohesive group practice culture. Moreover, in contrast with the prepaid group practice model of HMO, the IPA model creates the types of frustrating experiences encountered by Dr. Byrne. A PCP, who may see patients from several HMOs and participate in more than one IPA, often finds that a specialist or hospital participates in the physician panel for one HMO or IPA but not another, causing disruption and confusion when it comes to figuring out which specialist or hospital is eligible to accept a referral.

Most IPAs use the gatekeeper concept described in Chapter 6, requiring patients to sign up with a PCP who must initiate and coordinate all of the patient's medical care. The gatekeeper role in contemporary managed care organizations in the United States has tended to emphasize the PCP as an instrument of cost containment, with financial incentives to act more as a "gateshutter" than as a gatekeeper who can facilitate access to needed specialty services and promote coordination and continuity of care.

Another structure that is rising in prominence is the integrated medical group. Integrated medical groups have a tighter organizational structure than IPAs, consisting of groups in which physicians no longer own their practices and office assets but become employees of an organization that owns and manages their practice. Some modern-day integrated groups are survivors of the original breed of multispecialty group practices, such as the Mayo and Palo Alto Clinics described earlier. Others lack these clinics' historical genesis and consist of new organizations created in the managed care era. Many of these newer organizations were created by large, for-profit companies buying up the practices of formerly independent physicians and hiring these same physicians to work as employees of the medical group (Robinson and Casalino, 1996). Similar to IPAs, integrated medical groups contract with multiple managed care plans and often use bonus payments (see Chapter 5) to create incentives for their physicians to restrict services.

IPAs and integrated medical groups represent an alternative to the vertically integrated HMO. As shown in Figure 7–2, managed care relationships involving IPAs and medical groups consist of a network of contractual links between HMOs and autonomous physician groups, hospitals, and other provider units, rather than the "everything-under-one-roof" model of vertical integration. Observers have dubbed the IPA and medical group forms of managed care organization "virtual integration," signifying an integration of services based on contractual relationships rather than unitary ownership (Robinson and Casalino, 1996). In these virtually integrated systems, HMOs do not directly provide health services through their own hospitals and physician organizations, but rather serve as a middleman for negotiating contracts with providers.

For many years, policy analysts predicted that the organizational efficiency and coherence of vertically integrated, first-generation HMOs would position these systems of care to prevail as health care entered a more competitive era. These predictions have not come true, as enrollment in virtually integrated systems has surpassed that in traditional HMOs. Premium prices for many virtually integrated HMOs have dropped below those for Kaiser and other older HMOs. Some observers have attributed this competitive success to the greater flexibility of these newer HMOs. These HMOs respond more rapidly to a changing health care market by swiftly renegotiating contracts and by driving hard bargains with hospitals and physician groups that are operating in a "buyer's market" in which health plans can extract considerable concessions in fees (Robinson and Casalino, 1996). These HMOs are also

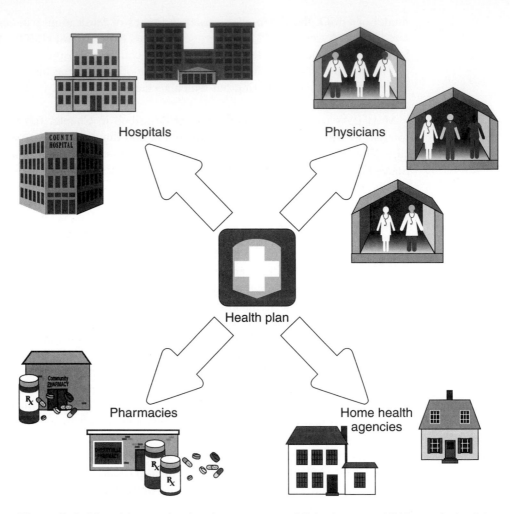

Figure 7–2. Virtual integration involves contractual links between HMOs and physician groups, hospitals, and other provider units.

spared the long-term investment costs that come with actually owning the "bricks and mortar" of hospitals and physician practices.

A variety of other organizational arrangements have arrived on the United States health care scene. In response to the reluctance of many patients to be "locked into" a limited panel of physicians and hospitals in conventional HMO plans, insurers have developed an HMO hybrid known as a point of service (POS) plan. Under the POS plan, a patient can use a care giver who is not in the HMO's provider panel, but at the cost of paying a large share of the payment out of pocket. (Under a conventional HMO policy, the patient would have to pay the full cost of services from an out-of-plan provider.) An even looser arrangement is found in preferred provider organization health plans, or PPOs. Like POS plans, PPOs pay much of the cost of using providers within the plan's selected panel and require higher out-of-pocket payments for using out-of-plan providers. However, unlike POS plan HMOs, PPOs pay their contracted panels of providers on a fee-for-service basis and do not shift much financial risk to physicians and hospitals. Providers in the PPO panel agree to accept discounted fees from the health plan with the hope that being listed by the health plan as a "preferred" provider will attract more patients to their practice.

WILL THE HMO ERA BRING PRIMARY CARE–BASED REGIONALIZED MEDICAL CARE?

Tensions have been intensifying between medical practice as a "cottage industry" of small, independent providers and the "corporate" form of practice based on larger, integrated systems of care. The use of the term "corporate" does not necessarily imply that medical practices need be owned by commercial, profit-seeking corporations. Many early prepaid group practices were developed along a cooperative, consumer-controlled model. Corporate, in this sense of the word, refers to organizational structures in health care delivery that achieve sufficient size and administrative scope to qualify as institutions rather than as loose collections of independent offices. Corporate organizations may range from a community health center staffed by a dozen health professionals, to an HMO with thousands of employees and ownership of several hospitals, to even the entirety of the British National Health Service (NHS). One of the fundamental concerns with more corporate models of medical care is that small may be better when it comes to delivering a personal service such as health care. Among the most valued features of quality health care is the relationship between an individual care giver and a patient. Fears abound that as health care becomes organized into larger entities, care will become more impersonal. Clinic and HMO switchboard operators and voicemail systems may replace the familiar receptionist at the end of the line when a family calls about a child with a fever. Once the call is answered, the child may then be scheduled with the urgent care "doc of the day" instead of with the family's personal physician.

Sociologist David Mechanic (1976) captured some of the trade-offs that may occur as systems move into larger organizational structures such as HMOs:

> HMOs can be thought of as large chain stores, like Sears, Penneys, or Wards, that market medical services rather than consumer goods. As their customers know, there are advantages and disadvantages to shopping at chain stores. Customers feel some confidence that such stores sell products at prices that are generally competitive. Moreover, many different products can be purchased at the same location . . . Nevertheless, it is often difficult to find store personnel to ring up a sale, salespersons tend to be ignorant about the products they market, and consumers may waste some time and experience frustration. (Mechanic D: The Growth of Bureaucratic Medicine. John Wiley & Sons, 1976.)

The department store criticism is not without some justification. Studies of patient preferences have found that satisfaction is highest when care is received in small offices rather than larger clinic structures (Rubin et al, 1993). A recent study found that patients gave higher ratings to fee-for-service, office-based physicians than to prepaid group practice HMOs and IPA plans as to accessibility, continuity, and comprehensiveness of care (Safran et al, 1994). For physicians, more organized systems of care offer the benefit of more regular work hours and less hassle with the business of medicine, but at the expense of loss of control over the conditions of one's work and the opportunity to "be your own boss."

Chapter 6 pictured the British NHS as an organizational model that typifies a primary care–based, regionalized structure of health care (see also Chapter 14). Although not without its troublesome bureaucratic aspects, the NHS has in many ways minimized the department store ambiance by providing primary care through small, decentralized groups of general practitioners and other care givers for the first tier of care.

The traditional dispersed model of United States medical care, featuring small, office-based, fee-for-service practice, has run its course. The uncontrollable expense of such a system is the major force leading to its demise. Will the HMOs of the twenty-first century bring to the United States health care system the positive principles of health care organization elaborated in Chapter 6? Will patients be cared for at the proper level of care—primary, secondary, and tertiary? Will the flow of patients among these levels be constructed in an orderly way within each geographic region—a regionalized structure? Will a sufficient number of primary care providers—generalist physicians, physician assistants, and nurse practitioners—be available so that everyone in the United States can have a regular source of primary care that allows for continuity and coordination of care? Will HMOs begin to take responsibility for the health of their enrollee population through community-oriented primary care, or will they be content to care only for whoever walks in the door? Will the skills of non-physician care givers be used to their maximum extent through the development of multidisciplinary health care teams, or will the provision of health care be controlled by cost-driven physicians and HMO executives?

What is an ideal health delivery system? Different people would have different answers. One vision is a system in which people choose their own primary care providers in small, decentralized, prepaid group practices that would be linked to community hospitals, including specialists' offices providing secondary care. Difficult cases could be referred to the academic tertiary care center in the region. In the primary care practices, teams of health care givers would endeavor to provide medical care to those people seeking attention, and would also concern themselves with the health status of the entire population served by the practice. Whether the monumental changes now taking place in health care delivery will allow for such a vision is a question that only future events can answer.

REFERENCES

Abel-Smith B: The rise and decline of the early HMOs: Some international experiences. Milbank Mem Fund Q 1988;66:694.

The Committee on the Costs of Medical Care. (Editorial.) JAMA 1932;99:1950.

Dye NS: Mary Breckinridge, the Frontier Nursing Service and the introduction of nurse-midwifery in the United States. Bull Hist Med 1983;57:485.

Ellwood PM et al: Health maintenance strategy. Med Care 1971;9:291.

Garfield SR: The delivery of medical care. Sci Am 1970;222(4):15.

Geiger HJ: Community health centers: Health care as an instrument of social change. In: Reforming Medicine. Sidel VW, Sidel R (editors). Pantheon Books, 1984.

Kepford AE: The Greater Community Association at Creston, Iowa. Mod Hosp 1919;12:342.

Luft HS: Health Maintenance Organizations: Dimensions of Performance. Transaction Books, 1987.

Mechanic D: The Growth of Bureaucratic Medicine. John Wiley & Sons, 1976.

Robinson JC, Casalino LP: Vertical integration and organizational networks in health care. Health Aff 1996;15(1):7.

Rothman SM: Woman's Proper Place: A History of Changing Ideals and Practices, 1980 to the Present. Basic Books, 1978.

Rubin HR et al: Patients' ratings of outpatient visits in different practice settings. JAMA 1993;270:835.

Safran DG, Tarlov AR, Rogers WH: Primary care performance in fee-for-service and prepaid health care systems. JAMA 1994;271:1579.

Schauffler HH, Wolin J: Community health centers under managed competition: Navigating uncharted waters. J Health Polit Policy Law 1996;21:461.

Shenkin BN: The independent practice association in theory and practice: Lessons from experience. JAMA 1995;273:1937.

Silver GA: Group practice: What it is. Med Care 1963;1:94.

Starr P: The Social Transformation of American Medicine. Basic Books, 1982.

Stevens R: In Sickness and in Wealth: American Hospitals in the Twentieth Century. Basic Books, 1989.

Stoeckle JD, Candib LM: The neighborhood health center: Reform ideas of yesterday and today. N Engl J Med 1969;280:1385.

Painful Versus Painless Cost Control

8

Dr. Joshua Worthy is chief of neurology at a large staff model health maintenance organization (HMO) and serves as the physician representative to the HMO's executive committee. Other members of the executive committee include the hospital and HMO plan chief executive officers (CEOs), representatives of nursing and other staff, and members of the HMO's consumer board of directors. A national health plan has just been enacted that imposes mandatory cost controls. The HMO's budget for the coming year will be frozen at the current year's level. In past years, the annual growth in the HMO's budget has averaged 12%.

The health plan CEO begins the committee meeting by groaning, "These cuts are draconian! To meet these new budget limits we'll have to cut staff and ration life-saving technologies. Patients will suffer." A consumer member responds, "We all know there's fat in the system. Why, in the newspaper just the other day there was an article about how rates of back surgery in our city are twice the national average. And if we're going to talk about cuts, maybe we should start by looking at your salary and the number of administrators working here. I'm not so sure patients have to suffer just because we're adopting the kind of reasonable spending limits that they have in most countries."

Dr. Worthy remains silent for much of the meeting. He wonders to himself, "Is the CEO right? Is cost containment inevitably a painful process that will deprive our patients of valuable health services? Or could we be doing a better job with the resources we're already spending? Is there a way that our HMO could implement these cost controls in a relatively painless fashion as far as our patients' health is concerned?" Interpreting Dr. Worthy's silence as an indication of great wisdom and judgment, the committee assigns him to chair the HMO's task force charged with developing a cost control strategy to meet the new budgetary realities.

Concerns about the rise of health care costs dominate the health policy agenda in the United States. The other most pressing health policy concern—lack of adequate insurance and access to care for tens of millions of people—is in part attributable to the problem of rising costs. The feverish pace of health care inflation has made health insurance and health services unaffordable to many families and employers.

In recent years, private and public payers in the United States have taken aim at health care inflation and discharged volleys of innovative strategies attempting to curb expenditure growth, such as creating new approaches to utilization review, encouraging HMO enrollment, devising diagnosis-related group (DRG) systems and other reforms of payments to providers (see Chapter 4), and a multitude of other measures. Until recently, these approaches had little noticeable impact on the rate of

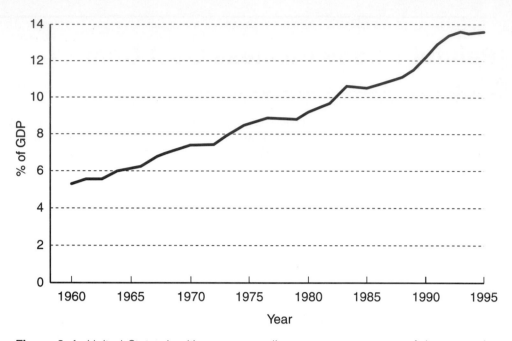

Figure 8–1. United States health care expenditures as a percentage of the gross domestic product. (Data extracted from Levit KR et al: National health expenditures, 1995. Health Care Fin Rev 1996;18(4):157.)

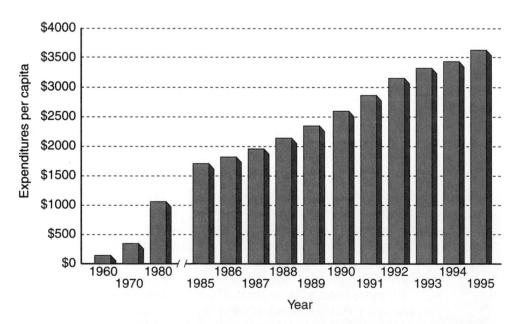

Figure 8–2. United States per capita health care expenditures. (Data extracted from Levit KR et al: National health expenditures, 1995. Health Care Fin Rev 1996;18(4):157.)

growth of health care costs in the United States. National health care expenditures as a percentage of gross domestic product increased from 8.9% in 1980 to 13.4% in 1992, with the dollar value exceeding $830 billion, or $3145 per person in 1992 (Figures 8–1 and 8–2). However, the rate of health care expenditure growth in the United States slowed substantially between 1992 and 1995. Expenditures as a percentage of gross domestic product rose only slightly, from 13.4% in 1992 to 13.6% in 1995, with the per capita expenditure reaching $3621 in 1995 (Levit et al, 1996).

Although doubts remain about whether the recent stabilization of health care costs in the United States will be a sustained or a transient phenomenon, health care providers are discovering that they have to adjust to the prospect of practicing in an era of finite resources. Like Dr. Worthy, physicians and other health care givers need to deliberate about how constraints on expenditure growth may affect patients' health. Must cost control necessarily be "painful," leading to rationing of beneficial services? Or is there a "painless" route to containing costs, reached by eliminating unnecessary medical treatments and administrative expenses?

In this chapter, the painful–painless cost control debate will be explored. First, a model will be constructed describing the relationship between health care costs and benefits in terms of improved health outcomes. Then, different general approaches to cost containment and their potential for achieving painless cost control will be discussed. Chapter 9 will describe specific cost control measures in more detail.

HEALTH CARE COSTS & HEALTH OUTCOMES

> Before entering medical school, Dr. Worthy worked in the Peace Corps in a remote area in Central America. At the time he first arrived in the region, the infant mortality rate was quite high, with many deaths due to infectious gastroenteritis. Dr. Worthy participated in the creation of a sewage treatment system and clean well-water sources for the region, as well as a program for implementing oral rehydration techniques for infants. By the end of Dr. Worthy's 2-year stay, the infant mortality rate had dropped by nearly 25%. The cost for the entire program amounted to 15 cents per capita, paid for by the World Health Organization.

> Conditions have been very different for Dr. Worthy as a practicing neurologist in the United States. In the past 5 years, over a dozen new MRI scanners have been installed in the city in which his HMO is located, an urban area with a population of 800,000. Dr. Worthy has found that MRI scans provide images better than those of CT scans, allowing him to more accurately diagnose conditions such as multiple sclerosis in earlier stages. He is less certain about the extent to which these superior images always make for superior outcomes for his patients.

From society's point of view, the value of health care expenditures lies in purchasing better health for the population. The concept of "better health" is a broad one, encompassing improved longevity and quality of life, reduced mortality and morbidity rates from specific diseases, relief of pain and suffering, enhanced ability to function independently for those with chronic illnesses, and reduction in fear of illness and death. It is important, then, to know whether investing more resources in health care buys improved health outcomes for society and, if so, what the magnitude of the improvement in outcomes may be relative to the amount of resources invested.

Figure 8–3, drawn from the work of Robert Evans (1984), illustrates a theoretic relationship between health care resource input and health care outcomes. Initially, as health care resources increase, these outcomes improve, but above a certain level, the slope of the curve diminishes, signifying that increasing investments in health care yield more marginal benefits. In terms of Dr. Worthy's experiences, the Central American region in which he worked lay on the steep slope of this cost–benefit curve: A small investment of resources to create more sanitary water supplies and to administer inexpensive hydration therapy yielded dramatic improvements in health. On the other hand, purchasing MRI scanners to supplement CT scanners represents a health care system operating on the flatter portion of the curve: Large investments of resources in new technologies may produce more marginal and difficult-to-measure improvements in the overall health of a population.

Naturally, different medical interventions lie on steeper (childhood immunizations) or on flatter (the costly prolongation of life for an anencephalic infant) portions of the curve. The curve in Figure 8–3 may be viewed as an aggregate cost–benefit curve for the functioning of a health care system as a whole. The system may be an entire nation or a smaller entity such as an HMO, with its defined population of enrollees.

Overall, the United States health care system currently operates somewhere along the flatter portion of the curve. Let us assume that Dr. Worthy's HMO system lies at point A on the curve in Figure 8–3, with average total health care expenditures per HMO enrollee being the same as the average overall per capita health care cost in the United States (roughly $3600 in 1995). If stringent new cost containment policies forced the HMO to virtually freeze spending at point A rather than increasing annual expenditures at their usual clip to move to point B, then Figure 8–3 implies that the

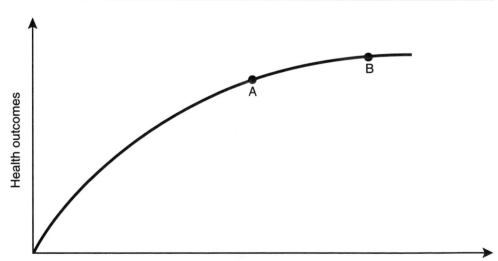

Figure 8–3. A theoretic model of costs and health outcomes. Moving from point A to point B on the curve is associated with both higher costs and better health outcomes.

HMO would sacrifice improving the health of its enrollees by an amount equal to the distance between points A and B on the vertical axis.

Such an analysis would confirm the opinion of those who argue that cost containment requires painful choices that affect the health of the population. Among the most forceful proponents of this view are Aaron and Schwartz (1984 and 1990), who have described cost containment as a "painful prescription" requiring rationing of beneficial care. In Figure 8–3, the distance between points A and B on the y axis measures how much health "pain" accompanies the decision to limit spending at point A instead of advancing to point B. Some degree of pain is inherent in the curve. As Evans (1984) observes, "if its slope is everywhere positive, then in a world of finite resources, unmet needs are inevitable." No matter where we sit on the curve, it will always be true that if we spent more we could do a little better.

In Figure 8–3, the distance between points A and B on the y axis is small, given the relatively flat slope of the curve at these points. But reassurances about relatively mild cost containment pain bring to mind the physician, scalpel in hand, hovering over a patient and declaring that "it will only hurt a little bit." A little pain, necessary as it may be, is not the same as no pain; or as Fuchs (1993) puts it, " 'low yield' medicine is not 'no yield' medicine."

Before allowing ourselves (and Dr. Worthy) to become overly chagrined at the inevitable painfulness of cost containment, let us add the new dimension of efficiency. We can picture a point C (Figure 8–4) at which spending is the same as that at point A but outcomes improve. How does the model account for point C, a point off the curve?

The move to point C requires a shifting of the curve (Figure 8–5), signifying a new, more efficient (or productive) relationship between costs and health outcomes (Donabedian, 1988). There are numerous possible routes to greater efficiency. For example, almost one in four births in the United States occurs by cesarean delivery, a rate nearly

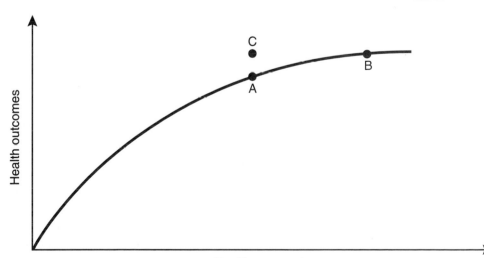

Figure 8–4. Moving off the curve. Point C represents achievement of better health outcome without increased costs.

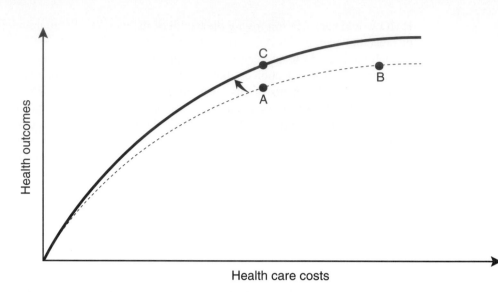

Figure 8–5. Shifting the curve. The shift of the curve represents moving to a more efficient relationship between costs and health outcomes.

twice that of most other Western industrialized nations. Many studies have suggested that the high rates of cesarean section in the United States add to the costs of care without improving overall neonatal or maternal birth outcomes. Reducing the number of unnecessary cesarean sections could save over $1 billion from averted surgical costs and prolonged postpartum hospital stays while simultaneously improving the quality of obstetric care (Stafford, 1990). In the remainder of this chapter, we will examine in greater detail the various possible methods that Dr. Worthy's cost control task force could consider, such as reducing unnecessary surgery, in order to achieve more health "bang" for the health care "buck." Before turning to this discussion, however, it is necessary to make explicit three assumptions about this model of costs and outcomes.

(1) Implicit in the model is the notion that the relevant outcome of interest is the overall health of a population rather than of any one individual patient. A number of authors have recently emphasized the need for physicians to broaden their perspective to encompass the health of a general population as well as their narrower traditional focus on providing the best possible care for each of their patients (Eddy, 1991; Greenlick, 1992). The population-oriented model of costs and outcomes depicted in Figures 8–3 to 8–5 may not fit easily with many physicians' experiences of caring for a particular patient. At the level of the individual patient, the outcome may be all or nothing (eg, the patient will almost certainly live if he or she receives an operation and die without it) and not easily thought about in terms of curves and slopes. Rather than focusing on any one particular intervention or patient, the curve attempts to represent the overall functioning of a health care system in the aggregate for the population under its care. (The ethical issues of the population health perspective are discussed in Chapter 13).

(2) The model assumes that it is possible to quantitate health at a population level. Traditionally, health status at this level has been measured relatively crudely, using

vital statistics such as life expectancy and infant mortality rates. While an index such as infant mortality rates may be a sensitive, meaningful way of evaluating the impact of health care and public health programs in rural Central America, many analysts have questioned whether such crude indicators accurately gauge the impact of health care services in wealthier industrialized nations. In these latter nations, much of health care focuses on "softer" health outcomes such as enhancement of functional status and quality of life in individuals with chronic diseases—aspects more difficult to monitor at the population level than death rates and related vital statistics. In other words, it may be difficult to conceptualize a scale on the y axis of Figures 8–3 to 8–5 that can register both the effects of managing gastroenteritis in a poor nation and the addition of MRI scanners in a United States city.

(3) When evaluating population health, it is difficult to disentangle the effects of health care on health from the effects of such basic social factors as poverty, education, lifestyle, and social cohesiveness (see Chapter 3). Susser (1993) has offered a taxonomy in which he defines *medical care* as "clinical and therapeutic measures that health professionals and medical systems provide for sick people." *Health care* consists of medical care plus "preventive measures and public health." Ultimately, the health status of a population is determined not only by health care, including its medical care component, but by such other powerful influences as standard of living and culture. For the purpose of our discussion of cost control, we view the curves depicted in Figures 8–3 to 8–5 as representing the workings of the health care system (including public health) per se rather than of the broader economic and social milieu. We therefore use the term *health outcomes* to describe the y axis, a term intended to suggest that we are evaluating those aspects of health status directly under the influence of health care. The x axis correspondingly represents expenditures for formal health care services.

Prices & Quantities   We have shown that painless cost control is theoretically possible. But can efficiency be improved in the real world? What strategies could Dr. Worthy's task force propose to move the HMO from point A to point C on the curve? An answer to these questions requires further scrutiny of resource costs in the health care sector.

Costs may be described by the equation

$$\text{Cost} = \text{Price} \times \text{Quantity}$$

Price refers to such items as the hospital daily room charge or the physician fee for a routine office visit. *Quantity* represents the volume and intensity of health service use (eg, the length of stay in an intensive care unit, or the number and types of major diagnostic tests performed during a hospitalization). Lomas and colleagues (1989), noting this distinction between prices (Ps) and quantities (Qs), refer to cost containment as "minding the Ps and Qs" of health care costs.

Let us look at an example of the $C = P \times Q$ equation:

> Blue Shield pays Dr. Morton $400 for 10 office visits at a fee of $40 per visit. The next year, the insurer pays Dr. Morton $480 for 10 visits at $48 per visit.

> Prudential pays Dr. Norton $400 for 10 office visits, and the next year pays $480 for 12 visits at the same $40 fee. An identical cost increase is a price rise for Dr. Morton but an increase in quantity of care for Dr. Norton.

Changes in prices and quantities have different implications for patients and providers (Reinhardt, 1987). In the example above, both physicians increase their income (and both insurance plans increase their expenditures) by $80, though in the case of the price increase, the additional income does not require a higher volume of work. To the patient, however, only the additional $80 spent on a greater number of visits purchases more health care services. (For simplicity's sake, we assume that all visits are identical and that the price rise does not reflect increased quality of service but simply a higher price for the same product.) A cost increase that merely represents higher prices without additional quantities of health care is an inefficient use of resources from the patient's point of view. Returning to the diagrams in Figures 8–3 and 8–4, if real costs in a health care system were rising only because medical price inflation was exceeding general price inflation while the quantity of care per capita remained static, then increased health costs would not bring about improved health outcomes, and the overall curve would become absolutely flat.

COST CONTROL STRATEGIES

Controlling Price Inflation

> After intense deliberation, Dr. Worthy's task force submits a plan for "painless cost containment" to the HMO executive committee. The first proposal calls for the HMO to aggressively seek discounts on the prices paid for supplies, equipment, and pharmaceuticals by having the HMO selectively contract with suppliers for bulk purchases and stock a more limited variety of product lines and drugs within the same therapeutic class. The proposal also calls for a 10% reduction in salaries for all HMO employees earning over $100,000 per year, as well as a 10% reduction in the capitation fee paid to the HMO's physician group. The executive committee never gets beyond this part of the plan, as furious argument erupts over the proposed income cuts.

Price inflation has been a major contributor to the rise of health care costs in recent decades. Between 1947 and 1987, United States health care costs rose 2.5% per year faster than the growth in the overall economy. Two-thirds of this higher growth rate, or 1.6%, was due to health care prices rising more rapidly than prices in the overall economy. The remaining 0.9% differential was due to differences in the rate of increase of quantities of health care relative to increases in the overall quantity of goods and services (Fuchs, 1990).

The rapid rise of health care prices manifests itself in such ways as physician net incomes rising more rapidly in the United States than average worker earnings, and prices for prescription drugs in the United States often being over 50% higher than prices for the same products sold in other nations. Limiting this type of price inflation is one way to restrain expenditures without inflicting "pain" on the public's health. (The effect on physician and other provider incomes is another matter.) (Table 8–1.)

Table 8–1. Examples of painless cost control.

Controlling fees and provider incomes
Cutting the price of pharmaceuticals and other supplies
Reducing administrative waste
Eliminating medical interventions of no benefit
Substituting less costly technologies that are equally effective
Increasing the provision of those preventive services that cost less than the illnesses they prevent

Eliminating Ineffective & Inappropriate Care

> After a brief hiatus to let the furor subside, the HMO executive committee reconvenes. Dr. Worthy introduces his task force's second recommendation—developing appropriateness of care guidelines—by recounting one of his own clinical experiences. When Dr. Worthy first came to the HMO, the neurologists were keeping their stroke patients at bed rest for 1 week before initiating physical therapy. Dr. Worthy, in contrast, began physical therapy and discharge planning for stroke patients the moment their neurologic status was stable. The average length of stay in the acute hospital for his stroke patients was 3 days, compared with 9 days for other neurologists. Dr. Worthy gave a grand rounds presentation demonstrating that 4 days of exercise are required to regain the strength lost from each day of bed rest, meaning that stroke patients would have better outcomes and use fewer resources—shorter acute hospital stays and less rehabilitation—under his care than under the care of his colleagues. Dr. Worthy cites this as merely one example of how the HMO may be devoting resources to ineffective, or even harmful, care.

If controlling prices is one approach to painless cost control, are there also ways to contain the "Q" (quantity) factor in a manner that does not sacrifice beneficial care? Earlier, we cited the unusually high rates of cesarean section in the United States as an example of a source of "inefficient" resource use in terms of quantities of services that add to costs without, in many cases, adding health benefits. A number of researchers have found convincing evidence of substantial amounts of unnecessary care in the United States (Eisenberg, 1986; Brook and Lohr, 1986; Leape, 1992). Recent studies affirm that physicians in the United States perform large numbers of inappropriate procedures (Chassin et al, 1987; Greenspan et al, 1988), and that much of what constitutes "appropriate" standards of practice (see Chapter 12) lacks proved efficacy (Wennberg, 1987; Roper et al, 1988; Grimes, 1993). The slope of the cost–benefit curve would become more favorable if a system could eliminate those components of rising expenditures that have flat slopes (no medical benefit) or negative slopes (harm exceeding benefit, as in the case of inappropriate cesarean sections or prolonged bed rest after strokes). Inducing physicians and patients to selectively eliminate unnecessary care is no easy matter, however.

Administrative Waste

> The third item on Dr. Worthy's painless cost containment plan targets the HMO's administrative costs. The task force

proposes eliminating the HMO's TV and radio advertising budget, laying off 25% of all HMO administrative personnel, and reassigning 25 of the 50 staff members in the department that handles contracts with employers to a new department to develop a program for ensuring that the HMO provides up-to-date child immunizations and adult preventive care services for 100% of plan enrollees. The HMO's marketing director patiently explains to Dr. Worthy that although he in principle agrees with these recommendations, he does not consider it in the HMO's best interest to cut costs in a way that jeopardizes the plan's ability to maintain its market share of enrollees.

Not all quantities in the health care cost equation are clinical in nature. The tremendous administrative overhead of the United States health care system has come under increasing scrutiny in recent years as a source of inefficiency in health care expenditures. Woolhandler and Himmelstein (1991) have estimated that as much as 24 cents of every dollar of United States health care spending goes for such quantities of administrative services as insurance marketing, billing and claims processing, and utilization review, rather than for actual clinical services. United States administrative costs are over twice as high proportionately as those in nations such as Canada, and have been rising 30% more rapidly than the rate of overall national health care inflation. While some level of administrative service is necessary for health care financing and related activities such as quality assurance, few argue that the burgeoning administrative and marketing activities translate into meaningful improvement in patients' health. Reducing administrative services is another route to painless cost containment.

Eliminating purely wasteful quantities of health care services, be they ineffective clinical services or administrative activities, is a relatively straightforward approach to painless cost control. The motto of this approach is: Stop doing things of no clinical benefit. More complicated are approaches to efficiency that involve not simply ceasing completely unproductive activities, but doing things differently. Examples of this latter approach include innovations that substitute less costly care of equal benefit, preventive care, and redistribution of resources from services with some benefit to services with greater benefit relative to cost.

Let us examine each of these examples in turn.

Innovation and Cost Savings: Much of the process of innovation in health care involves the search for less costly ways of producing the same, or better, health outcomes. A new drug is developed that is less expensive but equally efficacious and well tolerated as a conventional medicine. Services provided by highly paid physicians can often be delivered with the same quality by nurses, nurse practitioners, or physician assistants. A clinical trial documents that infusion of chemotherapy for many cancer treatments may be done safely on an outpatient basis, averting the expense of hospitalization. Often, new technologies are introduced in hopes that they will ultimately prove to be less costly than existing treatment methods.

New technologies often fail to live up to cost-saving expectations, however (Schwartz, 1987). A recent case in point is that of laparoscopic cholecystectomy. Through the use of fiberoptic technology, the gallbladder may be surgically removed using a much smaller abdominal incision than that required for traditional cholecystectomy, thereby significantly shortening the time required for postoperative recuperation in the hospital. The shorter length of hospital stay reduces the overall cost of the operation, with, if anything, improved outcomes due to less postoperative pain and disability—seemingly a classic case of "efficient substitution" that lowers costs and improves health outcomes. There's a catch, however. The necessity of gallbladder surgery is not always clear-cut for patients with gallstones. Many patients have only occasional, mild symptoms, and prefer to tolerate these symptoms rather than undergo an operation. Studies have found that rates of cholecystectomy have increased dramatically following the advent of the laparoscopic technique, apparently because gallbladder surgery is being performed on patients with milder symptoms. In one HMO, the cholecystectomy rate increased by 59% between 1988 and 1992 after the introduction of the laparoscopic technique. Even though the average cost per cholecystectomy declined by 25%, the total cost for all cholecystectomies in the HMO rose by 11% because of the increased number of procedures done (Legorreta et al, 1993).

Ounces of Prevention: If an ounce of prevention is worth a pound of cure, then replacement of expensive end-stage treatment with low-cost prevention would appear to be an ideal candidate for the "painless cost controller award." Investing in prevention sometimes generates this type of efficiency in health care spending (eg, providing prenatal care or childhood vaccinations costs less than caring for premature newborns or children with life-threatening infections) (White et al, 1985; Institute of Medicine, 1988). The prevention story is not always so simple, however. In many cases, the cost of implementing a widespread prevention program may exceed the cost of caring for the illness it aims to prevent. For example, screening the general population for elevated blood pressure and providing long-term treatment for those with mild to moderate hypertension to prevent strokes and other cardiovascular complications has been found to cost more than the expense of treating the eventual complications themselves (Stason, 1987). For some diseases, this is the case because the complications are rapidly, and inexpensively, fatal, while successful prevention leads to a long life with high medical costs, perhaps for a different illness, required at some point. Similarly, a program of routine mammography screening and biopsy following abnormal test results costs more than it saves by detecting breast cancers at earlier stages. Blood pressure and breast cancer screening programs result in the improved health of the population but require a net investment in additional resources.

Prioritization and Analysis of Cost Effectiveness:

> A fourth recommendation of Dr. Worthy's task force involves the diagnosis and treatment of colon cancer. Many HMO physicians suggest periodic screening sigmoidoscopy for their patients over age 50 for early detection of colon cancer. All the HMO's oncologists strongly recommend chemotherapy for patients who develop metastatic colon cancer. Analysis of cost effectiveness has demonstrated that screening sigmoidoscopy saves many more years of life per dollar spent than chemotherapy for metastatic colon cancer. Yet chemotherapy allows occasional patients with metastatic disease to enjoy an extra 6–12 months of life. The task force takes the position that the HMO's physicians

should do screening sigmoidoscopies but that the HMO insurance plan should not cover chemotherapy for metastatic colon cancer.

The most controversial strategy for making health care more efficient is the redistribution of resources from services with some benefit to services with greater benefit relative to cost. This approach is commonly guided by cost effectiveness analysis, which, as defined by Eisenberg (1989),

> measures the net cost of providing a service (expenditures minus savings) as well as the outcomes obtained. Outcomes are reported in a single unit of measurement, either a conventional clinical outcome (eg, years of life saved) or a measure that combines several outcomes on a common scale. (Eisenberg JM: Clinical economics. JAMA 1989; 262:2879.)

An example is a cost effectiveness analysis of different strategies to prevent heart disease, showing that the cost per year of life saved (in 1984 dollars) was approximately $1000 for brief advice about smoking cessation during a routine office visit, $24,000 for treating mild hypertension, and nearly $100,000 for treating elevated cholesterol levels with drugs (Cummings et al, 1989). In order to get the most "bang" for the health care "buck," this analysis suggests that a system operating under limited resources would do better by maximizing resources for smoking cessation before investing in cholesterol screening and treatment.

Cost effectiveness analysis must be used with caution. If the data used are inaccurate, the conclusions may be incorrect. Moreover, cost effectiveness analysis may discriminate against people with disabilities. Researchers are likely to assign less worth to a year of life of a disabled person than does the person himself or herself; thus, analyses using "quality-adjusted life years" may have a built-in bias against persons with less capacity to function independently (Menzel, 1992).

Dr. David Eddy (1991, 1992, 1993), in a series of provocative articles in the *Journal of the American Medical Association,* has discussed the practical and ethical challenges of applying cost effectiveness analysis to medical practice. Two of the essays involve the case of an HMO trying to decide whether to adopt routine use of low-osmolar contrast agents, a new type of dye for special x-ray studies with a lower risk of provoking allergic reactions than the cheaper conventional dye. With use of this new agent for all x-ray dye studies, 40 nonfatal allergic reactions would be avoided annually and the cost to the HMO would be $3.5 million more per year, compared with costs for use of the older agent in routine cases and use of the newer dye only for patients at high risk of allergy. The same $3.5 million dollars invested in an expanded cervical cancer screening program in the HMO would prevent approximately 100 deaths from cervical cancer per year.

In discussing how best to deploy these resources, Eddy highlights several points of particular relevance to clinicians.

(1) It must be agreed upon that resources are truly limited. Although the cost effectiveness of low-osmolar contrast dye and cervical cancer screening is quite different, both programs offer some benefit (ie, they are not flat-of-the-curve medicine). If no constraints on resources existed, the best policy would be to invest in both services.

(2) If resources are limited and trade-offs based on cost effectiveness considerations are to be made, these trade-offs will have professional legitimacy only if it is clear that resources saved from denying services of low cost effectiveness will be reinvested in services with greater cost effectiveness, rather than siphoned off for ineffective care or higher profits.

(3) Ethical tensions exist between maximizing health outcomes for a group or population as opposed to the individual patient. The radiologist experiences the trauma of patients having severe allergic reactions to the injection of contrast dye. Preventing future deaths from cervical cancer in an unspecified group of patients not directly under the radiologist's care seems an abstract and remote benefit from his or her perspective—one that may be perceived as conflicting with the radiologist's obligation to provide the best care possible to his or her patient.

Many analysts, including those who question the methods of cost effectiveness analysis, share Eddy's conclusion: Physicians must broaden their perspective to balance the needs of individual patients directly under their care with the overall needs of the population served by the health care system, whether the system is an HMO or the nation's health care system as a whole (see Chapter 13). Professional ethics will have to incorporate social accountability for resource use and population health, as well as clinical responsibility for the care of individual patients (Greenlick, 1992; Hiatt, 1975).

> The final recommendation of Dr. Worthy's task force is for the HMO to hire a consultant to advise the HMO on the relative cost effectiveness of different services offered by the HMO, in order to prioritize the most cost effective activities. While waiting for the consultant's report, the task force suggests that the HMO begin implementing this strategy by allocating an extra 5 minutes to every routine medical appointment for patients who smoke, so that the physician, nurse practitioner, or physician assistant has time to counsel patients on smoking cessation, as well as by setting up 2 dozen new community-based group classes in smoking cessation for HMO members. The costs of these new activities are to be funded from the HMO's existing budget for coronary artery bypass surgery, and the number of these operations is to be restricted to a dozen fewer than the number performed during the current year. The day following the executive committee meeting, the HMO's health education director buys Dr. Worthy lunch and compliments him on his "enlightened" views. On the way back from lunch, the chief of cardiology accosts Dr. Worthy in the corridor and says, "Why don't you just take my dozen patients with severe coronary artery disease out and shoot them? Get it over quickly, instead of denying them the life-saving surgery they need."

CONCLUSION

The relationship between health outcomes and health care costs is not a simple one. The "cost–benefit" curve has a diminishing slope as increasing investment of resources yields more marginal improvements in the health of the population. The curve itself may shift up or down, depending on the efficiency with which a given level of resources is deployed.

The ideal cost containment method is one that achieves progress in overall health outcomes through the "painless" route of making more efficient use of an existing level of resources. Examples of this approach include restricting price increases, reducing administrative waste, and eliminating inappropriate and ineffective services. "Painful" cost containment represents the other extreme, when controls on expenditures are accomplished only by sacrificing quantities of medically beneficial services. Making trade-offs in services based on relative cost effectiveness may be felt as painless or painful, depending on one's point of view; some individuals may experience the pain of being denied potentially beneficial services, but at a net gain in health for the overall population through more efficient use of the resources at hand.

Cost containment in the real world tends to fall somewhere between the entirely painless paragon and the completely painful pariah (Ginzberg, 1983; Platt, 1983). As the experiences of Dr. Worthy reveal, putting painless cost control into practice may be impeded by political, organizational, and technical obstacles. Price controls may make economic sense but risk intense opposition from providers. Administrative savings may be largely beyond the control of any single HMO or group of providers and require an overhaul of the entire health care system. Identifying and modifying inappropriate clinical practices is a daunting task, as is prioritizing services on the basis of cost effectiveness. But while painless cost control may be difficult to achieve, few would argue that the United States health care system currently operates anywhere near a maximum level of efficiency. Although data on health status are limited, indices such as infant mortality and life expectancy rates suggest that the nation's prolific degree of spending on health care has not been matched by a commensurate level of excellence in the health of the population (Schieber et al, 1993). Making better use of existing resources must be the priority of cost control strategies in the United States.

REFERENCES

Aaron H, Schwartz WB: The Painful Prescription: Rationing Hospital Care. Brookings Institution, 1984.

Aaron H, Schwartz WB: Rationing health care: The choice before us. Science 1990;247:418.

Brook RH, Lohr KN: Will we need to ration effective health care? Issues Sci Tech 1986;3(1):68.

Chassin MR et al: Does inappropriate use explain geographic variations in the use of health care services? JAMA 1987;258:2533.

Cummings SR, Rubin SM, Oster G: The cost-effectiveness of counseling smokers to quit. JAMA 1989;261:75.

Donabedian A: Quality and cost: Choices and responsibilities. Inquiry 1988;25(Spring):90.

Eddy DM: Applying cost-effectiveness analysis. JAMA 1992;268:2575.

Eddy DM: Broadening the responsibilities of practitioners. JAMA 1993;269:1849.

Eddy DM: The individual vs. society: Is there a conflict? JAMA 1991;265:1446.

Eisenberg JM: Clinical economics. JAMA 1989;262:2879.

Eisenberg JM: Doctors' Decisions and the Cost of Medical Care. Health Administration Press, 1986.

Evans RG: Strained Mercy: The Economics of Canadian Health Care. Butterworths, 1984.

Fuchs VR: The health sector's share of the gross national product. Science 1990;247:534.

Fuchs VR: No pain, no gain: Perspectives on cost containment. JAMA 1993;269:631.

Ginzberg E: Cost-containment: Imaginary and real. N Engl J Med 1983;308:1220.

Greenlick MR: Educating physicians for population-based clinical practice. JAMA 1992;
267:1645.

Greenspan AM et al: Incidence of unwarranted implantation of permanent cardiac pacemakers
in a large medical population. N Engl J Med 1988;318:158.

Grimes DA: Technology follies: The uncritical acceptance of medical innovation. JAMA
1993;269:3030.

Hiatt HH: Protecting the medical commons: Who is responsible? N Engl J Med 1975;293:235.

Institute of Medicine: Prenatal Care: Reaching Mothers, Reaching Infants (Summary and Recommendations). National Academy Press, 1988.

Leape LL: Unnecessary surgery. Ann Rev Public Health 1992;13:363.

Legorreta AP et al: Increased cholecystectomy rate after the introduction of laparoscopic
cholecystectomy. JAMA 1993;270:1429.

Levit KR et al: National health expenditures, 1995. Health Care Fin Rev 1996;18(4):157.

Lomas J et al: Paying physicians in Canada: Minding our Ps and Qs. Health Aff 1989;8(1):80.

Menzel PT: Oregon's denial: Disabilities and the quality of life. Hastings Center Rep
1992;22(6):21.

Platt R: Cost-containment: Another view. N Engl J Med 1983;309:726.

Reinhardt UE: Resource allocation in health care: The allocation of lifestyles to providers.
Milbank Mem Fund Q 1987;65(2):153.

Roper WL et al: Effectiveness in health care: An initiative to evaluate and improve medical
practice. N Engl J Med 1988;319:1197.

Schieber GJ, Poullier J, Greenwald LM: Health spending, delivery, and outcomes in OECD
countries. Health Aff 1993;12(2):120.

Schwartz WB: The inevitable failure of current cost-containment strategies. JAMA 1987;
257:220.

Stafford RS: Alternative strategies for controlling rising cesarean section rates. JAMA
1990;263:683.

Stason WB: Economics in hypertension management: Cost and quality trade-offs. J Hypertension 1987;5(Suppl):S55.

Susser M: Health as a human right: An epidemiologist's perspective on the public health. Am
J Public Health 1993;83:418.

Wennberg JE: The paradox of appropriate care. JAMA 1987;258:2568.

White CC, Koplan JP, Orenstein WA: Benefits, risks, and costs of immunization for measles,
mumps, and rubella. Am J Public Health 1985;75:739.

Woolhandler S, Himmelstein D: The deteriorating administrative efficiency of the U.S. health
care system. N Engl J Med 1991;324:1253.

Mechanisms for Controlling Costs   9

In Chapter 8, we discussed the general relationship between costs and health outcomes and explored the tension between "painful" and "painless" approaches to cost containment. In this chapter, we examine specific methods for controlling costs. Our emphasis is on distinguishing among the different types of cost control mechanisms and understanding their intent and rationale. We briefly cite evidence about how these mechanisms may affect cost and health outcomes.

Financial transactions under private or public health insurance (see Chapter 2, Figures 2–2, 2–3, and 2–4) may be divided into two components:

(1) **Financing,** the flow of dollars (premiums or taxes) from the payers (individuals and employers) to the health insurance plan (private health insurance or government programs), and

(2) **Reimbursement,** the flow of dollars from insurance plans to physicians, hospitals, and other providers.

Cost control strategies can be divided into those that target the financing side versus those that impact the reimbursement side of the funding stream (Figure 9–1, Table 9–1).

FINANCING CONTROLS

Cost controls aimed at the financing of health insurance attempt to limit the flow of funds into health insurance plans, with the expectation that the plans will then be forced to modify the "outflow" of reimbursement. Financing controls come in two basic flavors—regulatory and competitive.

Regulatory Strategies

> Dieter Arbeiter, a carpenter in Berlin, Germany, is enrolled in one of his nation's health insurance plans, the "sick fund" operated by the Carpenter's Guild. Each month, Dieter pays 6% of his wages to the sick fund and his employer contributes an equal 6%. The German federal government regulates these payroll tax rates. When the government proposes raising the rate to 7%, Dieter and his coworkers march to the parliament building to protest the increase. The government backs down, and the rate remains at 6%. As a result, physician fees do not increase that year.

In nations with tax-financed health insurance, government regulation of taxes serves as a control over public expenditures for health care (Glaser, 1991). This regulatory control is most evident when certain tax funds are earmarked for health insurance, as in the case of the German health insurance plans (see Chapter 14) or Medicare Part A in the United States. Under these types of social insurance systems, an increase in expenditures for health care requires explicit legislation to raise the rate of

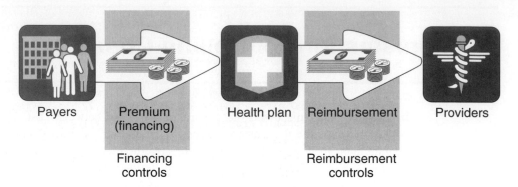

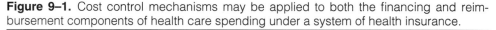

| Payers | Premium (financing) | Health plan | Reimbursement | Providers |

| | Financing controls | | Reimbursement controls | |

Figure 9–1. Cost control mechanisms may be applied to both the financing and reimbursement components of health care spending under a system of health insurance.

earmarked health insurance taxes. Public antipathy to tax hikes may serve as a political anchor against health care inflation.

President Clinton's 1994 health care proposal called for government regulation of health care costs. Unlike the process in most nations, the President's plan would have attempted to control financing not by limiting tax rates but rather through government regulation of premiums paid to private health insurance plans (Starr and Zelman, 1993).

Competitive Strategies An alternative United States proposal for containing health costs attempts to control the financing flow through a competitive strategy rather than through regulation. The basic premise of competitive financing strategies is to make payers more cost-conscious in their purchasing decisions. Health insurance plans would be encouraged to compete on the basis of price, with lower-cost plans being rewarded with a greater number of enrollees. Instead of having a government agency regulate financing by controlling tax rates for publicly financed insurance or by regulating the premiums charged by private insurance plans, the competitive market would pressure plans to restrain their premium prices and overall costs.

> Giovanni Costa works for General Auto (GA). It is 1985, and he and his family have Blue Cross health insurance that

Table 9–1. Categories of cost controls.

Financing controls
    Regulatory: limits on taxes or premiums
    Competitive
Reimbursement controls
    Price controls
        Regulatory
        Competitive
    Utilization (quantity) controls
        Aggregate units of payment: capitation, DRGs, global budgets
        Patient cost sharing
        Utilization management
        Supply limits
Mixed controls

covers most services provided by the health care provider of his choice, with no deductible. Giovanni does not know how much his health plan costs, because GA pays the premium. Once Giovanni asked his friend in the employee benefits department whether the company was worried about the costs of health insurance. "It's a problem," Giovanni was told, "but it's not too bad because our health insurance premiums are tax deductible for the company. Also, if we gave you higher wages you'd have to pay taxes on those wages, but if we give you better health care coverage, you don't pay taxes on the value of that coverage. So we're both better off by providing generous health care benefits. When it comes right down to it, the government's paying a portion of those premiums."

When considering competitive strategies that attempt to make purchasers more price-sensitive, it is important to consider who the purchaser of health insurance really is. For employment-based health insurance, is the purchaser the employer selecting which health plans to offer employees? Or is it the individual employee deciding to enroll in a specific plan? As in the case of Giovanni Costa and GA, the answer is often "both": GA selects which plans to offer employees and what portion of the premium to subsidize, and Giovanni chooses a particular plan from those offered by GA.

Historically, several factors have blunted both employers' and employees' consideration of price in the purchase of health insurance (Enthoven, 1993). For employees, the fact that employers usually write the check to purchase employees' private health insurance has insulated insured employees from the costs of insurance. Employees view health insurance premiums as an expense to the employer rather than as a cost borne by themselves. In fact, many employees might receive higher wages if the costs of health insurance were lower, but employees do not generally perceive health insurance benefits as foregone wages.

Moreover, the federal policy of treating health care benefits as nontaxable to both employee and employer makes it in the employee's financial interest to receive generous health care benefits and reduces the burden of paying for such benefits for the employer. A dollar contributed directly by the employer to a health plan goes farther toward the purchase of health insurance than a dollar in wages that is first taxed as income and then spent by the employee for health insurance. This dynamic has shielded employees from the real price of health insurance and given employees little incentive to be cost-conscious consumers when selecting an insurance plan.

For employers, inflation of health insurance premiums was an acceptable part of doing business when the economy was booming and health insurance costs consumed only a small portion of overall business expenses. However, as health insurance costs continued to spiral upward and economic growth slowed in the 1980s, employers became more active in their approach to health insurance (see Chapter 16).

It is 1995, and GA now offers Giovanni Costa three choices of health insurance plans. The health maintenance organization (HMO) plan costs $200 per month, with GA paying 80% and Giovanni paying 20%. The preferred provider organization (PPO) plan is worth $300 per month, and the fee-for-service plan runs at $400. If Giovanni chooses the HMO plan, GA pays $160 (80%) and Giovanni pays $40 (20%). If Giovanni signs up for the $300 PPO plan, GA still pays $160 (80% of the lowest-cost plan) and Giovanni must pay $140. If Giovanni wants to choose the fee-for-service plan, GA only pays $160 and Giovanni pays $240. GA has negotiated with all 3 of its health plans that premium levels will be frozen at their current 1995 rates for the next 3 years. A fourth plan formerly offered by GA refused to agree to this stipulation. GA dropped this plan from its portfolio of employee benefits.

The competitive approach to health insurance financing, now unfolding in the United States, encourages price-sensitive purchasing by both employer and employee. For employers, the competitive strategy calls for businesses to become more aggressive in their negotiations with health plans over premium rates. Employers bargain more actively with health plans and offer employees only plans that keep their rates below a certain level. Moreover, employers make employees more cost-aware when selecting a health plan by limiting the amount of the insurance premium that the employer will pay. Rather than paying all or most of the premium, many employers offer a fixed amount of insurance subsidy—often indexed to the cost of the cheapest health plan—and compel employees selecting more costly plans to pay the extra amount. Economist Alain Enthoven, one of the chief proponents of the competitive approach, has called this strategy "managed competition" (Enthoven and Kronick, 1989).

Is the evolving competitive approach succeeding at controlling costs? As noted in Chapter 8, the rate of growth of overall United States health care costs slowed between 1992 and 1995 during a period when many employers (and some government agencies) were adopting a more competitive approach to financing health insurance. Growth in insurance premiums appears to have been slower in more competitive markets within the United States (Zwanziger and Melnick, 1996). Some large employers in states such as California extracted concessions from major HMOs to lower their premiums in the mid-1990s (Enthoven and Singer, 1996). To be consistent with the spirit of making employees more "price-sensitive" by shouldering a greater portion of the premium cost, employers are subsidizing less of their employees' premiums; the percentage of insured employees with premiums fully paid by their employer dropped from 72% in 1980 to 45% by 1991 (Merlis, 1992). However, in late 1997 it appeared that costs may once again be on the upswing and that the 1992 to 1995 experience may have been a temporary phenomenon. Much of the competition occurring in the United States appears to be of an "unmanaged" variety, with little choice for employees, few ground rules for health plans, and scant data to help employers distinguish whether lower-cost plans are more efficient or are simply more successful at skimming off healthy enrollees.

Critics of competition argue that insurance companies will inevitably behave in ways that will defeat the market's ability to produce a more efficient and less costly health care system. These critics believe that insurance plans will continue to find it easier to compete by "gaming" the market through selection of low-cost enrollees rather than by disciplining providers to deliver a lower-cost, higher-quality "product." A marketplace dominated by a few large HMO conglomerates is viewed as creating a health insurance company "oligopoly" that will have the upper hand in price negotiations with employers and other purchasers and preclude true competition (Relman, 1993; Rice et al, 1993).

If competition could succeed at containing costs, would the outcome be painful or painless cost control? A fundamental concern about market-oriented reforms is that whatever "pain" may be produced in terms of compromised health status would be experienced most acutely by individuals with lower incomes. Under competition, individuals with higher incomes would be the ones most likely to pay the extra premium costs to enroll in more expensive health plans, while individuals of lesser means could not afford the extra premiums and would be relegated to the lower-cost plans. If the differential in premium prices across plans were large, enrollees in low-cost plans might experience inferior quality of care and health outcomes.

The Weaknesses of Financing Controls   For cost controls—whether regulatory or competitive—on the financing side of the health care equation to be successful, these strategies ultimately must produce reductions in the flow of funds on the reimbursement side. A government may try to limit the level of taxes earmarked for health care. However, if payments to physicians, hospitals, and other providers continue to grow at a rapid clip, the imbalance between the level of financing and level of reimbursement will produce budget deficits and ultimately force the government to raise taxes. Similarly, under competition, health insurers and HMOs will attempt to hold down premium increases in order to gain more customers, but if these health plans cannot successfully control what they pay to hospitals, physicians, pharmacies, and other providers, then insurers will be forced to raise their premiums and competitive relief from health care inflation will prove elusive. It is on the reimbursement side of the equation that the rubber meets the road in health care cost containment. Governments in nations with publicly financed insurance programs do not simply regulate health care financing but are actively involved in controlling provider reimbursement. Competition would place the onus on private health insurance plans—rather than a public agency—to regulate reimbursement costs. We now turn to an examination of the options available to private insurers or government for controlling the flow of funds in the reimbursement transaction.

REIMBURSEMENT CONTROLS

In Chapter 8, we distinguished between the "Ps" and "Qs" of health care costs: prices and quantities. Because cost equals price multiplied by quantity

$$C = P \times Q,$$

strategies to control costs on the reimbursement side can primarily target either prices or quantities (see Table 9–1).

Price Controls

> Under California's fee-for-service Medicaid program, Dr. Vincent Lo's reimbursement for a routine office visit has remained at $16 for the past five 5 years.

> The Medicare program reduced Dr. Ernesto Ojo's fee for cataract surgery from $1600 to $900.

> Instead of paying all hospitals in the area the going rate for MRI brain scans ($1200), Apple a Day HMO contracts with only those hospitals who agree to perform scans for $800, and will not allow its patients to receive MRIs at any other hospital.

> Metropolitan Hospital wants a contract with Apple a Day HMO at a per diem rate of $1400. Because Apple a Day can hospitalize its patients at Crosstown Hospital for $1100 a day, Metropolitan has no choice but to reduce its per diem rate to Apple a Day to $1100 in order to get the contract. In turn, to make up the $300 per day shortfall, Metropolitan increases its charges to several other private insurers.

In Canada and most European nations, a public or quasi-public agency regulates a uniform fee schedule for physician and hospital payments. Often, negotiations occur between the payers and professional organizations in establishing these fee schedules (Glaser, 1991; Evans et al, 1989). Payer-determined fee schedules have been less common in the United States, although as discussed in Chapter 4, Medicare, Medicaid, and many private insurance plans have replaced "usual, customary, and reasonable" physician fee screens with predetermined prices for particular services. Competitive approaches to controlling prices have also been attempted in the United States. In the 1980s, California initiated competitive bidding among hospitals for Medicaid contracts, with contracts awarded to hospitals offering lower per diem charges. Many private insurance plans have also used competitive bidding to bargain for reductions in physician and hospital fees.

Controlling prices has produced some limited success at restraining the growth of overall health care expenditures. The slower rate of increase in physician costs in Canada compared with that of the United States has been attributed to the regulation of physician fees in Canada (Evans et al, 1989; Hughes, 1991; Welch et al, 1996). In the United States, states with either highly regulated or highly competitive approaches to controlling the prices of hospital services have experienced slower rates of overall hospital cost inflation than states with neither type of cost containment strategy (Robinson and Luft, 1988; Zwanziger and Melnick, 1996). Two major problems limit the potency of price controls for containing overall costs, however, particularly when prices are regulated at the fee-for-service level.

(1) The first problem occurs when price controls are implemented in a piecemeal fashion by different payers. Providers, like Metropolitan Hospital, often respond to price controls imposed by one payer by increasing charges to other payers with less restrictive policies on fees—a phenomenon known as "cost shifting." The cost-shifting problem may be avoided when a uniform fee schedule is used by all payers (as in Germany) or by a single payer (as in Canada). Cost shifting may also be attenuated by a highly competitive market in which payers are equally intent on negotiating lower prices, limiting the number of plans willing to absorb higher prices to offset discounts awarded to other payers.

(2) Even under uniform fee schedules, increases in quantities may continue to drive up costs. Moreover, there is evidence that the volume and intensity of services increase particularly rapidly when prices are strictly controlled, leading some analysts

to conclude that providers respond to fee controls by "inducing" higher use of services in order to maintain earnings (Rice and Labelle, 1989).

Price controls have the appeal of being a relatively painless form of cost control insofar as they do not limit the quantity of services provided. Lack of uniformity, however, in the application of fee schedules may compromise access to care for certain populations; Medicaid fee-for-service rates to physicians are far below private insurance rates in most states, making it difficult for many Medicaid patients to find private physicians willing to care for them. In nations with uniform fee schedules, concerns have been voiced that unmitigated ratcheting down of fees could result in "patient churning" (high volumes of brief visits), with a consequent deterioration in quality of care and patient satisfaction.

Utilization (Quantity) Controls Because the effectiveness of price controls is limited by inflationary pressures from increases in the quantity of services, payers need to consider methods for containing the actual use of services. As indicated in Table 9–1, there are a variety of methods for attempting to control use. We begin by examining one strategy, changing the unit of payment, that we introduced in our review of physician and hospital reimbursement (Chapter 4). We then describe additional mechanisms that attempt to restrain the quantity of services.

Changing the Unit of Payment

> Dr. John Wiley is upset when the PPO reduces his fee from $35 to $30 per visit. In order to maintain his income, Dr. Wiley lengthens his day by half an hour so he can schedule more patient visits.

> Dr. Jane Stuckey is angry when the HMO reduces her capitation payment from $12 to $10 per patient per month. She is unable to maintain her income by seeing more patients because more patient visits do not bring her any more money. She hopes that more HMO patients will enroll in her practice so that she can receive more capitation payments.

One simple way to get a handle on the quantity factor is by redefining the unit of payment. In Chapter 4, we discussed how services may be bundled into more aggregate units of payment, such as capitated physician payment and diagnosis-related group (DRG) "episode of care" hospital payment. The more bundled the unit of payment, the more predictable the quantity tends to be. For example, in the case of Dr. Wiley receiving fee-for-service payment, there is a great potential for costs to rise due to increases in the number of physician visits, surgical procedures, and diagnostic tests. When the unit of payment is capitation, as in the case of Dr. Stuckey, the quantity factor is not the number of visits but rather the number of individuals enrolled in a practice or plan. From a health plan's perspective, the $C = P \times Q$ formula still applies when paying physicians by capitation, but now the "P" is the capitation fee and the "Q" is the number of individuals covered. Other than by raising birth rates, physicians have little discretion in inducing a higher volume of "quantities" at the capitation level for the health care system as a whole. Similarly, under global budgeting of hospitals, P represents the average global budget per hospital and Q is the number of hospitals.

Shifting the unit of payment to a more aggregated unit has obvious appeal as a way for third-party payers to counter cost inflation due to the quantity factor. Life is never so simple, however. In Chapter 4, we discussed how more aggregate units of payment shift financial risk to providers of care. Another way of describing this shifting of risk is that one person's solution to the quantity problem becomes another person's new quantity problem. A hospital paid by global budget instead of by fee-for-service now must monitor its own internal quantities of service lest these quantities drive hospital operating costs over budget. To the extent that providers are unsuccessful in managing resources under more global forms of payment, pressures mount to raise the prices paid at these more aggregated payment units.

Changes in policies for units of payment rarely occur independent of other reforms in cost control strategies, making it difficult to isolate the specific effects of changing the unit of payment. For example, physician capitation usually occurs in the context of other organizational and cost control features within a managed care plan. One large study of nearly 300 HMOs used statistical techniques to attempt to isolate the effects of different units of physician payment from the effects of other HMO characteristics (Hillman et al, 1989). The study found that compared with fee-for-service reimbursement, both capitation and salaried forms of payment were associated with lower HMO hospitalization rates. Most well-controlled studies of physician payment have tended to find that physicians practice a less costly style of medicine when paid by capitation rather than by fee-for-service (Hellinger, 1996).

For hospital payment, there is some evidence that changing Medicare hospital payments from a fee-for-service to an episode-of-care unit under the DRG-based prospective payment system in 1983 resulted in a modest slowing of the rate of increase in Medicare Part A expenditures (Russell and Manning, 1989). Some of these savings were offset by a shifting of costs to the outpatient and nursing home sector, however, blunting the ultimate effectiveness of this strategy for overall cost control. Many analysts consider that the Canadian and European strategy of global hospital budgeting has been a key element of these nations' relative success at containing hospital costs—or at least maintaining a slower rate of growth than that in the United States (Evans et al, 1989; U.S. General Accounting Office, 1991; Glaser, 1991).

The health care system in Germany and in some Canadian provinces has countered the open-ended dynamic of fee-for-service payment by introducing global budgeting, called expenditure caps, for physician payment (U.S. General Accounting Office, 1991; Barer et al, 1996). Under Canadian expenditure caps, a budget is established for all physician services in a province. Although individual physicians continue to bill the provincial health plan on a fee-for-service basis, if increases in the use of services cause overall physician costs to exceed the budget, fees are reduced (or fee increases for the following year are sacrificed) to stay within the expenditure cap. The intent is to create an incentive for physicians to cooperate in restraining the quantity of services provided, lest fees be reduced across the board to all physicians. In the United States, the Medicare program has adopted a less stringent version of an expenditure cap for physician fees, known as the "volume performance standard."

The types of regional expenditure caps for physician payments used in Germany and some Canadian provinces in effect allow the payer to focus on the aggregate "C" part of the equation—in this case, the total regional physician budget. A large portion of the responsibility for "solving" the right side of the equation—balancing the Ps of physician fees and the Qs of volume of services to remain within the expenditure cap—falls to physicians and their professional associations. Evidence from Canada suggests that implementation of expenditure caps has been associated with stabilization of physician costs in the mid-1990s (Barer et al, 1996).

No studies have measured the independent effect on health outcomes of changing the unit of payment to physicians. More scrutiny has been directed at the Medicare system of DRG hospital payment. A study in one state found that hip fracture patients received less physical therapy and experienced more prolonged nursing home stays after the enactment of the DRG system (Fitzgerald et al, 1988). However, a more recent and far more comprehensive study determined that quality of hospital care and health outcomes actually improved slightly from the pre-DRG to post-DRG period, although concerns remained that patients were being discharged in less stable condition in the post-DRG period (Rogers et al, 1990).

One final aspect of cost containment bears mentioning in the context of changing the unit of payment. As discussed in Chapters 4 and 5, many managed care plans in the United States not only have changed the unit of payment (eg, shifted from fee-for-service to capitation payment for physicians), but they also have incorporated additional financial incentives into physician payment in the form of income bonuses indexed to performance in holding down costs for referral services, hospital care, and related items. There is little evidence about the degree to which these financial incentives actually reduce use of services, much less about how they affect patient outcomes (Hellinger, 1996). The large (but somewhat dated) study of different units of physician payment cited earlier concluded that HMOs were more likely to "break even" financially if they used bonus incentives (Hillman et al, 1989).

Patient Cost Sharing

> Randy Payton has an insurance policy with a $1000 deductible and 20% copayment for all services; if he incurs medical expenses of $6000, he pays the first $1000 plus 20% of $5000, for a total of $2000.
>
> Joseph Mednick's insurance does not cover prescription drugs; suffering from diabetes, hypertension, and coronary artery disease, his multiple medications cost him $1200 per year.

Cost sharing refers to making patients pay directly out of pocket for some portion of their health care. In managed competition, cost sharing occurs as part of the financing transaction *at the point of purchasing a health insurance plan.* In this section, we discuss the more traditional notion of cost sharing—using deductibles, copayments, and uncovered services as part of the reimbursement transaction to make patients pay a share of costs *at the point of receiving health care services.* Cost sharing at the point of service reintroduces the process of out-of-pocket payments directly from the patient to the provider of care, bypassing the "third party" insurance plan (see Chapter 2).

The intent of cost sharing at the point of service is to discourage patients' demand for services. As discussed in Chapter 3, when individuals have insurance coverage, they are more likely to use services than when they have no insurance. While protection against individual financial risk is one of the essential benefits of insurance, insurance coverage removes the market restraint on costs that occur in a system of out-of-pocket payment. The goal of cost sharing is to reintroduce a sufficient degree of out-of-pocket payment to make individuals more "cost conscious" in their use of services while preserving a role for insurance coverage to protect against major or "catastrophic" out-of-pocket expenses.

Cost sharing at the point of service has been one of the few cost containment devices subjected to the rigorous evaluation of a randomized, controlled experiment. In the Rand Health Insurance Experiment, individuals were randomly assigned to health insurance plans with varying degrees of cost sharing. Individuals with cost-sharing plans made about one-third fewer visits and were hospitalized one-third less often than individuals randomized to the plan with no cost sharing (Newhouse et al, 1981).

Although the randomized, controlled trial provides an excellent laboratory for scrutinizing the effect of a single cost containment mechanism, some observers have cautioned that these types of "in vitro" analyses may produce results that cannot be generalized to the "in vivo" world of health policy. For example, the United States has one of the highest levels of cost sharing of any nation and also the highest overall costs. Studies have found that when cost sharing begins to produce lower use of services for a large population of patients rather than for a small number of patients in an experiment, providers may adjust their practices to keep busy and increase the volume of services provided to patients more able to pay or with better insurance coverage (Beck and Horne, 1980; Fahs, 1992).

The Rand experiment also evaluated the influence of cost sharing on appropriateness of care and health outcomes. Cost sharing did not reduce medically inappropriate use of services selectively, but equally discouraged use of appropriate and inappropriate services (Siu et al, 1986). The studies by Rand and others, cited in Chapter 3, demonstrate that people (especially those with low incomes) whose insurance plans require cost sharing, receive less preventive services and have poorer hypertension control than people without cost sharing (Brook et al, 1983). These studies suggest that cost sharing is not a "painless" form of cost control. More recent studies have examined cost sharing for emergency department care in two large HMOs (Selby et al, 1996; Magid et al, 1997); cost sharing reduced inappropriate use of emergency services without adversely affecting appropriate use or patients' health outcomes. The authors of these studies suggested that cost sharing may be a painless form of cost control when modest in amount, not applied to low-income patients, and designed to encourage patients to use lower-cost alternative sources of care (eg, clinics instead of emergency departments) rather than to discourage use of services altogether.

Utilization Management (UM)

> Thelma Graves suffers from a severe hyperthyroid condition; she and her physician agree that she will undergo thyroid surgery. Before scheduling the surgery, the physician has to call Ms. Graves' insurance company to obtain preauthorization, without which the insurer will not pay for the surgery.

> Fred Brady is hospitalized for an acute myocardial infarction. The hospital contacts the utilization management

(UM) firm for Mr. Brady's insurer, which authorizes 5 hospital days. On the fourth day, Mr. Brady develops a heart rate of 36 beats/min, requiring the insertion of a temporary pacemaker and prolonging the hospital stay for 10 extra days. After the fifth hospital day, Mr. Brady's physician has to call the UM firm every 2 days to justify why the insurer should continue to pay for the hospitalization.

Derek Jordan has juvenile onset diabetes and at age 42 becomes eligible for Medicare due to his permanent disability from complications of his diabetes. He is admitted to the hospital for treatment of a gangrenous toe. Under Medicare's DRG method of payment, the hospital receives the same payment for Derek's hospitalization regardless of whether it lasts 2 days or 12 days. Therefore, the hospital wants Derek's physician to discharge Derek as soon as possible. Each day, a hospital UM nurse reviews Derek's chart and suggests to the physician that Derek is no longer acutely ill and no longer requires acute hospitalization. The hospital keeps computerized profiles on physician practice patterns, and those doctors whose average patient length of stay exceeds the expected number of days are warned and placed under even tighter UM inspection.

Utilization management involves the surveillance of and intervention in the clinical activities of physicians for the purpose of controlling costs. Long a feature of Medicare and Medicaid, in recent years UM has become one of the rapidly growing cost containment mechanisms used by private managed care insurance plans (Grumbach and Bodenheimer, 1990). In contrast to cost sharing, which attempts to restrict health care use by influencing patient behavior, UM seeks to influence physician behavior. The mechanism of influencing physician decisions is simple and direct: denial of payment for services deemed unnecessary.

UM is related to the unit of payment in the following way: Whoever is at financial risk (see Chapter 4) performs UM. Under fee-for-service reimbursement, insurance companies perform UM to reduce their payments to hospitals and physicians. The DRG system induces hospitals, at risk for losing money if their patients stay too long, to perform UM. Under an HMO capitation contract with a primary physician group, the physicians conduct UM such that more of the capitation fee goes to primary care physician incomes rather than to laboratory or specialist fees. If an HMO pays a hospital a per diem rate, the HMO may send a UM nurse to the hospital each day to review whether the patient is ready to go home. If an HMO pays a hospital by capitation, the hospital, rather than the HMO, is at risk and performs UM.

Micromanage, Inc., performs UM for several insurance companies. Each day, Rebecca Hasselbach reviews the charts of each patient hospitalized by these insurers to determine whether the patients might be ready for discharge. In some cases, Ms. Hasselbach discusses the case with her medical director and with the patient's attending physician. Usually, if the attending physician wants the patient to remain in the hospital, his or her opinion is honored. By pushing for early discharges, Ms. Hasselbach, her Micromanage colleagues around the country, and the medical director

save their insurers about $500,000 each year. The annual
cost of the UM operation is $495,000.

Although a few case studies of UM have shown some short-term reduction in rates
of hospitalization and surgery, there is little evidence that this approach yields substantial savings overall on a long-term basis, particularly when the overhead of administering the UM program itself is taken into account (Wickizer, 1990). UM, if
successful at containing costs, would appear to be a painless form of cost control because it intends to selectively reduce inappropriate or unnecessary care. However,
studies have shown that authorization decisions are not reliably based on objective,
standardized evaluations of the appropriateness of care. Reviewers often make decisions on a case-by-case basis without explicit guidelines or criteria, with the result
that decisions are frequently inconsistent both between different reviewers for the
same case and among the same reviewer for different cases (Dippe, 1989; Light,
1994; Kerr et al, 1995).

UM has come under fire as a process of "micromanagement" of clinical decisions
that intrudes into the physician–patient relationship and places an unwelcome administrative hassle on physicians and other care givers. Physicians in the United States
have been called the most "second-guessed and paperwork-laden physicians in western industrialized democracies" (Lee and Etheredge, 1989). Substantial physician
time goes into appealing denials and persuading insurers on the appropriateness of
services delivered. Some physicians write long notes in the patient chart with the purpose not of documenting a medical condition and treatment but of justifying reimbursement. Many physicians feel that UM is turning the United States health care
system into a giant game of "Mother May I?"

Several approaches to UM have been developed that attempt to avoid some of the
onerous features of case-by-case utilization review. Practice profiling, rather than focusing on individual cases, uses summary data on practice patterns to identify physicians whose overall use of services significantly deviates from the standard of other
physicians in the community (Welch et al, 1994). Physician outliers identified by
practice profiling are then subject to various interventions. In Canada and Germany,
these interventions consist of educational and monitoring activities performed by regional medical societies (Glaser, 1991). In the United States, some managed care
plans use practice profiling to "economically credential" physicians, offering contracts only to those whose practice patterns accord with the plan's cost control objec-
tives.

Establishing a primary care "gatekeeper" may also be viewed as a different approach to UM (see Chapter 6). Under managed care, it is difficult to disentangle the
effect of having a physician to coordinate care from the many financial incentives
that are often associated with gatekeeping arrangements. Nevertheless, the coordination function in and of itself, even in a financially neutral environment, might reduce
inappropriate self-referral for specialist services. Studies of United States insurance
plans, however, have failed to find that simply assigning patients to a gatekeeper produces major reductions in overall costs (Moore et al, 1983).

The least intrusive forms of UM involve general educational activities and feedback on practice patterns without attendant disciplinary measures. In general, these
voluntary approaches have not been shown to have a measurable impact on containing costs (Greco and Eisenberg, 1993). Because the provision of inappropriate quan-

tities of care, whether too much or too little, often has quality of care implications (see Chapter 12), UM and quality improvement activities often overlap.

Supply Limits

> Harry is a patient enrolled in the Kaiser Health Plan in Los Angeles. He develops back pain, has several visits to his family physician, but wants an MRI of his spine to rule out a herniated intervertebral disc. His physician refuses his request because, given the limited number of MRI scanners for Kaiser's enrolled population, Harry's physical findings are not sufficiently severe to warrant an MRI scan under Kaiser's criteria.
>
> Larry sustains a football injury causing intense back pain with radiation to the leg. He goes to Kaiser's urgent care clinic and is found to have loss of sensation, strength, and the deep tendon reflex in his left leg. The Kaiser physician prescribes complete bed rest and arranges for an urgent MRI scan in 3 days.
>
> Bob is a patient in the Canadian province of Alberta. He develops back pain, and after several visits to his family physician requests an MRI of his spine to rule out disk disease. His physician, who does not suspect a disk herniation, agrees to place him on the waiting list for an MRI, which for non-urgent cases is 5 months long.
>
> Rob lives in Alberta and, after lifting an 80-pound load at work, experiences severe lower back pain radiating down his right leg. Finding a positive straight-leg-raising test on the right with loss of the right ankle reflex, his family physician calls the radiologist and obtains an emergency MRI scan within 3 days.

Supply limits are controls on the number of physicians and other care givers and on specific material resources such as the number of hospital beds or MRI scanners. Supply limits can take place within a specific institution such as an HMO in the United States (the example of Harry and Larry), or for an entire geographic region such as a Canadian province (the example of Bob and Rob).

There is evidence that the quantity of services provided correlates with the supply of physicians, a phenomenon known as "supplier-induced demand" (Evans, 1984; Rice and Labelle, 1989). A greater number of surgeons in a geographic area, for example, has been associated with more operations performed in that area (Bunker, 1970; Wennberg and Gittelsohn, 1973). Controlling physician supply may reduce use of physician services and thereby contribute to cost containment.

The principle of supplier-induced demand pertains to material capacity as well as to physician supply. Some studies have shown that hospital days per capita are higher in geographic areas with more per capita hospital beds; the maxim that "empty beds tend to become filled" has been known as "Roemer's law" (Roemer and Shain, 1959). Conversely, strictly regulating the number of centers allowed to perform open heart surgery establishes a limit to the total number of cardiac operations that can be performed. In situations of limited supply, physicians must determine which patients are most in need of the limited supply of services. Ideally, those truly in need gain access to appropriate services, with physicians possessing the wisdom to distinguish those patients truly in need (Larry and Rob) from those not requiring the service (Harry and Bob). In less ideal circumstances, the supply of resources cannot accommodate all needy patients, and physicians and other care givers are forced to prioritize patients based on degree of medical need (see Chapter 13).

Most of the evidence that limiting supply succeeds in controlling costs derives from observational studies that compare different geographic regions and demonstrate that use of services is related to the availability of physicians, hospital beds, and technologies (Wennberg and Gittelsohn, 1973; Wennberg et al, 1987). In some cases, research has failed to detect a strong association between supply and costs (Folland and Stano, 1990). Although there may not always be a directly linear relationship between supply and use of services, there are clear instances in which limitations of capacity restrain use. For example, international comparisons demonstrate large variations in use of coronary artery bypass surgery with a relatively low rate of surgery in the United Kingdom, an intermediate rate in Canada, and the highest rate in the United States. These rates correspond to the degree to which these nations regulate (minimal in the case of the United States) the number of centers performing cardiac surgery (McPherson, 1989; Rublee, 1994). Studies in the United States have found that patients admitted with myocardial infarction (MI) receive different treatments, depending on whether they are admitted to hospitals with cardiac catheterization and surgery units. Those admitted to hospitals with such units are far more likely to receive coronary artery angiography or bypass surgery than MI patients who are admitted to hospitals without such units (that must transfer patients to other facilities to perform these procedures) (Blustein, 1993; Every et al, 1993).

A few studies have examined how supply constraints may affect health outcomes. One of the studies of MI patients mentioned above found that outcomes were as good for patients admitted to hospitals without cardiac catheterization units as for those admitted to hospitals with this capability, despite the lower use of cardiac procedures for the former group of patients (Every et al, 1993). A "natural experiment" in supply restriction took place in a hospital when a nursing shortage abruptly reduced the number of staffed intensive care unit beds from 18 to eight (Singer et al, 1983). For patients admitted to the hospital for chest pain, physicians became more accurate in admitting to the intensive care unit only those patients who actually suffered MIs. Limiting use of intensive care unit beds did not result in any adverse health outcomes for patients admitted to non-intensive care unit beds, including those few non-intensive care unit patients who actually sustained MIs. These studies suggest that physicians, when faced with supply limits, may be able to prioritize patients on clinical grounds in a manner that selectively reduces unnecessary services. Establishing supply limits that require physicians to prioritize services based on the appropriateness and urgency of patient need represents a very different (and less intrusive) approach to containing costs than UM, which relies on external parties to authorize or deny individual services in a setting of relatively unconstrained capacity.

Controlling the Type of Supply: A specific form of supply control is regulation of the *types (rather than the total number)* of providers. Chapter 6 explored the balance between the number of generalist and specialist physicians in a health care system.

Increasing the proportion of generalists may yield savings for two reasons (Grumbach and Lee, 1991). First, generalists earn lower incomes than specialists. Second, and of greater impact for overall costs, generalists appear to practice a less resource-intensive style of medicine and generate lower overall health care expenditures, including lower use of hospital and laboratory services (Greenfield et al, 1992). Studies have also indicated that nurse practitioners and physician assistants can effectively perform many of the tasks of the primary care provider at a lower cost than physicians (Greenfield et al, 1978; Mundinger, 1994).

MIXED CONTROLS

In the real world, cost containment strategies are applied not as isolated phenomena in a static system but as an array of policies concerned with modes of financing, patterns of medical care delivery, and cost control all mixed together. We now turn to two case studies that exemplify a mixture of cost containment methods: United States managed care and the Canadian health care system.

Managed Care in the United States   "Managed care" refers to a heterogeneous array of health insurance plans that differ to greater or lesser degree from traditional health insurance. Previously (see Chapters 4, 5, and 7), we have discussed how managed care plans may be characterized in terms of their organizational structures and methods for reimbursing providers. Yet, another vantage point from which to categorize managed care plans is their approach to cost containment (Table 9–2).

PPO plans differ the least from traditional "unmanaged" health insurance. To control costs, PPOs rely on measures such as utilization management and price discounts for fee-for-service payments to physicians and hospitals. Individual practice association (IPA) forms of HMOs often alter the unit of payment to a more bundled level as an additional cost containment strategy, usually in association with the requirement that patients select a primary care gatekeeper who may practice an "economical" style of medicine.

Group and staff model HMOs, by dint of their more fundamental reorganization of the delivery system, wield additional cost control weapons. Because of their more integrated relationship with physicians and hospitals, these plans tend to pay providers

Table 9–2. Managed care cost control strategies.

Preferred Provider Organization
    Price controls
    Utilization management
    Patient cost sharing
Independent Practice Association HMOs
    Price controls
    Utilization management
    Gatekeeping
    Changing unit of payment to capitation
    Regulating supply via selective contracting
Group and staff model HMOs
    Changing unit of payment to salary and global budgets
    Supply controls
    Administrative simplicity

using the most aggregated units of payment possible (ie, salaries for physicians and global budgets for hospitals). These HMOs also introduce supply controls as a major cost containment device. Most group and staff model HMOs plan their hospital bed and physician supply on the basis of explicit targets for bed-to-enrollee and physician-to-enrollee ratios; they may also limit the number of costly resources such as MRI scanners.

Effect on Costs: One of the most contentious issues in contemporary health policy in the United States is whether managed care health plans truly control costs more effectively than do non-managed care plans. Research on this topic is beset with methodological problems, including difficulties in measuring differences in underlying medical risk among plan enrollees; accounting fully for all spending, including administrative overhead and out-of-pocket expenses by patients; standardizing benefits covered by different plans; and tracking costs over time. There is general agreement that, compared with traditional non-managed insurance plans, HMOs use fewer resources for hospital care, because of lower hospitalization rates. Although many studies have found that outpatient services are used more frequently in HMOs, this higher rate of use does not appear to fully offset reductions in inpatient care (Luft, 1978; Miller and Luft, 1994).

Attempting to avoid some of the methodologic problems, the Rand Health Insurance Experiment randomly assigned individuals to an HMO or a traditional insurance plan. The Rand study found that overall costs were about 25% lower for individuals enrolled in the HMO (Manning et al, 1984). Many analysts caution against generalizing from the Rand study because the experiment included only a single HMO plan, Group Health Cooperative of Puget Sound. A staff model HMO founded in 1947 as a consumer cooperative, Group Health is not representative of most of the managed care plans that proliferated during the 1980s.

A comprehensive review of managed care performance concluded that the research "does not provide policy makers with adequate bottom-line estimates of expenditure differences per enrollee compared with indemnity [traditional insurance] plans," but only suggests possible cost savings among managed care plans (Miller and Luft, 1994). A U.S. General Accounting Office (1993) analysis similarly determined that "empirical evidence of employers' cost savings from managed care is inconclusive." The possible reductions in overall costs in managed care plans resulting from lower use of hospital services may produce only a "one time" savings. Premiums for managed care plans have been rising at the same rate as those for indemnity plans (Newhouse et al, 1985; Gabel, 1992). One recent study in a single state found that a higher HMO market share in an area was associated with lower overall rate of growth of insurance premiums (Wickizer and Feldstein, 1995).

Effect on Outcomes: The results of the Rand Health Insurance Experiment are emblematic of the ambiguous findings that often occur in studies of costs and outcomes. Health outcomes such as reduction in cholesterol levels were better for higher-income people without health problems at the start of the study if they received care from the Group Health Cooperative of Puget Sound HMO. For low-income people with initial health problems, however, the health status of HMO patients ended up worse than that of patients in fee-for-service practice (Ware et al, 1986).

More recent studies have tended to find results similar to the Rand Health Insurance Experiment. The most rigorously conducted studies indicate that for the general population, outcomes are comparable in managed care and non–managed care plans. However, for patients with chronic illnesses who are elderly or low income, several studies suggest that outcomes are worse in managed care plans (Miller and Luft, 1994; Miller and Luft, 1997). These latter findings have caused concern that managed care may perform less well for patients with the greatest medical needs. Enrollees in managed care plans also tend to be less satisfied with the perceived quality of care and patient–physician interactions but more satisfied with the financial protection offered by the managed care plans, suggesting a potential trade-off between the values of quality and affordability (Miller and Luft, 1994; Miller and Luft, 1997).

The Canadian Health Care System   Canada has a single-payer system of national health insurance administered by the provincial governments (see Chapter 14). The Canadian approach to cost containment emphasizes regulation of prices, payment by global budgets, and supply limits (Evans et al, 1989) (Table 9–3). Patient cost sharing and utilization management have not featured prominently in the Canadian cost control strategy. Fee-for-service is the dominant method of paying physicians, with provincial plans using fee controls as a strategy for containing growth in physician expenditures. Work force policies have not (until recently) strictly limited the overall number of physicians, but have regulated residency training positions in order to achieve close to a 50:50 balance in specialist and generalist physician supply. Payments to hospitals occur by global budgeting of operating costs. Provincial plans also regulate all new capital projects as a means of controlling the supply of major technologies, resulting in lower per capita supply of cardiac surgery centers, lithotripsy machines, and CT scanners, compared with levels in the United States.

Effect on Costs: From 1970, about the time that Canadian national health insurance became fully implemented, to 1995, overall health care costs as a proportion of the gross domestic product (GDP) grew by 33% in Canada and by 92% in the United States (see Chapter 14). (GDP is the total output of goods and services produced within a country, valued at market prices.) Between 1970 and 1990, inflation-adjusted per capita health care spending (known as "real expenditures") increased at an average annual rate of 5.0% in Canada and 5.5% in the United States (Organisation for Economic Cooperation and Development, 1992).

A number of studies have compared trends in health care costs in the United States and Canada in greater detail. One of the most dramatic differences between the two nations is the level of administrative expenses, which is as high as 25% of total health care costs in the United States and only 11% in Canada (Woolhandler and Himmelstein, 1991). This difference in administrative costs accounts for almost half of the difference in overall health care expenditures in the two nations. The single-payer approach to health insurance yields administrative savings on both the financing and re-

Table 9–3. Canadian cost control strategies.

Price controls
Changing the unit of payment
    Hospitals: global budgets
    Physicians: expenditure caps
Supply controls
Administrative simplicity

imbursement sides of the cost equation. On the financing side, a unitary, tax-financed government insurance plan obviates the need for insurer marketing expenses, permits simplification of the eligibility and enrollment process, collects insurance revenues using existing tax collection agencies, and eliminates the profits of investor-owned private insurance intermediaries. On the reimbursement side, claims processing becomes streamlined for fee-for-service physician services and is eliminated for payment of hospitals under global budgets. Avoidance of case-by-case utilization management also keeps overhead costs lean for both provincial insurance plans and providers.

In addition to minimizing administrative expenses, Canada has adopted specific measures to contain physician costs. Government regulation in Canada has slowed growth in physician fees relative to trends in the United States (Hughes, 1991). A lower proportion of Canadian physicians practice in higher-income specialty fields. Because of the differences in fee levels and specialty mix, overall Canadian expenditures per capita on physician services are almost 40% lower than those in the United States, even though Canadians use 20% more physician services (Fuchs and Hahn, 1990; Welch et al, 1996). Although physician costs are lower in Canada than in the United States, Canadian physicians retain a higher share of their total earnings as net income, because of lower overhead expenses.

Although the Canadian system has had relative success at controlling expenditures for physician services, the rate of growth of physician costs remains a concern in Canada. As discussed earlier in this chapter, several provinces have begun to counter the open-ended dynamic of fee-for-service payment through the imposition of global expenditure caps on physician costs (Barer et al, 1996). Global expenditure caps in Canada appear to have slowed the rate of growth in the volume of some types of physician services, in addition to maintaining control of physician fees (Katz et al, 1997a). The Canadian system has also begun to focus on the growing physician-to-population ratio as an impediment to cost containment and has adopted new measures to control the overall supply of physicians (Barer et al, 1996).

Analyses of hospital costs in the United States and Canada reveal that the combination of global budgeting and regulation of new technology has kept per capita hospital expenditures 20% lower in Canada. Unlike the case of physician expenditures, price differences do not explain the difference in costs. Wages for nurses and other hospital labor and material supplies are comparable in the two nations. Nor does there appear to be a major difference in the quantity of clinical services in most instances. Hospitalization rates and length of stay are higher in Canada, overall rates of surgery are similar for most procedures (including transplantation), and general patterns of use of inpatient diagnostic tests appear comparable in both nations (Redelmeier and Fuchs, 1993; Anderson et al, 1989).

Coronary artery disease is one of the few clinical conditions for which studies have documented less intensive use of major procedures in Canada. Overall rates of coronary artery bypass surgery are much higher in the United States than in Canada, largely due to greater use among the elderly in the United States (Anderson et al, 1993). Several comparative studies of patients with MI have shown that patients in the United States are up to three times more likely to have coronary angiography performed and about five times as likely to have coronary angioplasty or bypass surgery following their infarction, with relative differences even larger among the elderly (Rouleau et al, 1993; Mark et al, 1994; Tu et al, 1997).

Effect on Outcomes: Data comparing health outcomes among different nations are scarce. Public health indices, such as infant mortality and life expectancy rates, are significantly better in Canada than in the United States (Schieber et al, 1993). However, as discussed in Chapter 3, these indices are influenced by many socioeconomic factors, not just medical care, and therefore may not accurately reflect the relative performances of the health care systems. Few studies have carefully evaluated the outcomes of care in the United States and Canada for similar types of patients. One study comparing outcomes for patients with severe mental illness in Vancouver, British Columbia, and Seattle, Washington, found that those in Vancouver received more mental health services and showed greater clinical improvement over time (Beiser et al, 1985). A more recent, larger study also showed that patients with the greatest need—those with low incomes and moderate-to-severe mental illness—were much more likely to receive mental health services in Canada than in the United States (Katz et al, 1997b). Comparisons of patients in Canada and the United States with MI have failed to detect significant differences in survival and rates of reinfarction despite more aggressive treatment in the United States; however, patients in the United States were less likely to experience activity-limiting angina following their infarctions (Rouleau et al, 1993; Mark et al, 1994; Tu et al, 1997). Although it is difficult to draw firm conclusions from limited data, these studies may be reasonably representative of the ways in which health care differs between Canada and the United States. The Canadian system is geared more toward improving population health outcomes affected by primary care. Its strengths may be particularly apparent in the area of mental illness; whereas comprehensive mental health benefits are included in all provincial health plans, most insurance plans in the United States offer limited coverage for mental health services, and access to adequate care in the United States is a particularly pressing problem for the mentally ill. On the other hand, no nation can match the United States for availability of high technology cardiac care. While the more widespread use of cardiac services may not offer a major improvement in mortality rates, these services may enhance functional status and quality of life.

CONCLUSION

There is no perfect mechanism for controlling health care costs. Strategies must be judged by their relative success at containing costs and doing so in as "painless" a manner as possible—without compromising health outcomes. In the view of Dr. John Wennberg, the key to cost control in the United States

> is not in the micromanagement of the doctor-patient relationship but the management of capacity and budgets. The American problem is to find the will to set the supply thermostat somewhere within reason. (Wennberg JE: Outcomes research, cost containment, and the fear of health care rationing. N Engl J Med 1990;323:1202.)

Although United States managed care plans and Canadian provincial health plans are often viewed as diametrically opposed paradigms for health care reform, both the Canadian plans and United States group and staff model HMOs base their cost control approaches on what Wennberg terms "the management of capacity and budgets." In Canada, this management is under public control through regulation of physician supply, physician and hospital budgets, and technology. In the United States, privately administered HMOs adjust their own "thermostats" by setting their own budgets and numbers of physicians, hospital beds, and high-cost equipment.

If there is a lesson to be learned from attempts to control health care costs in the United States over the past decades, it is that cost containment policies affecting provider reimbursement need to focus more on macromanagement and less on micromanagement (Luft and Grumbach, 1994). Trying to manage costs at the level of individual patient encounters (ie, regulating fees for each service, reviewing daily practice decisions, or imposing cost sharing for every prescription and visit to the physician) is a cumbersome and largely ineffectual strategy for containing overall expenditures. Moreover, one payer lowering its costs by shifting expenses to another payer does not produce system-wide cost savings. Payers in the future must increasingly emphasize more global cost containment tools (ie, paying by capitation or other aggregate units, limiting the size and specialty mix of the physician workforce, and concentrating high-technology services in regional centers). The future debate over cost containment in the United States will center on whether these cost containment tools are best wielded by private managed care plans operating in a price competitive market or by public regulation of health care providers.

REFERENCES

Anderson GA, Newhouse JP, Roos LL: Hospital care for elderly patients with diseases of the circulatory system. A comparison of hospital use in the United States and Canada. N Engl J Med 1989;321:1443.

Anderson GA et al: Use of coronary artery bypass surgery in the United States and Canada: Influence of age and income. JAMA 1993;269:1661.

Barer ML et al: Re-minding our Ps and Qs: Cost controls in Canada. Health Aff 1996;15(2):216.

Beck RG, Horne JM: Utilization of publicly insured health services in Saskatchewan before, during and after copayment. Med Care 1980;18:787.

Beiser M et al: Does community care for the mentally ill make a difference? A tale of two cities. Am J Psychiatry 1985;137:1047.

Blustein J: High-technology cardiac procedures: The impact of service availability on service use in New York State. JAMA 1993;270:344.

Brook RH et al: Does free care improve adults' health? N Engl J Med 1983;309:1426.

Bunker J: Surgical manpower. N Engl J Med 1970;282:135.

Dippe SE et al: A peer review of a Peer Review Organization. West J Med 1989; 151:93.

Enthoven A, Kronick R: A consumer choice health plan for the 1990s: Universal health insurance in a system designed to promote quality and economy. (Parts 1 and 2.) N Engl J Med 1989;320:29, 94.

Enthoven AC: The history and principles of managed competition. Health Aff 1993 (Suppl);12:24.

Enthoven AC, Singer SJ: Managed competition and California's health care economy. Health Aff 1996;15(1):39.

Evans RG: Strained Mercy: The Economics of Canadian Health Care. Butterworths, 1984.

Evans RG et al: Controlling health expenditures: The Canadian reality. N Engl J Med 1989;320:571.

Every NR et al: The association between on-site cardiac catheterization facilities and the use of coronary angiography after acute myocardial infarction. N Engl J Med 1993;329:546.

Fahs MC: Physician response to the United Mine Workers' cost-sharing program: The other side of the coin. Health Serv Res 1992;27:25.

Fitzgerald JF, Moore PS, Dittus RS: The care of elderly patients with hip fracture: Changes since implementation of the prospective payment system. N Engl J Med 1988;319:1392.

Folland S, Stano M: Small area variations: A critical review of propositions, methods, and evidence. Med Care Rev 1990;47(4):419.

Fuchs VR, Hahn JS: How does Canada do it? A comparison of expenditures for physicians' services in the United States and Canada. N Engl J Med 1990;323:884.

Gabel JR: Witness to a thousand stories: A look at insurance data. Health Aff 1992;11(4):186.

Glaser WA: Health Insurance in Practice. Jossey-Bass, 1991.

Greco PJ, Eisenberg JM: Changing physicians' practices. N Engl J Med 1993;329:1271.

Greenfield S et al: Efficiency and cost of primary care by nurses and physician assistants. N Engl J Med 1978;298:305.

Greenfield S et al: Variations in resource utilization among medical specialties and systems of care. JAMA 1992;267:1624.

Grumbach K, Bodenheimer T: Reins or fences: A physician's view of cost containment. Health Aff 1990;9(3):120.

Grumbach K, Lee PR: How many physicians can we afford? JAMA 1991;265:2369.

Hellinger FJ: The impact of financial incentives on physician behavior in managed care plans: A review of the evidence. Med Care Res Rev 1996; 53:294.

Hillman AL, Pauly MV, Kerstein JJ: How do financial incentives affect physicians' clinical decisions and the financial performance of health maintenance organizations? N Engl J Med 1989;321:86.

Hughes JS: How well has Canada contained the costs of doctoring? JAMA 1991;265:2347.

Katz SJ et al: The growth of physician services for the elderly in the United States and Canada: 1987–1992. Med Care Res Rev 1997a;54:301.

Katz SJ et al: Mental health care use, morbidity, and socioeconomic status in the United States and Ontario. Inquiry 1997b;34(Spring):38.

Kerr EA et al: Managed care and capitation in California. Ann Intern Med 1995;123:500.

Lee PR, Etheredge L: Clinical freedom: Two lessons for the UK from US experience with privatisation of health care. Lancet 1989;1:263.

Light DW: Life, death, and the insurance companies. N Engl J Med 1994;330:498.

Luft HS: How do health maintenance organizations achieve their savings? N Engl J Med 1978;317:1743.

Luft HS, Grumbach K: Global budgets and the competitive market. In: Critical Issues in U.S. Health Reform. E Ginzberg (editor). Westview Press, 1994.

Magid DJ et al: Absence of association between insurance copayments and delays in seeking emergency care among patients with myocardial infarction. N Engl J Med 1997; 336:1722.

Manning WG et al: A controlled trial of the effect of a prepaid group practice on the use of services. N Engl J Med 1984;310:1505.

Mark DB et al: Use of medical resources and quality of life after acute myocardial infarction in Canada and the United States. N Engl J Med 1994;331:1130.

McPherson K: International differences in medical care practices. Health Care Fin Rev 1989;Ann Suppl:9.

Merlis M: CRS Issue Brief, Health Insurance. Congressional Research Service, 1992.

Miller RH, Luft HS: Does managed care lead to better or worse quality of care? Health Aff 1997;16(5):7.

Miller RH, Luft HS: Managed care plan performance since 1980: A literature analysis. JAMA 1994;271:1512.

Moore SH, Martin DP, Richardson WC: Does the primary-care gatekeeper control the costs of health care? N Engl J Med 1983;309:1400.

Mundinger MO: Advanced-practice nursing: Good medicine for physicians? N Engl J Med 1994;330:211.

Newhouse JP et al: Are fee-for-service costs increasing faster than HMO costs? Med Care 1985;23:960.

Newhouse JP et al: Some interim results from a controlled trial of cost sharing in health insurance. N Engl J Med 1981;305:1501.

Organisation for Economic Cooperation and Development: U.S. Health Care at the Cross-Roads. Health Policy Studies No. 1. Organisation for Economic Cooperation and Development, 1992.

Redelmeier DA, Fuchs VR: Hospital expenditures in the United States and Canada. N Engl J Med 1993;328:772.

Relman AS: Controlling costs by managed competition: Would it work? N Engl J Med 1993;328:133.

Rice T, Brown R, Wyn R: Holes in the Jackson Hole approach to health care reform. JAMA 1993;270:1357.

Rice TH, Labelle RJ: Do physicians induce demand for medical services? J Health Polit Policy Law 1989;14:587.

Robinson JC, Luft HS: Competition, regulation, and hospital costs, 1982 to 1986. JAMA 1988;260:2676.

Roemer MI, Shain M: Hospital Utilization Under Insurance. American Hospital Association, 1959.

Rogers WH et al: Quality of care before and after implementation of the DRG-based prospective payment system. JAMA 1990;264:1989.

Rouleau JL et al: A comparison of management patterns after acute myocardial infarction in Canada and the United States. N Engl J Med 1993;328:779.

Rublee DA: Medical technology in Canada, Germany, and the United States: An update. Health Aff 1994;13(4):113.

Russell LB, Manning CL: The effect of prospective payment on Medicare expenditures. N Engl J Med 1989;320:439.

Schieber GJ, Poullier J-P, Greenwald LM: Health spending, delivery, and outcomes in OECD countries. Health Aff 1993;12(2):120.

Selby JV et al: Effect of a copayment on use of the emergency department in a health maintenance organization. N Engl J Med 1996;334:635.

Singer DE et al: Rationing intensive care: Physician responses to a resource shortage. N Engl J Med 1983;309:1155.

Siu AL, Sonnenberg FA, Manning WG: Inappropriate use of hospitals in a randomized trial of health insurance plans. N Engl J Med 1986;315:1259.

Starr P, Zelman WA: Bridge to compromise: competition under a budget. Health Aff 1993;12(Suppl):7.

Tu JV et al: Use of cardiac procedures and outcomes in elderly patients with myocardial infarction in the United States and Canada. N Engl J Med 1997;336:1500.

U.S. General Accounting Office: Health Care Spending Control: The Experience of France, Germany, and Japan. 1991.

U.S. General Accounting Office: Managed Health Care: Effect on Employers' Costs Difficult to Measure. 1993.

Ware JE et al: Comparison of health outcomes at a health maintenance organization with those of fee-for-service care. Lancet 1986;1:1017.

Welch HG, Miller ME, Welch WP: Physician profiling: An analysis of inpatient practice patterns in Florida and Oregon. N Engl J Med 1994;330:607.

Welch WP et al: A detailed comparison of physician services for the elderly in the United States and Canada. JAMA 1996;275:1410.

Wennberg JE: Outcomes research, cost containment, and the fear of health care rationing. N Engl J Med 1990;323:1202.

Wennberg JE, Freeman JL, Culp WJ: Are hospital services rationed in New Haven or over-utilised in Boston? Lancet 1987;1:1185.

Wennberg JE, Gittelsohn A: Small area variations in health care delivery. Science 1973;182:1102.

Wickizer TM: The effect of utilization review on hospital use and expenditures: A review of the literature and an update on recent findings. Med Care Rev 1990;47(3):327.

Wickizer TM, Feldstein PJ: The impact of HMO competition on private insurance premiums, 1985–1992. Inquiry 1995;33:241.

Woolhandler S, Himmelstein DU: The deteriorating administrative efficiency of the U.S. health care system. N Engl J Med 1991;324:253.

Zwanziger J, Melnick G: Can managed care plans control health care costs? Health Aff 1996;15(2)185.

Long-Term Care

10

Eddie Taylor awoke one morning at his home in California unable to speak or to move the right side of his body, but able to understand other people around him. After 3 terrifying days in a hospital and 3 frustrating weeks in a stroke rehabilitation center, Mr. Taylor failed to improve. Because he no longer required hospital-level care, he became ineligible for Medicare hospital coverage. Since Mrs. Taylor was wheelchair bound with crippling rheumatoid arthritis and unable to care for him, he was transferred to a nursing home. Medicare did not cover the $115 per day cost. After 2 years, Medicaid began to pick up the nursing home bills. The family's life savings—earned during the 50 years Mr. Taylor worked in a men's clothing store—had been spent down to $66,000, the amount that California Medicaid allows the spouse of a nursing home resident to keep. Because Medicaid paid only $80 per day, few recreational activities were offered, and Mr. Taylor spent each day lying in bed next to a demented patient, who screamed for hours at a time. Unable to voice his complaints at the inhuman conditions of his life, he became severely depressed, stopped eating, and within 3 months was dead. After his death, the state placed a lien on Mrs. Taylor's home; when she sold the house, the state took $30,000 from the sale as reimbursement for her husband's Medicaid costs.

On high school graduation night, Lyle celebrated with a few drinks and drove to his girlfriend's house. He lost control of the car, hit a tree, and suffered a fractured cervical spine, unable to move his arms or legs. After 9 months in a rehabilitation unit, Lyle remained quadriplegic. He returned home, with a home care agency providing total 24-hour-a-day care at a cost of $160 per day, not covered by insurance. Lyle's father, a businessman, became increasingly angry at his wife, the principal flutist in the city's professional orchestra, because she refused to leave the orchestra to care for Lyle. After 1 year and $60,000 in long-term care expenses, Lyle's parents were close to divorce. One night Lyle's father awoke in a cold sweat; in his dream, he had placed a plastic bag over Lyle's head and suffocated him.

Time and again, physicians and other care givers witness the tragedy of chronic illness compounded by the failure of the nation's health care system to meet the social needs created by the illness. The crisis of long-term care is twofold: thousands of families each year lose their savings to pay for the chronic illness of a family member, and care for the chronically ill often takes place in dehumanized institutions that rob their occupants of the last remaining vestiges of independence.

Long-term care includes those health, social, housing, transportation, and other supportive services needed by persons with physical, mental, or cognitive limitations

Table 10–1. Activities requiring assistance in long-term care.

Activities of daily living (ADLs) (basic human functions)
    Eating
    Dressing
    Bathing
    Toileting
    Getting in and out of bed or chair
Instrumental activities of daily living (IADLs) (activities necessary to remain independent)
    Doing housework and laundry
    Preparing meals
    Shopping for groceries
    Using transportation
    Managing finances
    Taking medications
    Telephoning

sufficient to compromise independent living. The need for long-term care services is usually determined by evaluating a person's impairment in activities of daily living (ADLs) (eg, eating, dressing, bathing, toileting, and getting in or out of bed or a chair) and in instrumental activities of daily living (IADLs) (eg, laundry, housework, meal preparation, grocery shopping, transportation, financial management, taking medications, and telephoning) (Table 10–1). Between 9 and 11 million people in the United States require assistance with one or more ADLs or IADLs, and can therefore be considered as needing long-term care services. Of these, about 4 million are disabled people below age 65. Several special populations require long-term care services, including persons with AIDS, Alzheimer's and other dementias, or chronic mental illness (Pepper Commission, 1990).

Projections of growth for the elderly population in the United States are startling. In 1990, the population 65 years of age and older numbered 32 million; this figure is expected to reach 53 million by the year 2020. Three million were 85 years and older in 1990, making up the fastest-growing age-group. The number of residents 85 years and older will double to 6 million by the year 2020. Those 85 years and older are most likely to need long-term care because about half are disabled or need help performing one or more ADLs (U.S. Bureau of the Census, 1997).

As more and more people need long-term care, the answers to two questions become increasingly urgent: How shall the nation finance long-term care? Should most long-term care be delivered through institutions or in people's homes and communities?

WHO PAYS FOR LONG-TERM CARE?

> Phoebe McKinnon was in good health until she fell, broke her hip, and suffered a postoperative joint infection. She was placed on complete bed rest, with oral antibiotics, for 3 months, after which time she would have another surgery. Widowed, Ms. McKinnon lived alone; her only daughter lived 1500 miles away. Because Ms. McKinnon required 24-hour-a-day help, the social worker, after carefully researching the financial options, reluctantly suggested that Ms. McKinnon spend the 3 months in a nursing home. Ms. McKinnon and her daughter agreed but were shocked when

Table 10–2. Long-term care financing, 1995.[1]

	Out-of-Pocket	Private Insurance	Medicare	Medicaid	Other
Nursing home care	37%	3%	9%	46%	5%
Home care	21%	12%	41%	14%	12%
Total long-term care[2]	33%	6%	18%	38%	5%

[1] Data extracted from Levit KR et al: National health expenditures, 1995. Health Care Fin Rev 1996;18(1):175.
[2] These figures do not include long-term care items such as adult day care, other community-based services, durable medical equipment, or unpaid care provided by family members at home.

> the social worker explained that the cost would be $120 a day, for a total bill of $11,000.

The United States spent $107 billion on long-term care in 1995, including $78 billion on nursing home care. A 1-year nursing home stay in 1995 cost $46,000 (Levit et al, 1996).

Direct out-of-pocket payments by patients and their families finance 33% of long-term care services in the United States. A frequent scenario is that of Eddie Taylor: After a portion of their life savings are spent for long-term care, families finally become eligible for Medicaid long-term care coverage. Medicaid pays for 38% of United States long-term care expenditures (Table 10–2).

Many people expect the Medicare program to pay for nursing home stays and, like Phoebe McKinnon and her daughter, are surprised and shocked when they find that Medicare will not assist them (Kane and Kane, 1987). Only 18% of long-term care costs are financed by Medicare.

Out-of-pocket expenses for health care paid by the elderly amounted to 21% of family income in 1995 (Physician Payment Review Commission, 1997). One-third of these expenses went to nursing homes. For poor, minority, and female elders, health costs are an even greater proportion of income. Single older women living alone may spend up to 42% of their income for health care, including long-term care (U.S. House Select Committee on Aging, 1990).

What are the precise roles of Medicare, Medicaid, and private insurance in the financing of long-term care services?

Medicare Long-Term Coverage

> Glenn Whitehorse, who was a diabetic, developed gangrene of his right leg, requiring an above-the-knee amputation. He was transferred from the acute care hospital to the hospital's skilled nursing facility, where he received physical therapy services. Because he was generally frail, he was unable to move from bed to chair without assistance. Mr. Whitehorse's physical and occupational therapists felt he might do better at home, where he could receive home physical therapy and nursing care. All these services were covered by Medicare.
>
> Mrs. Whitehorse had Parkinson's disease and was unable to assist her husband in bathing, getting out of bed, and going to the bathroom; she was forced to hire someone to assist

> with these custodial functions, which were not covered by
> Medicare. When Mr. Whitehorse no longer showed any po-
> tential for improvement, Medicare discontinued coverage of
> his home health services. The situation became too difficult,
> and he was placed in a nursing home for custodial care.
> Medicare did not cover the nursing home costs.

Which services provided in a nursing facility or at home are covered by Medicare?
The key distinction is between "skilled care," for which Medicare pays, and "custodial care," which is usually not covered. A related issue is that of postacute versus
chronic care: Medicare usually covers services needed for a few weeks or months after an acute hospitalization, but often does not pay for care required by a stable
chronic condition. Medicare health maintenance organizations (HMOs) tend to cover
the same long-term care services as traditional Medicare.

What are some examples of skilled care versus custodial services? Registered
nurses in a hospital nursing facility, nursing home, or home care agency provide a
wide variety of services, such as changing the dressing on a wound, taking blood pressures, listening to the heart and lungs to detect heart failure or pneumonia, reviewing
patient compliance with medications, and providing patient education about diabetes,
hypertension, heart failure, and other illnesses. Physical and occupational therapists
work with stroke, hip fracture, and other patients to help them reach their maximum
potential level of functioning. Speech therapists perform the difficult task of teaching
stroke patients with speech deficits how to communicate. These are all skilled services, usually covered by Medicare.

Custodial services involve assistance with ADLs and IADLs rather than treatment
or rehabilitative care related to a disease process; these are tasks such as cooking,
cleaning house, shopping, or helping a patient to the toilet. These services, usually
provided by nurses' aides, home health aides, homemakers, or family members, are
considered unskilled and are often not covered by Medicare. But, to cloud the skilled
versus custodial distinction, assistance by home health aides for 1–2 hours per day
may be covered by Medicare if the aide performs personal care (eg, bathing a patient)
as well as cleaning the house or cooking a meal, and if skilled services are also being
provided. In the past few years, Medicare has relaxed its home care coverage criteria
and is paying for more long-term custodial care (Welch et al, 1996).

Medicaid Long-Term Coverage

> Willie Robinson, who lived alone, suffered from deforming
> degenerative arthritis and was unable to do anything more
> active than sitting in a chair. Because Mr. Robinson had no
> skilled care medical needs, Medicare would not provide any
> assistance. Medicaid and the county welfare agency paid
> for a homemaker to provide 20 hours of help per week, but
> that was not sufficient. Mr. Robinson had no choice but to
> enter a nursing home, because that was the only way he
> could obtain 24-hour-a-day help paid for by Medicaid.

Medicaid differs from Medicare in paying the costs of nursing home care. Medicaid's coverage of home health care, however, is far more limited; Medicaid generally does not cover 24-hour-a-day custodial services for people unable to care for
themselves. The completeness of Medicaid's nursing home coverage, in contrast to

the limited nature of Medicaid-financed home health care, forces many low-income disabled people like Willie Robinson to go into nursing homes, unless they have families capable of providing 24-hour-a-day custodial care.

In order to qualify for Medicaid nursing home coverage, families may be forced to spend their savings down to low levels, although in some states Medicaid allows spouses of nursing home residents to keep some of their assets. As in the case of Eddie Taylor, states may place liens on the homes of Medicaid-covered nursing home residents, so that when the spouse dies or moves out of the home, the state can seek reimbursement for the Medicaid bill from the sale of the home.

Private Long-Term Care Insurance

> Sue and Lew MacPherson, both age 72, were worried about their future. They remembered their cousin, who was turned down for private long-term care insurance because of his high blood pressure and later spent his entire savings on nursing home bills. Hoping to protect their $32,000 in savings, they decided to apply for long-term care insurance before an illness would make them uninsurable. Their insurance agent calculated the cost of two policies at $6000 per year, or 30% of their $20,000 per year income. At that price, Sue and Lew would spend most of their savings on insurance premiums within a few years. They declined the insurance and became active in the Gray Panthers, fighting for government-supported long-term care coverage.

Private insurance plays a minor role in long-term care financing. Less than 4 million people have private long-term care insurance, and only 6% of long-term care costs are covered by private policies (Levit et al, 1996).

Experience rating (see Chapter 2) has had a profound effect on the dynamics of private long-term care insurance. The largest market for this type of insurance is the elderly population. Under experience-rated insurance, the elderly are charged high premiums because they are at considerable risk of requiring long-term care services. Moreover, the elderly have an average income only 62% that of the general population. Thus, people requiring or likely to require long-term care either cannot afford experience-rated private insurance premiums or must pay more than younger people, even though their income is likely to be less. Given these realities, the private financing of long-term care presents difficulties for both private insurers and for those needing insurance (Bodenheimer and Estes, 1994).

For private insurers, it is difficult to sell long-term care policies. For the elderly, premiums must be high enough to cover costs but low enough to attract clients (Liu et al, 1990). Some insurers reject 30% of applicants, those with medical conditions that make them unacceptable risks (Ball and Bethell, 1989). The severely disabled under age 65 are uninsurable due to their chronic disease. The major attractive market for long-term care insurers is the younger employed population, but only a tiny fraction of this group is interested in long-term care insurance because the prospects of needing such care are so remote. Thus, long-term care insurers are forced to market high-cost policies to high-risk elderly individuals—an improbable task (Van Gelder and Johnson, 1991; Aaron, 1991; Cohen and Kumar, 1997).

Some people purchasing long-term care insurance find it to be a poor investment. Many private policies specify that a policyholder must be dependent in three or more

ADLs before receiving benefits for home health services (Kolb et al, 1991). Less than 10% of the population under 85, and less than 30% over 85, have impairment in three or more ADLs, which is considered severe disability. Yet many people with fewer than three ADL impairments need long-term care services; for these people, their insurance may pay nothing (Liu et al, 1990; Jennings and Porter, 1991).

Long-term care policies usually have a large deductible (measured in nursing home days) for nursing home care, and most policies pay a fixed daily fee rather than reimbursing actual charges. A typical policy provides $85 per day after a $60-day deductible. The 1995 average daily nursing home charge is $127, meaning that $42 would be the patient's responsibility. Thus, a year's stay would require out-of-pocket expenditures of $20,430 (60 days × $127 = $7620 plus 305 days × $42 = $12,810) over and above payment of the insurance premium. In 1994, the average annual premium for $85 per day of nursing home benefits with a 60-day deductible was $1500 (Cohen and Kumar, 1997). The U.S. General Accounting Office (1990) has concluded that long-term care insurance is affordable for only 20% of persons age 65–79 years.

WHO PROVIDES LONG-TERM CARE?

Informal Care Givers

> Since her husband died, Mrs. Dora Whitney has lived alone. At age 71, she became forgetful and one day left the gas stove on, causing a fire in the kitchen. Two months later she was unable to find her way home after going to the store and was found by the police wandering in the streets. Her daughter, Kimberly, brought her to the university hospital, where she was diagnosed with Alzheimer's dementia. After a team conference with her mother's physicians, nurses, occupational therapist, and social worker, Kimberly admitted that her only option was to abandon her career as a teacher to care for her mother. Kimberly refused to place her mother in a nursing home, and funds were not available to hire the needed 24-hour-a-day help.

About 85% of people needing long-term care services receive them from their family and friends. Three-quarters of this unpaid care is provided by women. For men, their wives often provide long-term care, and for women, their daughters are frequently care givers. A growing number of the elderly do not have family living near enough to them to provide informal care; the absence of an informal care giver is a common reason for nursing home placement. For 8 out of 10 informal, unpaid care givers, the amount of help they provide averages 4 hours a day, 7 days a week. One-third of informal care givers are over 65, one-third are poor or nearly poor, and one-third are not in good health themselves. Many unpaid care givers leave their jobs or reduce their work hours, thereby experiencing financial losses in addition to the emotional costs of handling the demands of family members who are ill, demented, incontinent, or awake during many hours of the night. Frequently, informal care givers must juggle the needs of the disabled elderly with those of children or grandchildren (The Pepper Commission, 1990; Council on Scientific Affairs, 1990).

Community-Based & Home Health Services

> Ana Dominguez insisted that her daughter Juana accept the Yale scholarship. Though Ms. Dominguez, at age 49, was bed and wheelchair bound with multiple sclerosis, she would feel too guilty if Juana remained in San Antonio, Texas, just to care for her. Before Juana left, she arranged with the home care agency to have her mother transported to an adult day health center 3 days a week; for nursing, physical, and occupational therapy 3 times a week; and for meals-on-wheels. Medicare paid for these services. But Ms. Dominguez needed someone in the home 24 hours a day, a service not covered by Medicare. For $10 a day, Juana was able to hire Vilma, an undocumented teenager from El Salvador, to live in the home. Adding Vilma's pay and the cost of her food, Juana figured they would spend $30,000 of their $42,000 in savings by the time she graduated from Yale.
>
> AIDS had devastated Brian Reynolds. He had survived three episodes of *Pneumocystis* pneumonia, but was unable to take the new protease inhibitor medications. He had lost 60 pounds, suffered racking headaches and constant diarrhea, and was in and out of the hospital. Brian's lover had died 3 months earlier, and his support system was crumbling. Brian was a fighter. But after a severe depression brought on by pain, weakness, and loneliness, he decided he had had enough. Brian's physician agreed with his decision, discontinued his intravenous medications, and referred him to a hospice program to provide Medicaid-financed home comfort care. But the hospice required that an unpaid care giver had to be with him 24 hours a day, and Brian had no one. While a social worker was searching for a nursing home that would accept an AIDS patient, Brian died at home without the comfort of hospice care.

Community-based long-term care is delivered through a variety of programs, such as home care, adult day care, home-delivered meals, board and care homes, hospice care for the terminally ill, mental health programs, and others.

Home health services are rapidly growing entities in the health care system. While the number of hospital beds declined and nursing home beds increased by 2% annually, the home health industry has grown from $2 billion to $29 billion between 1980 and 1995. In 1992, there were 8200 licensed home health care agencies, an enormous increase from 3000 in 1981. A growing number of these agencies are owned by for-profit corporate chains (Harrington, 1994).

During the 1970s, the independent living movement among disabled people created a strong push away from institutional (hospital and nursing home) care toward community-based and home care that fostered the greatest possible independence. During the 1980s, AIDS activists furthered the development of hospice programs that provide intensive home care services for people with terminal cancer and AIDS. The home is usually a far more therapeutic, comforting environment than the hospital or nursing home. One study of hospital versus home care for stroke patients showed that the home program resulted in a quicker return of function and a reduction in mortality rates. Other illnesses demonstrate similar outcomes (Batavia, 1993; Council on Scientific Affairs, 1990).

While home care is usually a preferable alternative to prolonged hospital care, a balance must be struck between the advantages and risks of keeping elderly patients with complicated medical conditions in the hospital versus the benefits and harms of sending them home. The diagnosis-related group (DRG) system of reimbursing hospitals (see Chapter 4), under which hospitals earn a greater net income by reducing the length of the hospital stay, has led to patients being discharged "quicker and sicker," thereby placing far more demands on home care agencies.

Many categories of health care givers function in teams to perform home care, including nurses, physical, occupational, speech, and respiratory therapists, social workers, home health aides, case managers, and drivers delivering meals-on-wheels. Yet, home care, designed to help fill the "low-tech" niche in the health care system that assists the disabled with ADLs and IADLs, has become increasingly specialized. Home care agencies now offer intravenous antibiotic infusions, morphine pumps, indwelling central venous lines, and home renal dialysis, administered by highly skilled intravenous and wound care nurses, respiratory therapists, and other health professionals. These developments are a major advance in shifting medical care from hospital to home, but they have not been matched by growth in paid personal custodial care needed to allow disabled people to remain safely in their homes. Similarly, hospice care, while providing excellent nursing services for patients with terminal illnesses, is limited in the ADL support it provides. Home care agencies will not accept terminal patients into hospice programs without an informal care giver in the home; thus, the people who may need home hospice services the most—those, like Brian Reynolds, who are alone—cannot receive them.

Because of the limitations of home care, many disabled individuals are released from hospitals in need of long-term care services to assist in their day-to-day functioning, unable to pay privately for such "custodial" care, yet unable to meet the eligibility requirements of community-based long-term care providers. These people have been described as living in the "no-care zone" (Estes et al, 1993).

Nursing Homes

> Each morning, more than one and a quarter million Americans awaken in nursing homes. Most of them are very old and very feeble. Most will stay in the nursing home for a long time. For most, it will be the last place they ever live . . . [Nursing home] residents live out the last of their days in an enclosed society without privacy, dignity, or pleasure, subsisting on minimally palatable diets, multiple sedatives, and large doses of television—eventually dying, one suspects at least partially of boredom. (Vladeck BC: Unloving Care: The Nursing Home Tragedy. Basic Books, 1980.)

Often, informal help and formal home health services are unable to provide the care required for severely disabled people. Such people may be placed in nursing homes with 24-hour-a-day care provided by health aides and orderlies under the supervision of nurses. Seventy-five percent of nursing home residents are women, who more often outlive their spouses. Frequently, after caring for a sick husband at home, women will themselves fall ill and be placed in a nursing home because no one is left to care for them at home. Men over 65 have a 30% chance of entering a nursing home at some time in their lives, while for women the chance is 52% (U.S. House Select Committee on Aging, 1990).

Less than half of nursing home residents can walk unassisted, more than 30% are incontinent, more than 60% need assistance with bathing and dressing, and half are demented. There are two main differences between the chronically ill inside and outside nursing homes: nursing home residents have no family able to care for them, and a larger proportion of nursing home patients suffer from dementia, a condition whose care is extremely difficult to provide at home by family members (Vladeck, 1980).

Nursing homes vary widely in quality. A United States Senate report (1986) found that as many as one-third of nursing homes provide substandard quality care, and a 1993 report revealed continuing and frequent severe deficiencies (Harrington, 1996). For the affluent with long-term care insurance or the ability to pay their own way, lodgings can be quite pleasant, with reasonably good food, plenty of assistance, and daily group activities. But lower-income people, whose nursing home bill is invariably paid by Medicaid at a low rate of reimbursement, are housed in close quarters with several other patients and become totally dependent on an underpaid, inadequately trained staff. Hour after hour may be spent lying in bed or sitting in a chair in front of a TV. While quality of life varies between one nursing home and another, placement in a nursing home almost always thwarts the human yearning for some degree of independence of action and for companionship. A sense of futility overwhelms many nursing home residents, and the desire to live often wanes.

As summarized in the Institute of Medicine's (1986) report on nursing homes,

> Residents are often treated with disrespect; they are frequently denied any choices of food, of roommates, of the time they rise and go to sleep, of their activities, or the clothes they wear, and of when and where they may visit with family and friends. (Reprinted, with permission, from Improving the Quality of Care in Nursing Homes. Copyright 1986 by the National Academy of Sciences. Courtesy of the National Academy Press, Washington, D.C.)

To keep down costs, most care in nursing homes is provided by nurse's aides, who are paid very little, receive minimal training, are inadequately supervised, and are required to care for more residents than they can properly serve. The job of the nursing home aide is very difficult, involving bathing, feeding, walking residents, cleaning them when they are incontinent, lifting them, and hearing their complaints. Staffing levels for nursing personnel are extremely low and have not improved significantly since 1985 (Harrington, 1996). The turnover rate for nurse's aides is very high, perhaps 75% per year, and pay is very low, starting at $13,000 per year in 1997. Quality of life is intimately related to the quality of staff-resident interactions and to the issue of privacy. Most rooms are not single occupancy, and this makes the quality of life highly dependent on roommates, who may have behavior problems, talking or screaming for hours, day or night.

Seventy-one percent of all nursing homes are under for-profit ownership, many operated by large corporate chains. For-profit ownership has been associated with lower staffing levels and poorer quality of care compared with nonprofit ownership (Harrington, 1996).

Nursing homes are regulated by federal law. Those not in compliance could be denied Medicaid or Medicare funding, which would be a major blow to many nursing homes. States also have a regulatory function over nursing homes. However, regulations are never an adequate tool to ensure respectful, dignified, friendly staff–resident and resident–resident interactions, which are so key to the nursing home quality of life.

To offer a humane existence to a group of severely disabled people housed together in close quarters is a nearly impossible task. One view of nursing home reform holds that only the abolition of most nursing homes and the development of adequately financed home and community-based care can solve the nursing home problem.

IMPROVING LONG-TERM CARE

Financing Long-Term Care

> Boomer was mad. As a self-employed person, his family's HMO coverage was costing $400 each month, in addition to his out-of-pocket dental bills. To make matters worse, a big chunk of his social security payments went to Medicare each year, not to mention federal and state income taxes and sales taxes going to finance Medicare and Medicaid, so that other people could get health care. While spending all this money, Boomer was healthy and had not seen a doctor for 6 years.
>
> One day Boomer's father, Abraham, suffered a devastating stroke. After weeks in the hospital, largely paid for by Medicare, Abraham was transferred to a nursing home. Because Medicare does not cover most long-term care, Boomer's mother paid the bills out of her savings, until most of the money ran out. Abraham then became eligible for Medicaid, which took care of the nursing home bills. After Abraham's illness, Boomer stopped complaining about his social security and tax payments going to medical care. Even though Boomer was paying more than he was receiving, Abraham was receiving far more than he was paying. Boomer was grateful for the care his father received and figured that he might be in Abraham's shoes some day.

In the early 1960s, it was recognized that private insurance was unable to solve the problem of health care financing for people over 65. The costs of health care for the elderly were too great, making experience-rated health insurance premiums unaffordable for most elderly people. Accordingly, Medicare, a social insurance program, was passed (see Chapter 2). An identical problem confronts long-term care financing: As shown earlier in this chapter, most people who might wish to purchase long-term care insurance are unable to afford an adequate policy. Table 10–3 lists some proposals for improving long-term care.

The most influential recent analysis of long-term care financing came from the Pepper Commission (1990), a body created by the United States Congress and composed chiefly of members of Congress from both political parties. The 1990 Pepper Commission report recommended that the nation follow the example of Medicare and institute a social insurance program to finance long-term care. This program, like Medicare Part A, could be financed by an increase in the rate of social security contributions by employers and employees. It would pay for care givers to provide those

Table 10–3. Proposals for improving long-term care.

Developing social insurance to finance long-term care
Shifting from nursing home care to community-based care by improved financing of community-based care
Training and supporting family members as care givers
Expanding the number of comprehensive acute and long-term care organizations modeled on
On Lok Senior Health Services, which reduce costs by keeping the elderly out of the hospital as much as possible

services not currently covered by Medicare, especially in-home help in feeding, dressing, getting in and out of bed, bathing, toileting, laundry, housework, grocery shopping, transportation, and other assistance with ADLs and IADLs.

What is social insurance? Insurance can be divided into private insurance, which is voluntary, and social insurance, which is compulsory. The insuring institution is a private company in the case of private insurance and usually a public agency in the case of social insurance (Bodenheimer and Grumbach, 1992). Because its coverage is compulsory, social insurance spreads the financial risk of illness among the entire population and does not concentrate the risk within the elderly population. Rather than a small number of people paying large amounts, a large number of people pay relatively small amounts to finance the program. Social insurance contributions differ from general taxation and resemble private insurance premiums in the sense that they are earmarked for a particular use. Social insurance represents a transfer of income from younger employed people to older people or to people who become prematurely disabled, which places it in the long-term self-interest of contributors, many of whom will require its benefits as they grow older.

Providing Long-Term Care

> Mei Soon Wang was desperate to go home. Since a brain tumor had paralyzed her left side and left her incontinent, she had been confined to a nursing home because she had no family in San Francisco to care for her. Her daughter, visiting from Portland, heard of the On Lok program in Chinatown, which cared for the disabled elderly in their homes. On Lok accepted Ms. Wang, placed her in adult day care, arranged for meals to be delivered to her home, and paid for part-time help on evenings and weekends.

Because a reasonable quality of life and personal independence, within the confines of a patient's illness, are so difficult to achieve in the nursing home environment, long-term care reformers often advocate that most long-term care be provided in the home. The first step toward deinstitutionalizing long-term care is a financing mechanism that pays for more comprehensive community-based and home long-term care services. The Pepper Commission (1990), accordingly, encouraged the provision of long-term care in home and community settings by restricting its coverage of nursing home care.

The ideal long-term care givers are the patient's family and friends; thus, it can be argued that long-term care reform should support, assist, and pay informal care givers, not replace them. Teams of nurses, physical and occupational therapists, physicians (who often know the least about long-term care), social workers, and attendants can train and work with informal care givers, and personnel can be available to provide respite care so informal care givers can have some relief from the 24-hour-a-day, 7-day-a-week burden. If informal care givers are not available, all possible efforts can still be made to deliver long-term care in people's homes rather than in nursing homes (Harrington et al, 1991).

A number of innovative long-term care programs have sprung up around the United States, including social health maintenance organizations (which extend the HMO concept of comprehensive, prepaid financing for acute care to include a variety of long-term care services), continuing care retirement communities, congregate living, and assisted living centers (Rivlin and Wiener, 1988; Miller, 1991; Harrington et al, 1993). A program that has achieved great success over a number of years is the On Lok Senior Health Services program in San Francisco.

Translated from Chinese, *On Lok* means peaceful, happy abode. Begun in 1971 in San Francisco's Chinatown, On Lok merges adult day services, in-home care, home-delivered meals, housing assistance, comprehensive medical care, respite care for care givers, hospital care, and skilled nursing care into one program. The average age of On Lok participants is 81, three-fourths are Chinese, 64% live alone, and 30% live with a spouse or relative. Over 70% are incontinent, and the average participant has 5.4 serious medical diagnoses (Miller, 1991). Persons eligible for On Lok have chronic illness sufficiently severe to qualify them for nursing home placement, but only 15% ever spend time in a nursing home. Some participants live in On Lok House, a 54-unit facility with a central dining area and day health center; most live at home, but may occasionally stay for 2 weeks at On Lok House to give their families and care givers a rest. Services for each participant are organized by a multidisciplinary team, including physicians, nurses, social workers, rehabilitation and recreation therapists, and nutritionists. The team uses case management to tailor care to each participant and to control costs.

In 1983, On Lok became the first organization in the United States to assume full financial risk for the care of a frail elderly population, receiving monthly capitation payments from Medicare and Medicaid to cover all services. Individuals not fully eligible for Medicaid contribute on a sliding scale. All payments are integrated into a single fund, so that the program is not subject to Medicare or Medicaid payment restrictions. The comprehensiveness of On Lok's community-based program reduces hospital and nursing home use; since 1980, the number of days the average On Lok patient spent in the hospital decreased from 9.9 to 3.3 per year. During the 1980s, On Lok's costs were 8–19% lower than costs of traditional care, while its patients appeared to enjoy a better quality of life than similar patients not in the program (Miller, 1991). By providing coordinated acute and long-term care to the frail elderly in their own community, the On Lok program has become a model that is being replicated in other settings around the United States.

REFERENCES

Aaron HJ: Serious and Unstable Condition: Financing America's Health Care. The Brookings Institution, 1991.
Ball RM, Bethell TN: Because We're All in This Together. Families USA Foundation, 1989.
Batavia AI: Health care reform and people with disabilities. Health Aff 1993;12(1):40.

Bodenheimer T, Estes CL: Long-term care: Requiem for commercial private insurance. In: The Nation's Health. Lee PR, Estes CL (editors). Bartlett & Jones, 1994.

Bodenheimer T, Grumbach K: Financing universal health insurance: Taxes, premiums, and the lessons of social insurance. J Health Polit Policy Law 1992;17:439.

Cohen MA, Kumar AKN: The changing face of long-term care insurance in 1994. Inquiry 1997;34:50.

Council on Scientific Affairs: Home care in the 1990s. JAMA 1990;263:1241.

Estes CL et al: The Long-term Care Crisis: Elders Trapped in the No-Care Zone. Sage Publications, 1993.

Harrington C: The nursing home industry: Public policy in the 1990s. In: Perspectives in Medical Sociology. Brown P (editor). Waveland Press, 1996.

Harrington C: Quality, access, and costs: Public policy and home health care. In: Health Policy and Nursing. Harrington C, Estes CL (editors). Jones & Bartlett, 1994.

Harrington C, Lynch M, Newcomer RJ: Medical services in social health maintenance organizations. Gerontologist 1993;33:790.

Harrington C et al: A national long-term care program for the United States: A caring vision. JAMA 1991;266:3023.

Institute of Medicine: Improving the Quality of Care in Nursing Homes. National Academy Press, 1986.

Jennings MC, Porter M: The changing elderly market. Topics Health Care Fin 1991;17(4):1.

Kane RA, Kane RL: Long-Term Care: Principles, Programs, and Policies. Springer, 1987.

Kolb DS, Veysey PJ, Gocke JL: Private long-term care insurance: Will it work? Topics Health Care Fin 1991;17(4):9.

Levit KR et al: National health expenditures, 1995. Health Care Fin Rev 1996;18(1):175.

Liu K, Manton KG, Liu BM: Morbidity, disability, and long-term care of the elderly: Implications for insurance financing. Milbank Mem Fund Q 1990:68(3):445.

Miller JA: Community-Based Long-Term Care. Sage Publications, 1991.

The Pepper Commission: A Call for Action. U.S. Government Printing Office, 1990.

Physician Payment Review Commission: Annual Report to Congress. 1997.

Rivlin AM, Wiener JM: Caring for the Disabled Elderly. The Brookings Institution, 1988.

U.S. Bureau of the Census: www.census.gov. June 1997.

U.S. General Accounting Office: Long-Term Care Insurance: Proposals to Link Private Insurance and Medicaid Need Close Scrutiny. Sept 1990.

U.S. House Select Committee on Aging: Emptying the Elderly's Pocketbook: Growing Impact of Rising Health Care Costs: A Report by the Chairman. U.S. Government Printing Office, March 1990.

U.S. Senate: Special Committee on Aging. Nursing Home Care: The Unfinished Agenda. U.S. Government Printing Office, 1986.

Van Gelder S, Johnson D: Long-Term Care Insurance: A Market Update. Health Insurance Association of America, Jan 1991.

Vladeck BC: Unloving Care: The Nursing Home Tragedy. Basic Books, 1980.

Welch HG et al: The use of Medicare home health care services. N Engl J Med 1996;335:324.

The Prevention of Illness

11

WHAT IS PREVENTION?

> In 1995, the United States spent $1 trillion on health care.
> Three percent of this total was dedicated to government
> public health activities designed to prevent illness.

The renowned medical historian, Henry Sigerist, writing in 1941, listed the main items that must be included in a national health program. The first three items were free education, including health education, for all; the best possible working and living conditions; and the best possible means of rest and recreation. Medical care rated only fourth on his list (Terris, 1992a). For Sigerist (1941), medical care was

> A system of health institutions and medical personnel, available to all, responsible for the people's health, ready and able to advise and help them in the maintenance of health and in its restoration *when prevention has broken down.* (Sigerist HE: Medicine and Human Welfare. Yale Univ Press, 1941.)

Many people working in the fields of medical care and public health believe that "prevention has broken down" too often; sometimes because modern science has insufficient knowledge to prevent disease, but more often because society has dedicated insufficient resources and commitment to prevent disease.

Prevention is often described as having three components.

(1) Primary prevention seeks to avert the occurrence of a disease or injury (eg, immunization against polio; tax on the sale of cigarettes to reduce their affordability and, thereby, their use).

(2) Secondary prevention refers to early detection of a disease process and intervention to reverse or retard the condition from progressing (eg, Pap smears to screen for premalignant and malignant lesions of the cervix; mammograms for early detection of breast cancer).

(3) Tertiary prevention is a term used to describe efforts to minimize the effects of disease and disability (eg, the use of physical therapy to prevent deformities associated with rheumatoid arthritis) (Last, 1986).

In truth, secondary and tertiary prevention are not prevention, but are medical care services designed to reduce morbidity and mortality rates once a disease has already occurred. We will use the term "secondary prevention" in this chapter because it does prevent disease progression, although not disease itself. We will not use the term "tertiary prevention" because it is only remotely related to true prevention.

Table 11–1. Strategies of prevention.

Strategy	Examples
1. Improvement in the standard of living	Job creation Increase in minimum wage
2. Public health interventions to reduce the incidence of illness in the population	Water purification systems in underdeveloped nations Increased tobacco taxes to reduce the purchase of cigarettes Mass education on the dangers of high-fat diets
3. Preventive medical care, performed by health care providers	Screening and treatment of hypertension Periodic breast examinations and mammograms Prenatal care

The promotion of good health and the prevention of illness encompass three distinct levels or strategies (Terris, 1986):

(1) The first and broadest level includes societal measures to improve the overall standard of living; as evidence presented in Chapter 3 shows, lower income is associated with higher morbidity and mortality rates. Improvement in the standard of living (eg, through job creation programs to reduce or eliminate unemployment) may have a greater impact on preventing disease than specific public health programs or medical care services.

(2) The second level of prevention involves public health interventions to reduce the incidence of illness in the population as a whole. Examples are water purification systems, the banning of cigarette smoking in the workplace, and public health education on HIV prevention in the schools. These strategies generally consist of primary prevention. The 3% figure cited in the opening paragraph represents these public health activities (Levit et al, 1996).

(3) The third level of prevention involves individual health care providers performing preventive interventions for individual patients; these activities can be either primary or secondary prevention. The Canadian Task Force on the Periodic Health Examination, the United States Preventive Services Task Force, and other organizations such as the American College of Physicians have established regular schedules for preventive medical care services (U.S. Preventive Services Task Force, 1996; Woolf et al, 1996). (Table 11–1).

THE FIRST EPIDEMIOLOGIC REVOLUTION

Until modern times, the conditions that produced the greatest amount of illness and death in the population were infectious diseases. The initial decline of infectious disease mortality rates took place even before the cause of these illnesses was understood. In the eighteenth and nineteenth centuries, food production increased markedly throughout the Western world. By the early nineteenth century, infectious disease mortality rates were dropping in England, Wales, and Scandinavia, probably due to improved nutrition that allowed individuals, particularly children, to resist infectious agents. Thus, the initial success of illness prevention took place through the improvement of overall living conditions rather than from specific public health or medical interventions (McKeown, 1990).

In the nineteenth century, scientists and public health practitioners discovered many of the agents causing infectious diseases. Comprehending the causes (such as bacteria and viruses) and the risk factors (eg, poverty, overcrowding, poor nutrition, and contaminated water and food supplies) associated with these illnesses, public health measures (such as water purification, sewage disposal, and pasteurization of milk) were implemented that drastically reduced their incidence. Dr. Milton Terris (1985) has called these successes the first epidemiologic revolution.

From 1870 to 1930, the death rate from infectious diseases fell rapidly. Medical interventions, whether immunizations or treatment with antibiotics, were introduced only after much of the decline in infectious disease mortality rates had taken place. The first effective treatment against tuberculosis, the antibiotic streptomycin, was developed in 1947; but its contribution to the decrease in the tuberculosis death rate since the early nineteenth century has been estimated to be a mere 3%. For whooping cough, measles, scarlet fever, bronchitis, and pneumonia, mortality rates had fallen to similarly low levels before immunization or antibiotic therapy became available. Pasteurization and water purification were probably the main reason for the decline in deaths resulting from gastroenteritis and the overall reduction in infant mortality rates (McKeown, 1990).

Some illnesses are exceptions to the rule that infectious disease mortality rates are influenced more by improved living standards and public health measures than by medical interventions. Immunization for smallpox and tetanus and antimicrobial therapy for syphilis had a substantial impact on mortality rates from those illnesses. Polio vaccination had a major effect on that disease. Considering infectious diseases as a group, however, medical measures probably account for less than 5% of the decrease in mortality rates for these conditions over the past century (McKeown, 1990; McKinlay et al, 1989).

As infectious diseases waned in importance during the first half of the twentieth century and as life expectancy increased, rates of noninfectious chronic illness grew rapidly. Eleven major infectious diseases accounted for 40% of the total deaths in the United States in 1900 but less than 10% in 1980. In contrast, heart disease, cancer, and stroke (cerebrovascular disease) caused 16% of the total deaths in 1900 but 64% in 1980 (McKinlay et al, 1989).

THE SECOND EPIDEMIOLOGIC REVOLUTION

Fifty years ago, epidemiologists did not understand the causes of the major noninfectious chronic diseases. According to Dr. Terris,

> Unable to prevent the occurrence of these diseases, we retreated to a second line of defense, namely, early detection and treatment—so-called secondary prevention. But secondary prevention has—with few exceptions—proved disappointing; it cannot compare in effectiveness with measures for primary prevention. The periodic physical examination, the cancer detection center, multiphasic screening, and a host of variations on these themes, have incurred enormous expenditures for relatively modest benefits . . .

Major exceptions are cancer of the cervix, for which early detection has proved dramatically effective, and, to a lesser extent, cancer of the breast.

Beginning in 1950, dramatic breakthroughs occurred in the epidemiology of the noninfectious diseases. During the next three decades, our epidemiologists forged powerful weapons to combat most of the major causes of death. In doing so, they initiated a second epidemiologic revolution which, if we act appropriately, will result in an enormous reduction in premature death and disability. (Terris M: Healthy lifestyles: The perspective of epidemiology. J Public Health Policy 1992b;13:186.)

During the second epidemiologic revolution, it was learned that the major illnesses in the United States have a few central causes and are in large part preventable. In 1993, 2.3 million people died (see Table 11–2). A surprisingly small number of risk factors are implicated in a large number—35%—of these deaths. It has been estimated that use of tobacco causes 400,000, a high-fat diet and inactivity contributes to 300,000, and alcohol is responsible for 100,000 deaths (McGinnis and Foege, 1993). By discovering and educating the population about the risk factors of smoking, rich diet, and lack of exercise, the second epidemiologic revolution has already had success among the well-educated portion of the population. From 1950 to 1987, age-adjusted mortality rates for coronary heart disease (CHD) declined by an astonishing 45%. This decline was associated with reduced rates of tobacco use and lowered mean serum cholesterol levels in the population. As with infectious diseases a century earlier, this decline has more to do with public health interventions regarding smoking and diet than with such medical advances as coronary care units and coronary bypass surgery (Goldman and Cook, 1984; Stamler, 1985). The unfortunate side of this success story is that those with the least education have experienced only a small reduction in CHD mortality (Terris, 1996).

Table 11–2. Causes of death in the United States, 1993.[1]

Total deaths	2,269,000
Top 10 causes	
Heart disease	743,000
Cancer	530,000
Cerebrovascular disease	150,000
Chronic obstructive pulmonary disease	101,000
Unintentional injuries	91,000
Pneumonia and influenza	83,000
Diabetes	54,000
HIV infection	37,000
Suicide	31,000
Homicide	26,000
Top 3 contributors to mortality	
Tobacco	400,000
Diet and inactivity	300,000
Alcohol	100,000

[1] Data extracted from U.S. Department of Health and Human Services. Health United States, 1995. 1996.

INDIVIDUAL OR POPULATION?

Chronic disease prevention may be viewed from two distinct perspectives, that of the individual and that of the population (Rose, 1985). The medical model seeks to identify high-risk individuals and offer them individual protection, often by counseling on such topics as smoking cessation and low-fat diet. The public health approach seeks to reduce disease in the population as a whole, using such methods as mass education campaigns to counter drinking and driving, the taxation of tobacco to drive up its price, and the labeling of foods to indicate fat and cholesterol content. Both approaches have merit (Breslow, 1990), but the medical model suffers from some drawbacks.

The individual-centered approach of the medical model may produce tunnel vision regarding the causation, and thus the prevention, of disease. Let us take the example of cholesterol.

Ancel Keys (1970) performed a famous study comparing CHD in different nations. In east Finland, CHD was common, 20% of diet calories came from saturated fat, and 56% of men age 40–59 years had cholesterol levels over 250 mg/dL. In Japan, coronary heart disease was rare, 3% of calories were provided by saturated fat, and only 7% of men age 40–59 years had cholesterol levels above 250 mg/dL. If we compared two individuals in east Finland who eat the same diet, one with a cholesterol level of 200 mg/dL and the other with a level of 300 mg/dL, we might conclude that the variation in cholesterol levels among individuals is caused by genetic or other factors, but not diet. If, on the other hand, we remove our individual blinders and look at entire populations, studying the average cholesterol level and the percentage of fat in the diet in east Finland and in Japan, we will conclude that high-fat diets correlate with high levels of cholesterol and with high rates of CHD.

Individual variations within each country are often of less importance than variations within an entire population between one nation and another. The clues to the causes of diseases "must be sought from differences between populations or from changes within populations over time" (Rose, 1985).

The medical model may also target its interventions to the wrong individuals. Let us continue with the cholesterol example. In the United States, most people with high cholesterol levels remain healthy for years, and some people with low levels have heart attacks at an early age. Why is this so? Because the risk of CHD for persons with high cholesterol or low cholesterol levels is not so different; even for the low-risk individual, CHD is the most likely cause of death. Everyone in the United States is at risk for this mass disease. A "low" cholesterol level of 180 mg/dL is low by United States standards but high in terms of heart disease risk. A large number of people at small risk for a disease may give rise to more cases of the disease than the smaller number of people who are at high risk (Brown et al, 1992). This fact limits the utility of the medical model's "high-risk" approach to prevention. A public health approach (eg, mass educational campaigns on the health effects of rich diets and the labeling of foods) strives to reduce the mean population cholesterol level. A 10% reduction in the serum cholesterol distribution of the entire population would do far more to reduce the incidence of heart disease than a 30% reduction in the cholesterol levels of those relatively few individuals with counts greater than 300 mg/dL.

A coherent ideology underlies the medical model of chronic disease prevention—the concept that in the arena of noninfectious chronic disease, individuals play a major role in causing their own illnesses by such behaviors as smoking, drinking alcohol, and eating high-fat foods. The corollary to this view is that chronic disease mortality rates can be reduced by persuading individuals to change their lifestyles. These statements are true, but they do not tell the whole story.

An alternative ideology, which fits more closely with the public health approach to chronic disease prevention, argues that modern industrial society, rather than the individuals living in that society, creates the conditions leading to heart disease, cancer, stroke, and other major chronic diseases of the developed world. Large-scale tobacco growing and advertising, processed high-fat, high-salt foods, easy availability of alcoholic beverages, societal stress, an urbanized and suburbanized existence that substitutes automobile travel for exercise, and a markedly unequal distribution of income and wealth are the substrates upon which the modern epidemic of chronic disease has flourished. Such a world view leads to an emphasis on societal rather than individual strategies for chronic disease prevention (Fee and Krieger, 1993).

Both the medical and the public health models (seeing responsibility as both individual and societal) must be joined to further implement the second epidemiologic revolution; medical care givers must attempt to change high-risk lifestyles of their individual patients, and society must search for ways to reduce the consumption of tobacco, alcohol, and rich foods.

One shortcoming of the United States health care system has been the lack of emphasis placed not only on public health prevention but also on preventive medical care services, with inadequate insurance coverage of such services and low reimbursement of providers performing preventive medical care. In addition, clinical training has not always emphasized preventive care. When seeing a patient, medical care providers are taught to ask themselves, "What is the diagnosis and what is the treatment?" Such an approach is insufficient. An additional question must be asked: "Why did this patient get this disease at this time?" (Rose, 1985). This query leads to the critical issue in the preventive clinician's mind: "What are the diseases to which this patient is susceptible and how can these diseases be prevented?" Current medical education and the prevention activities of some health maintenance organizations (HMOs) are beginning to address these problems.

MODELS OF PREVENTION

To provide examples of different approaches to preventing illness, we have chosen to discuss four serious health problems in the United States: coronary heart disease, breast cancer, interpersonal violence, and acquired immune deficiency syndrome (AIDS).

Coronary Heart Disease   CHD is associated with four major risk factors: the eating of a rich diet (the principal cause of the CHD epidemic); elevated levels of serum cholesterol; cigarette smoking; and hypertension (J. Stamler, 1992).

Primary prevention strategies are available for CHD because the causes of the disease are well understood. Primary CHD prevention involves risk factor reduction, including cessation of cigarette smoking, replacement of rich diets by low-fat diets, and

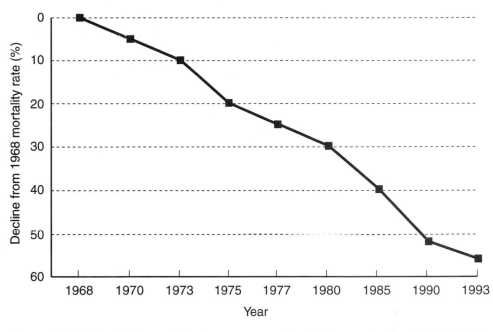

Figure 11–1. Trends in mortality from coronary heart disease in the United States, 1968–1993.

control of hypertension. These strategies have been largely responsible for the large decrease in CHD death rates (Figure 11–1).

Cigarette Smoking: Tobacco has been called the smallpox virus of chronic disease—a harmful agent whose elimination from the planet would benefit humankind (Fee and Krieger, 1993). Since the 1964 release of the first Surgeon General's Report on the Health Consequences of Smoking, the smoking behavior of the United States population has changed dramatically. Between 1965 and 1993, the age-adjusted percentage of men who were current smokers dropped from 52 to 28%; for women, the decline was from 34 to 23% (Figure 11–2). These reductions in smoking prevalence will have avoided an estimated 3 million deaths between 1964 and the year 2000—a major public health achievement (U.S. Department of Health and Human Services, 1996; Warner, 1989a).

Over 50 million people continue to smoke in the United States, however, and tobacco usage is still the leading cause of death. Antismoking campaigns have been relatively successful for well-educated middle class people, but have largely failed to reach people with less education, who also tend to be poorer. Between 1974 and 1987, cigarette smoking declined only 7% among the least educated persons, while it dropped 39% among the most educated. In 1987, 41% of the least educated persons smoked cigarettes, compared with only 17% of the most educated (Terris, 1992b; Pierce et al, 1989). Moreover, while smoking prevalence in adults has declined, it has increased slightly for adolescents. Of regular smokers, 80–90% start by age 18 years (Matzen and Lang, 1993; Kessler, 1995).

Since the 1969 ban on radio and television cigarette advertising, the tobacco industry has increased its advertising expenditures dramatically. In 1988, cigarettes were

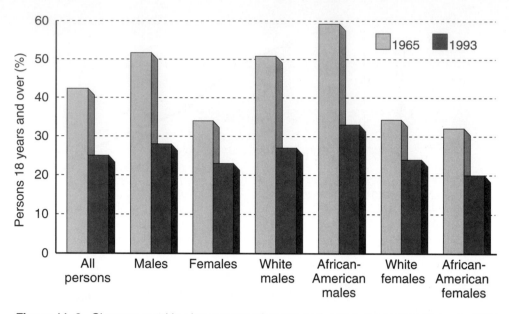

Figure 11–2. Cigarette smoking by persons 18 years and over in the United States in 1965 (shaded bars) and 1993 (black bars). Percentages are age adjusted. (Data extracted from U.S. Department of Health and Human Services: Health United States 1995. 1996.)

the most advertised product on billboards and the second most advertised in print media. The $6 billion spent on cigarette advertising in 1993 is 100% tax deductible. The principal target group for cigarette advertising is young people, with promotion also heavily focused upon minority populations (Broder, 1992; Warner et al, 1992; Bartecchi et al, 1994; Gilpin, 1997).

The antismoking campaign of the past 30 years has merged the medical and public health models of prevention. At least 70% of smokers visit a physician each year; controlled trials suggest that physician counseling can influence smokers to quit. Physician counseling is a relatively inexpensive intervention that adds years of life to those who stop smoking. The cost of brief advice given to smokers during routine office visits ranges from $705 to $988 per year of life saved for men and from $1204 to $2058 for women. However, 56% of smokers visiting a physician during the previous year reported never having been advised by their physician to stop smoking (Cummings et al, 1989). Thus, one of the most cost-effective preventive measures available to clinicians is underused.

Three public health interventions designed to reduce smoking have been effective: public education, cigarette taxes, and restriction of smoking in public places. Cigarette taxes have been particularly successful. A 10% increase in the price of cigarettes produces a reduction of 4% in the quantity of cigarettes smoked. For teenagers, the 10% price increase reduces consumption by 14% (Warner, 1984). It is estimated that the 8% increase in the cigarette tax legislated in 1982 caused 2 million adults to stop smoking and prevented 600,000 teenagers from starting. Yet, the United States still has the lowest tax (as a percentage of retail price) on cigarettes in the developed world (McKinlay et al, 1989; MacKenzie et al, 1994). Studies have also shown that prohibition of smoking in public areas and work places is correlated with a drop in cigarette consumption (Warner, 1989b).

Rich Diet: A rich diet is a diet high in fat, saturated fat, cholesterol, salt, and often alcohol, and with an elevated calorie level in relation to the amount of energy expended (J. Stamler, 1992). The rich diet produces CHD primarily by causing an increase in serum cholesterol, particularly its low-density-lipoprotein fraction. Lowering elevated serum cholesterol levels has been shown to reduce the risk of heart attacks caused by CHD.

In the late 1980s, a major national campaign was launched by the National Institutes of Health (NIH) to reduce serum cholesterol levels. The campaign is based on the medical model, with health care providers screening individuals for elevated cholesterol and treating hyperlipidemic patients with diet or cholesterol-lowering medications, or both (National Cholesterol Education Program, 1988).

Many public health analysts have criticized the NIH strategy as relying too heavily on a medical model of prevention that is expensive and of potentially limited effectiveness. The NIH approach attempts to lower cholesterol levels by 10–15% among individuals identified as having cholesterol levels in the top 20–25% of the population. However, it is difficult to achieve this level of cholesterol reduction simply by altering dietary consumption of fatty foods. Most studies of dietary interventions have found that they reduce cholesterol levels by only about 5%. Dr. Dean Ornish's program of massive lifestyle alteration—with very low fat, vegetarian diets, exercise, and stress reduction—is capable of lowering serum cholesterol levels by 24% and of reversing coronary artery pathologic changes (Ornish et al, 1990). For millions of people to adhere to such a program over decades of life span would require radical changes in people's lifestyle and in the fat content of foods available for purchase. Many people identified as having high cholesterol would therefore "fail" dietary interventions and qualify under the NIH primary prevention guidelines for drug treatment to reduce their cholesterol level.

Evidence about the effectiveness of drug treatment in primary prevention has been mixed, however. Some studies of the drugs initially developed to lower cholesterol levels demonstrated that drug treatment could reduce the incidence of nonfatal myocardial infarction and CHD deaths. However, these benefits were offset by many unpleasant drug side effects and by an unexpected increase in deaths from causes other than CHD (Grumbach, 1991). Only recently has a study shown that drug treatment for primary prevention using one of the newer cholesterol-lowering agents can actually reduce total mortality and not just nonfatal coronary events (Sheperd et al, 1995). However, the effectiveness of this drug for primary prevention of CHD is relatively modest. Over 40 patients would have to take the medication for 5 years to avert 1 patient experiencing a nonfatal myocardial infarction or death. The cost for this benefit is relatively steep, with some studies estimating costs of over $100,000 in medical costs for every year of life saved (Pharoah and Hollingworth, 1996; Goldman et al, 1991). Moreover, the benefits of drug treatment for primary prevention have only been demonstrated in middle-aged men. It is less clear that similar benefits would accrue in treating women or elderly individuals, since cholesterol is a less powerful predictor of CHD in these groups.

In contrast to the evidence on drug treatment as a mode of primary prevention, studies suggest that drug treatment to lower cholesterol levels may be effective as a form of secondary prevention, to reduce morbidity and mortality among patients diagnosed as having symptomatic CHD, such as angina or a past myocardial infarction (MI). These individuals are at excessive risk for experiencing future CHD events, having a risk much higher than that of individuals with high cholesterol levels without symptomatic CHD. Giving cholesterol-lowering drugs to patients with known CHD and high cholesterol levels can avoid about 1 nonfatal MI or death for every 10 patients treated, with costs in the range of $5000–$25,000 for every year of life saved (Pharoah and Hollingworth, 1996; Goldman et al, 1991). The medical model of prevention may be most suitable as a secondary rather than a primary preventive measure for cholesterol and CHD, targeting individuals who are already "patients" with CHD rather than medicalizing the lives of otherwise healthy individuals by subjecting these healthy individuals to many years of drug treatment, laboratory tests, and physician appointments.

The weakness of the NIH cholesterol reduction strategy highlights the paradox of primary prevention: Prevention within a population of healthy individuals may be better (and less expensively) served by broad public health efforts to reduce risk among the majority of people at moderate risk than by concentrating intensive medical interventions on the the smaller number of high-risk persons (Rose, 1985; Brown et al, 1992). The traditional orientation of physicians toward individual patients (the medical model) has led the medical profession and the NIH to emphasize identification and treatment of high-risk individuals with elevated cholesterol levels. Reducing the mean cholesterol level of the United States population rather than reducing the individual cholesterol counts of hyperlipidemic patients may have better long-term results for primary prevention. Studies have also shown that these population-wide approaches are a far more cost-effective form of primary prevention than the strict medical model. For example, an experimental campaign to educate people in a community about CHD risk factors has been calculated to cost approximately $3000 per year of life saved, a fraction of the cost per year of life saved using drug treatment of cholesterol as a primary prevention method (Tosteson et al, 1997).

Mass education on the danger of rich diets has been associated with reduced per capita consumption of animal fat during the 1970s and a 7% decline in the mean population total cholesterol level from 1960 to 1990. Yet, the food industry spends billions of dollars on advertising, a substantial proportion of which promotes high-fat "fast foods." During the 1980s, animal fat consumption began to rise again, and persons between 19 and 29 years of age are more likely to eat high-fat foods than older men and women. Whether mass education can compete with food industry advertising in order to permanently change the eating habits of the population is as yet unknown. Public health advocates were active in passing recent legislation to improve food product nutritional labeling, an important tool of public education. Regulation of food advertising is a public health strategy that has been considered (Goldman and Cook, 1984; J. Stamler, 1992; Bodenheimer, 1991).

Because mass education about diet may be an insufficient public health intervention, proposals have been made to copy the strategy used by tobacco prevention campaigns in reducing the availability of high-fat foods. Because food, as opposed to tobacco, is essential for human survival, such measures as taxing high-fat foods or limiting the number of candy vending machines and fast food franchises have not met with popular approval. Reduction in the high animal fat content of school lunch programs is a primary preventive measure that might gain public acceptance.

Hypertension: The cause of hypertension (high blood pressure) is as yet not clearly understood. Risk factors for hypertension include high salt intake, low potassium intake, high ratio of dietary sodium to potassium, obesity, and excess alcohol intake; other important risk factors likely exist. Prior to the advent of modern agriculture, intake of sodium was low and of potassium high, and few persons were overweight because of high levels of physical exertion.

CHD risk is associated with increased blood pressure, even at relatively moderate levels of blood pressure elevation. Individuals with systolic blood pressures of 130–140 mm Hg have almost twice the cardiovascular risk of those with systolic blood pressures less than 110 mm Hg. A quarter of hypertension-related cardiovascular deaths take place among borderline hypertensives, and in the United States, 90% of men age 35–57 have blood pressure levels creating excess cardiovascular risk. Thus, it can be said that high blood pressure as a risk factor for CHD is a problem for the entire population and not simply a problem for the 20–25% of the population with frank hypertension. Similar to the cholesterol situation, the greatest impact in reducing hypertension-related CHD mortality rates will come from a reduction in the blood pressure of the large number of borderline hypertensives rather than from sole focus on people with very high blood pressures.

Primary prevention of high blood pressure can be accomplished by a reduction in the dietary sodium–potassium ratio from 3 (commonly observed in United States diets) to 1, a reduction in average body weight of 10%, and the elimination of heavy alcohol intake.

These three measures would lower the mean systolic blood pressure of the population by 5.4 mm Hg, which in turn would reduce CHD deaths by 9% and stroke deaths by 14%. A 50% reduction in average salt intake would both reduce the mean blood pressure of the population and reduce the number of cases of overt hypertension (R. Stamler, 1992).

African Americans have a higher prevalence of high blood pressure than whites and tend to suffer from more severe hypertensive disease. These differences persist even after controlling for socioeconomic status (ie, education, occupation, and income). Diastolic blood pressure higher than 115 mm Hg (severe hypertension) is five times more common in African American men than white men and seven times more common in African American women than white women. African Americans have a 7.3 times greater risk of developing end-stage kidney disease produced by high blood pressure than whites. The reasons for the high prevalence and severity of high blood pressure among African Americans are unknown; a higher dietary sodium-potassium ratio in the African American diet has been proposed as one explanation (Last, 1986; Matzen and Lang, 1993). Research has also suggested that racism and related social stresses may contribute to the high prevalence of hypertension in African Americans (James et al, 1987). Hypertension is much less commonly encountered among populations residing in Africa, suggesting that genetics is unlikely to account for the elevated rates of hypertension among African Americans (Polednak, 1989).

Prevention of hypertension has focused on screening and early treatment of elevated blood pressure. These measures are considered secondary prevention (early diagnosis and intervention) with respect to high blood pressure as a disease, but are categorized as primary prevention (averting the occurrence) with respect to CHD as a disease.

> In the late 1960s and early 1970s, the formula—1/2-1/2-1/2—characterized the United States situation in regard to hypertension: about half those with HBP [high blood pres-

sure] undetected, about half the detected persons untreated, about half the treated persons still hypertensive, ie, only about 1 in 8 detected, treated, and controlled. Since the launching by the United States government in 1973 of the National High Blood Pressure Education Program, the situation has changed markedly. In the late 1970s and early 1980s, multiple surveys showed that a majority of the tens of millions with HBP were detected, treated, and controlled. (Stamler J: The marked decline in coronary heart disease mortality rates in the United States, 1968–1981: Summary of findings and possible explanations. Cardiology [Karger, Basel] 1985;72:11.)

Primary prevention of CHD by screening and treating severe hypertensives is far more effective than primary CHD prevention through drug treatment of high serum cholesterol. For patients with severe hypertension, five patients must be treated for 1.5 years to avert a death or nonfatal cardiac event; for patients with high cholesterol levels, 40 patients must be treated for 5 years to avert a nonfatal cardiac event. Though the precise reduction in CHD mortality rates produced by improved high blood pressure control is unclear, it is known that reducing blood pressures has helped to reduce stroke mortality rates by over 50% in the last 25 years (Leaf, 1993).

In summary, the medical model of primary CHD prevention has been effective in the area of hypertension. While the medical model has received major emphasis in the attempt to reduce cholesterol levels, the public health model may have greater potential for benefit. In the realm of smoking cessation, a combination of the two models has had considerable success.

Breast Cancer   Whereas mortality rates for cardiovascular disease declined since the late 1960s, cancer mortality rates continued to increase through 1991. Between 1991 and 1994, cancer mortality rates finally eased downward, probably as a result of reductions in cigarette smoking. However, the incidence (number of new cases) of cancer has continued to climb in all age groups (Doll, 1991; Bailar, 1997).

The designing of effective primary prevention for a disease generally depends on an understanding of the epidemiology of that disease. In the case of lung cancer, the discovery of the link with cigarette smoking allowed a widespread primary prevention program to be developed—the antismoking campaign. But the second epidemiologic revolution has thus far failed to uncover the precise causes of many cancers, thereby frustrating the use of primary prevention techniques to reduce incidence and mortality rates. Preventive strategies for many cancers, therefore, use secondary rather than primary prevention. Pap smears for early detection of cervical cancer and fecal occult blood testing and sigmoidoscopy for detection of colorectal cancer are examples of secondary prevention. Pap smears have been the most successful secondary prevention program, having contributed to a significant reduction in mortality rates from cervical cancer.

The incidence of breast cancer increased gradually for several decades until 1980, increased more steeply from 1980 to 1987, and leveled off from 1987 to 1992 (Kelsey and Bernstein, 1996). Breast cancer mortality rates have remained relatively constant over the past 50 years, with a slight decrease for white females since 1990. The combination of rising incidence and relatively stable mortality rates for breast cancer probably reflects an increase in the true incidence of cancer, "detection bias" related to screening for asymptomatic cancers, and improved effectiveness of treatment to improve survival among women with breast cancer. Breast cancer incidence rates are higher for white women than for African-Americans, but mortality rates from breast cancer are higher for African-American than for white women (U.S. Department of Health and Human Services, 1996) (Figure 11–3).

Multiple risk factors for breast cancer have been uncovered, of which the most important are age greater than 65, a prior diagnosis or a family history (especially in a first-degree relative) of breast cancer, a prior diagnosis of atypical hyperplasia on breast biopsy, and having been born in North America or Northern Europe. Less important risk factors include obesity, age over 30 years at first full-term pregnancy, no pregnancies, and prior radiation to the thorax. Women with more years of ovulatory menstrual cycles have a greater risk, indicating a hormonal influence on the disease (Matzen and Lang, 1993).

Unfortunately, analyzing these variables to construct a theory of breast cancer causation suffers from a major limitation: Only one-fourth of breast cancer cases can be accounted for by these risk factors. The differences between high and low age-adjusted breast cancer risk in the United States are small compared with the differences between such high-incidence nations as the United States and low-incidence (generally underdeveloped) nations. Perhaps, unknown agents related to modern industrialization are the primary causes of breast cancer, while such influences as female hormones, family history, and obesity are secondary promoters of the disease. What would such an unknown agent be?

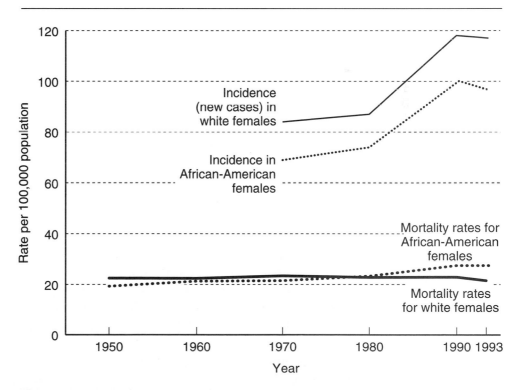

Figure 11–3. Incidence and mortality rates for breast cancer in the United States (age adjusted).

Dietary fat is one candidate, especially because nations with low fat intake also have low breast cancer incidence. Other factors related to industrialization might explain this association, however, and overall evidence linking fat to cancer of the breast is inconsistent and weak (Kelsey and Bernstein, 1996). Nonetheless, it is widely believed and recommended that women should reduce fat intake in order to protect themselves from breast cancer. Another view that has been inadequately studied holds that environmental carcinogens are a possible explanation for the rise in the incidence of breast and other cancers (Epstein, 1994; Sternglass and Gould, 1993). From the 1940s to the 1980s, industrial production of synthetic organic chemicals rose from 1 billion to 400 billion pounds annually, and the volume of hazardous wastes has also increased 400-fold during that period (Epstein, 1990). One study estimated that toxic chemicals encountered at workplaces are responsible for 20% of all human cancers (Landrigan, 1992). Estrogens have been used as additives to poultry and cattle feed, and pesticide residues contain estrogen-like compounds that may contribute markedly to breast cancer causation (Davis and Bradlow, 1995). In a study of 14,000 women published by the *Journal of the National Cancer Institute,* breast cancer was strongly associated with exposure to organochlorine insecticides, especially the principal metabolite of DDT, which remains in the fat for years following exposure (Wolff et al, 1993). Other studies, however, have failed to confirm this association.

The development of primary prevention programs for breast cancer is dependent on an understanding of its chief causes. If fat is the problem, dietary education and other public health measures to reduce the availability of high-fat foods are in order. If toxic chemical exposure is the culprit, primary prevention must attempt to eliminate the offending chemicals from the environment and protect humans from exposure to those chemicals. If the cause of breast cancer is multifactorial, primary prevention (ie, reducing the incidence of the disease) must find a strategy for each cause.

For breast cancer, lack of knowledge has forced modern medicine to retreat to secondary prevention (ie, early diagnosis through breast examinations and mammography) to reduce mortality rates in women with the disease. Thankfully, breast cancer, like cervical cancer, lends itself to secondary prevention techniques. Regular breast examinations by a health care provider plus periodic mammograms can reduce breast cancer mortality rates in women over age 50 by one-third. There is still controversy regarding how frequently to perform mammograms and at what age to start, but there is no disagreement about the overall secondary prevention strategy (Love, 1990).

Public debate regarding breast cancer in the United States has not focused on the issue of causation but has rather been reduced to controversies over the best means of secondary prevention. Opposing scientific panels and economic interest groups debate whether mammograms should be initiated at age 40 or age 50. Large sums of research monies are spent to determine whether tamoxifen, an antiestrogen medication, should be used to retard disease spread in all cases of proved breast cancer. These issues are important and have the potential to save thousands of lives. Yet, many breast cancer activists decry the relatively paltry sums going for basic epidemiologic research to determine the causes of breast cancer.

Interpersonal Violence   Interpersonal violence has become a major public health problem in the United States. Homicide is the second leading cause of death in persons 15–24 years of age and the leading cause for young African-Americans. Each year, over 25,000 people die from homicide. Alcohol is associated with more than half of all homicides and serious assaults. In 1985, an estimated 1.8 million women were physically assaulted by male partners. Over 1800 women are raped each day. While interpersonal violence includes a number of different crimes, such as homicide, robbery, assault, rape, and others, we will focus chiefly on homicide (Mason, 1992; Fagan, 1993; Rosenberg, 1997).

Firearms are responsible for 75% of homicides. Of total deaths occurring in teenagers, 20% are related to firearms. Each year, 100,000 nonfatal gunshot injuries occur (Kellerman, 1996). Approximately 200 million guns are owned by private citizens in the United States today. In contrast to cardiovascular disease and cancer, homicides are far more common in the United States than in other developed countries (Figure 11–4). From 1988 to 1991, homicides of males ages 15–24 were 10–40 times more common in the United States than in any other Western industrialized nation (Mason, 1992; Mercy et al, 1993; AMA Council on Scientific Affairs, 1992).

Research into the causes of interpersonal violence remains an inexact science, creating disagreements over the measures proposed to prevent violence. Three strategies for violence prevention include the criminal justice, the public health, and the broader sociologic approaches. Many criminal justice professionals tend to see violent behavior as an individual character flaw and thus advocate long prison terms to keep offenders quarantined from the rest of society; the other strategies place greater priority on societal as contrasted with individual responsibility for violence. Public health personnel point to the association of guns, alcohol, and illegal drugs with violence and propose solutions in the areas of gun control and alcohol and drug education and treatment (Moore, 1993).

Gun control experts have identified dozens of regulatory interventions, from outright bans on the manufacture and possession of guns to limited proposals involving the licensing of firearms or the imposition of waiting periods for the sale of guns. A

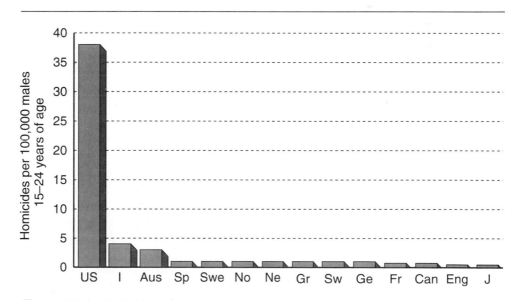

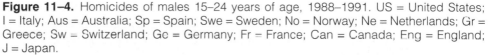

Figure 11–4. Homicides of males 15–24 years of age, 1988–1991. US = United States; I = Italy; Aus = Australia; Sp = Spain; Swe = Sweden; No = Norway; Ne = Netherlands; Gr = Greece; Sw = Switzerland; Ge = Germany; Fr = France; Can = Canada; Eng = England; J = Japan.

1976 District of Columbia law restricting handgun sale and possession was associated with an abrupt decline of almost 25% in the rate of homicides by firearm, an effect that persisted for 11 years (Teret and Wintemute, 1993). Over 80% of Americans support some form of government restriction on owning guns (Blendon, 1996). Gun control is growing as an important public health intervention to reduce homicides, though the existence of 200 million firearms in private homes makes effective gun control a daunting task.

One major opening for the public health approach to violence is control of alcohol consumption because alcohol, like firearms, is a factor in so many homicides. Per capita alcohol consumption rose 74% from 1950 to 1980, but fell from 1980 to 1992 (Muller, 1996). Not all ill effects of alcohol occur in people considered to be alcoholics; a substantial fraction of alcohol-related health problems involve moderate drinkers (Walsh, 1990). Just as a social drinker can become an alcohol-related fatality if the drinks are consumed just before driving an automobile, so can a moderate drinker commit murder if a few drinks are consumed in the course of a family, neighborhood, or gang-related altercation.

One strategy to prevent alcohol-related health problems is to restrict the availability of alcoholic beverages by raising the minimum drinking age, reducing the number of stores and bars where alcohol can be purchased, or increasing the price of alcohol. Many public health experts favor the third option as the most effective. The real price of alcohol has declined 28% since 1967 because alcohol tax rates have not risen as overall prices have inflated. A doubling of the federal tax on liquor, or a tax increasing the price of a six-pack of beer by 10 cents, has been shown to substantially reduce alcohol consumption (Mosher and Jernigan, 1989; Ashley and Rankin, 1988).

Another proposed public health intervention to reduce the homicide rate is the elimination of TV violence. The average child in the United States watches 8000 murders and 100,000 acts of violence on television before finishing elementary school (Shalala, 1993). Some studies have demonstrated a correlation between adult criminal violence and childhood exposure to TV violence (Centerwall, 1992), though this association has not been conclusively proved.

Complementing the criminal justice and public health approaches to interpersonal violence is the broader sociologic view that violence is related to economic and racial oppression. Risk factors for violence include minority status (particularly African-American), residence in large urban centers, and low income. The perpetrators of violence are seldom strangers to their victims; 60% of homicides of women are committed by someone known to the victim, usually a spouse or intimate acquaintance. Often, the murderer resembles the victim (eg, young African-American males tend to be murdered by other young African-American males). While much interpersonal violence is linked to poverty, some observers have noted that violence of a different type is perpetrated by the wealthy against the poor (Platt, 1978). Examples are promotion of cigarettes as safe products by tobacco companies, who for years have known but refused to admit their dangers and addictive properties (Glantz, 1995), or distribution of heroin and cocaine by wealthy drug pushers, with resultant drug-selling–related homicides in inner-city neighborhoods.

Several studies that have considered the striking difference in rates of homicide between the United States and other industrialized nations have suggested that socioeconomic inequality, economic discrimination against minority groups, and ethnic heterogeneity correlate with increased homicide rates. If these are significant variables, the criminal justice and public health approaches are likely to have only limited success in violence prevention; a far-reaching program would be needed to redistribute income and promote racial equality in the United States (Hawkins, 1993).

Acquired Immunodeficiency Syndrome (AIDS)

> AIDS seemed to appear out of historical context, at once entirely new, but also old; it properly belonged to a distant and less comfortable past, before economic and scientific progress had combined to banish the ancient plagues. (Fee E, Krieger N: Thinking and rethinking AIDS: Implications for health policy. Int J Health Serv 1993;23:323. Copyright 1993, Baywood Publishing Co.)

AIDS challenged the twentieth century dichotomy of infectious diseases in the underdeveloped world and chronic diseases in the industrialized nations. AIDS linked both worlds in a global plague, mimicking the epidemics of the past, such as cholera, yellow fever, leprosy, syphilis, and the plague (Fee and Krieger, 1993). Yet, AIDS is a different kind of plague: It is less communicable, and its course is more chronic. The prevention of AIDS, in a sense, belongs to both the first and the second epidemiologic revolutions.

The World Health Organization estimates that 40 million people worldwide will be infected with the human immunodeficiency virus (HIV) by the year 2000. In the United States, almost 1 million are infected; 37,000 died from HIV infection in 1993 (Figure 11–5). Controlling the AIDS epidemic requires primary preventive measures. Although great strides have been made in the secondary prevention of AIDS (ie, early detection and treatment to retard disease progression) through the use of potent medications that inhibit replication of HIV and forestall many of the complications of HIV infection, a true cure for AIDS remains elusive. The high cost of HIV medications (typically $10,000–$15,000 per year) also makes secondary prevention an unaffordable option for many developing nations, nations that have some of the highest rates of HIV infection in the world.

Educational efforts to promote safe sexual practices have been the major preventive tool employed in the United States. These efforts have two targets: the general population, and specific high-risk groups such as intravenous drug users and homosexuals.

AIDS education has enjoyed some success but is limited by the difficulty in changing behaviors over long time periods. In a national survey, only 17% of heterosexuals with multiple sexual partners reported that they used condoms all the time (Coates, 1993). Whereas the percentage of gay and bisexual men in San Francisco who reported engaging in unprotected anal intercourse dropped from about 65% to about 15% between 1984–1985 and 1987–1988, more recent data show that unprotected sexual practices have reemerged in the gay community in this city (Stall et al, 1990). Among HIV-negative persons, counseling and testing alone has a limited effect on reducing high-risk behaviors (Otten et al, 1993).

Another AIDS prevention strategy is to reduce the opportunity for viral spread from one person to another. An example was the closing of gay bathhouses in San Francisco, thereby eliminating a locus of promiscuous sexual practices among high-risk individuals (Shilts, 1987). HIV testing of the nation's blood supply has been ef-

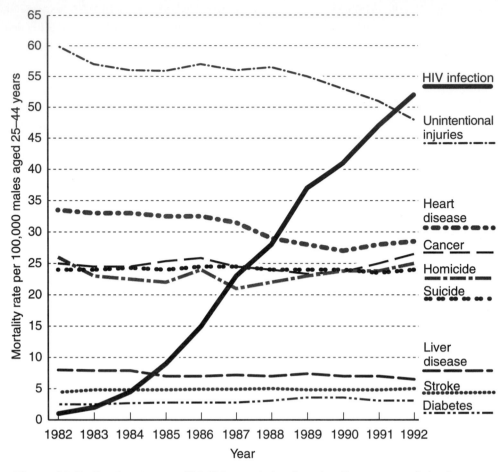

Figure 11–5. Death rates per 100,000 population from leading causes of death among men aged 25–44 years, by year in the United States, 1982–1992.

fective in reducing the spread of AIDS through transfusions. Needle exchange programs (providing sterile needles) for intravenous drug users are effective in reducing the spread of HIV infection (Coates and Feldman, 1997). These strategies must be closely associated with educational efforts.

Because education and measures to reduce viral spread are limited in their capacity to stop the spread of AIDS, the adoption of compulsory public health measures has been entertained. This approach has been employed in such programs as premarital syphilis serologies, childhood vaccination, involuntary hospitalization of people with mental health problems that could result in violence, and the government's right, which has been upheld in court cases, to confine people with active tuberculosis who constitute a danger to the health of others (Brandt, 1990; Annas, 1993).

The chief debate over a compulsory approach to AIDS prevention has focused on the mandatory testing of blood for evidence of HIV infection in certain subpopulations (eg, people seeking marriage licenses, people admitted to hospitals or scheduled for surgery, health care givers, pregnant women, and groups at high risk of infection). The proponents for such testing argue that health authorities and potential contacts have the right to know who carries a lethal communicable disease. But proposals for such testing present a serious problem of confidentiality. In public opinion polls taken in 1987, 81% of respondents believed that controlling the spread of AIDS should take precedence over the individual privacy of persons with AIDS. In the mid-1980s, 30% of the public believed that HIV-positive persons should be quarantined (Blendon and Donelan, 1990). Because of widespread fear of AIDS and prejudice against those groups at greatest risk for HIV infection, required HIV testing would likely lead to noncompliance by high-risk individuals, fear of seeking treatment, and a consequent worsening of the epidemic.

The most rigorous compulsory public health approach to prevention of AIDS is found in Cuba, where a large proportion of the population has been tested and HIV-positive persons have been confined in a sanatorium for a minimum of 6 months. Cuba's approach has limited the epidemic, with only 927 HIV-positive persons and 187 AIDS cases reported by 1993 for a population of over 10 million persons. New York City, with a similar population, has 43,000 people with AIDS. Cuba chose to restrict the human rights of infected persons in its attempt to protect the uninfected (Scheper-Hughes, 1993; Granich, 1995).

Summary   The examples of CHD, breast cancer, interpersonal violence, and AIDS illustrate different aspects of illness prevention. Primary prevention has been remarkably successful in reducing mortality rates for CHD. Secondary prevention has had some success in reducing breast cancer mortality rates, but the incidence of the disease continues to rise, and primary prevention is badly needed. For both interpersonal violence and breast cancer, the causes are not well understood, and primary prevention strategies are thus difficult to formulate. In the case of AIDS, the cause of the illness is known, but effective primary prevention continues to be elusive.

DOES PREVENTION REDUCE MEDICAL CARE COSTS?

It is generally true that effective prevention of illness can reduce the costs of health care to society. However, the influence of prevention on medical care costs is a complex one. As a rule, primary prevention using public health measures is far more cost effective than primary prevention through medical care; public health measures do not require many millions of expensive one-to-one interactions with medical care providers.

In the arena of individual medical care prevention, some measures save money and some do not. Every dollar spent on prenatal care saves $3.38 in newborn intensive care. Every dollar invested in measles, mumps, and rubella immunizations saves $13.40 in medical care costs (Harvey, 1990). Physician counseling on smoking cessation is a low-cost activity that can reduce the multibillion dollar cost of caring for people with tobacco-related illness. These preventive care activities do reduce health care spending in the long run. Cholesterol-lowering medical care interventions, in contrast, are unlikely to result in significant savings to the health care system, and for hypertension, only 22% of blood pressure treatment costs can be recovered through savings stemming from reduced rates of heart attacks and strokes (Weinstein and Stason, 1976).

Primary prevention through public health action can be enormously effective in reducing the burden of human suffering and the cost of treating disease. From 1900 to

1940, the nation's public health efforts achieved a 97% reduction in the death rate for typhoid fever, 97% for diphtheria, 92% for infectious diarrhea, 91% for measles, scarlet fever, and whooping cough, and 77% for tuberculosis (Winslow, 1944). The imposition of a $2 per pack increase in the tobacco tax can substantially reduce the $50 billion annual cost of tobacco-related disease while at the same time yielding tens of billions of dollars per year in tax revenues—an ideal preventive measure that actually earns money. If the three primary preventive methods known to reduce the incidence of coronary heart disease, cancer, and stroke (ie, reduction in smoking, cholesterol levels, and blood pressure) were intensified, the medical care costs of these illnesses could be reduced by 50%. These three illnesses account for 20% of personal health care costs in the United States (close to $200 billion in 1994), yielding a cost savings on the order of $100 billion per year (Terris, 1984).

It can be argued that money saved by preventing disease X will ultimately be spent on the treatment of disease Y or Z, which will strike those people spared from disease X. It is certainly true that disease prevention has had great success, with age-adjusted death rates from all causes dropping by 25% from 1970 to 1987 (Terris, 1992b). But has the burden of illness been reduced? Dr. James Fries has argued that there is a trend for morbidity from chronic diseases to be compressed into the later years of life; thus, people are healthy for a longer time and spend a shorter proportion of their lives sick (Fries, 1990). An alternate view suggests that while life expectancy is increasing, the proportion of life spent with significant disability is also rising (Guralnik and Schneider, 1990).

CONCLUSION

The goals of disease prevention are to delay disability and death and to maximize illness-free years of life. Improvements in living standards, public health measures, and preventive medical care have made enormous contributions toward the achievement of these goals. Producing further improvements in the overall health of society will likely depend on reducing the growing gap between rich and poor and shifting a greater proportion of the health dollar to disease prevention.

REFERENCES

AMA Council on Scientific Affairs: Assault weapons as a public health hazard in the United States. JAMA 1992;267:3067.

Annas GJ: Control of tuberculosis: The law and the public's health. N Engl J Med 1993;328:585.

Ashley MJ, Rankin JG: A public health approach to the prevention of alcohol-related health problems. Ann Rev Public Health 1988;9:233.

Bailar JC, Gornik HL: Cancer undefeated. N Engl J Med 1997;336:1569.

Bartecchi CE, MacKenzie TD, Schrier RW: The human costs of tobacco use (Part I). N Engl J Med 1994;330:907.

Blendon RJ, Donelan K: AIDS and discrimination: Public and professional perspectives. In: AIDS and the Health Care System. Gostin LO (editor). Yale Univ Press, 1990.

Blendon RJ et al: The American public and the gun control debate. JAMA 1996;275:1719.

Bodenheimer T: A public health approach to cholesterol: Confronting the "TV-auto-supermarket society." West J Med 1991;154:344.

Brandt AM: AIDS in historical perspective: Four lessons from the history of sexually transmitted diseases. In: The Nation's Health. Lee PR, Estes CL (editors). Jones & Bartlett, 1990.

Breslow L: A health promotion primer for the 1990s. Health Aff 1990;9(2):6.

Broder S: Cigarette advertising and corporate responsibility. JAMA 1992;268:782.

Brown EY, Viscoli CM, Horwitz RI: Preventive health strategies and the policy makers' paradox. Ann Intern Med 1992;116:593.

Centerwall BS: Television and violence: The scale of the problem and where to go from here. JAMA 1992;276:3059.

Coates TJ: Prevention of HIV-1 infection: Accomplishments and priorities. J NIH Res 1993;5:73.

Coates TJ, Feldman MD: An overview of HIV prevention in the United States. J Acquired Immune Deficiency Syndromes and Human Retrovirology 1997;14(Suppl 2):S13.

Cummings SR, Rubin SM, Oster G: The cost-effectiveness of counseling smokers to quit. JAMA 1989;261:75.

Davis DL, Bradlow HL: Can environmental estrogens cause breast cancer? Scientific American, Oct 1995:166.

Doll R: Progress against cancer: An epidemiologic assessment. Am J Epidemiol 1991;134:675.

Epstein SS: Environmental and occupational pollutants are avoidable causes of breast cancer. Int J Health Serv 1994;24:145.

Epstein SS: Losing the war against cancer: Who's to blame and what to do about it. Int J Health Serv 1990;20:53.

Fagan J: Interactions among drugs, alcohol, and violence. Health Aff 1993;12(4):65.

Fee E, Krieger N: Thinking and rethinking AIDS: Implications for health policy. Int J Health Serv 1993;23:323.

Fries JF: An introduction to the compression of morbidity. In: The Nation's Health. Lee PR, Estes CL (editors). Jones & Bartlett, 1990.

Gilpin EA et al: Are adolescents receptive to current sales promotion practices of the tobacco industry? Prev Med 1997;26:14.

Glantz SA et al: Looking through a keyhole at the tobacco industry. JAMA 1995;274:219.

Goldman L, Cook EF: The decline in ischemic heart disease mortality rates. Ann Intern Med 1984;101:825.

Goldman L et al: Cost-effectiveness of HMG-CoA reductase inhibition for primary and secondary prevention of coronary heart disease. JAMA 1991;265:1145.

Granich R et al: Cuba's national AIDS program. West J Med 1995;163:139.

Grumbach K: How effective is drug treatment of hypercholesterolemia? A guided tour of the major clinical trials for the primary care physician. J Am Board Fam Pract 1991;4:437.

Guralnik JM, Schneider EL: The compression of morbidity: A dream which may come true, someday! In: The Nation's Health. Lee PR, Estes CL (editors). Jones & Bartlett, 1990.

Harvey B: Toward a national child health policy. JAMA 1990;264:252.

Hawkins DF: Inequality, culture, and interpersonal violence. Health Aff 1993;12(4):80.

James SA et al: Socioeconomic status, John Henryism, and hypertension in blacks and whites. Am J Epidemiol 1987;126:664.

Kellerman AL et al: Injuries due to firearms in three cities. N Engl J Med 1996;335:1438.

Kelsey JL, Bernstein L: Epidemiology and prevention of breast cancer. Annu Rev Public Health 1996;17:47.

Kessler DA: Nicotine addiction in young people. N Engl J Med 1995;333:186.

Keys A: Coronary heart disease in seven countries. Circulation 1970;41(Suppl 1):11.

Landrigan PJ: Commentary: Environmental disease: A preventable epidemic. Am J Public Health 1992;82:941.

Last JM: Maxcy-Rosenau Public Health and Preventive Medicine. Appleton-Century-Crofts, 1986.

Leaf A: Preventive medicine for our ailing health care system. JAMA 1993;269:616.

Levit KR et al: National health expenditures, 1995. Health Care Fin Rev 1996;18:175.

Love SM: Dr. Susan Love's Breast Book. Addison-Wesley, 1990.

MacKenzie TD, Bartecchi CE, Schrier RW: The human costs of tobacco use (Part II). N Engl J Med 1994;330:975.

Mason J: Reducing youth violence: The physician's role. JAMA 1992;267:3003.

Matzen RN, Lang RS: Clinical Preventive Medicine. Mosby, 1993.

McGinnis JM, Foege WH: Actual causes of death in the United States. JAMA 1993;270:2207.

McKeown T: Determinants of health. In: The Nation's Health. Lee PR, Estes CL (editors). Jones & Bartlett, 1990.

McKinlay JB, McKinlay SM, Beaglehole R: A review of the evidence concerning the impact of medical measures on recent mortality and morbidity in the United States. Int J Health Serv 1989;19:181.

Mercy JA et al: Public health policy for preventing violence. Health Aff 1993;12(4):7.

Moore MH: Violence prevention: Criminal justice or public health? Health Aff 1993; 12(4): 34.

Mosher JF, Jernigan DH: New directions in alcohol policy. Ann Rev Public Health 1989;10:245.

Muller A: Alcohol consumption and community hospital admissions in the United States. Addiction 1996;91:231.

National Cholesterol Education Program: Report of the Expert Panel on Detection, Evaluation, and Treatment of High Blood Cholesterol in Adults. Arch Intern Med 1988;148:36.

Ornish D et al: Can lifestyle changes reverse coronary heart disease? Lancet 1990;336:129.

Otten MW et al: Changes in sexually transmitted disease rates after HIV testing and posttest counseling, Miami, 1988 to 1989. Am J Public Health 1993;83:529.

Pharoah PD, Hollingworth W: Cost effectiveness of lowering cholesterol concentration with statins in patients with and without pre-existing coronary heart disease. BMJ 1996; 312:1443.

Pierce JP et al: Trends in cigarette smoking in the United States: Educational differences are increasing. JAMA 1989;261:56.

Platt T: "Street" crime: A view from the left. Crime Soc Justice 1978;9:26.

Polednak AP: Racial and Ethnic Differences in Disease. Oxford Univ Press, 1989.

Rose G: Sick individuals and sick populations. Int J Epidemiol 1985;14(1):32.

Rosenberg ML et al: Applying science to violence prevention. JAMA 1997;277:1641.

Scheper-Hughes N: AIDS, public health, and human rights in Cuba. Lancet 1993;342:965.

Shalala DE: Addressing the crisis of violence. Health Aff 1993;12(4):30.

Sheperd J et al: Prevention of coronary heart disease with pravastatin in men with hypercholesterolemia: West of Scotland Coronary Prevention Study Group. N Engl J Med 1995;333:1301.

Shilts R: And the Band Played On. St. Martin's Press, 1987.

Sigerist HE: Medicine and Human Welfare. Yale Univ Press, 1941.

Stall R et al: Relapse from safer sex: The next challenge for AIDS prevention efforts. J Acquired Immune Deficiency Syndromes 1990;3:1181.

Stamler J: Established major coronary risk factors. In: Coronary Heart Disease Epidemiology. Marmot M, Elliott P (editors). Oxford Univ Press, 1992.

Stamler J: The marked decline in coronary heart disease mortality rates in the United States, 1968–1981: Summary of findings and possible explanations. Cardiology (Karger, Basel) 1985;72:11.

Stamler R: The primary prevention of hypertension and the population blood pressure problem. In: Coronary Heart Disease Epidemiology. Marmot M, Elliott P (editors). Oxford Univ Press, 1992.

Sternglass EJ, Gould JM: Breast cancer: Evidence for a relation to fission products in the diet. Int J Health Serv 1993;23:783.

Teret SP, Wintemute GJ: Policies to prevent firearm injuries. Health Aff 1993;12(4):96.

Terris M: The changing relationships of epidemiology and society: The Robert Cruikshank Lecture. J Public Health Policy 1985;6:15.

Terris M: Concepts of health promotion: Dualities in public health theory. J Public Health Policy 1992a;13:267.

Terris M: The development and prevention of cardiovascular disease risk factors: Socioeconomic influences. J Public Health Policy 1996;17:426.

Terris M: Healthy lifestyles: The perspective of epidemiology. J Public Health Policy 1992b;13:186.

Terris M: Prevention, the aged, and the costs of medical care. J Public Health Policy 1984;5: 157.

Terris M: What is health promotion? J Public Health Policy 1986;7:147.

Tosteson ANA et al: Cost-effectiveness of populationwide educational approaches to reduce serum cholesterol levels. Circulation 1997;95:24.

U.S. Department of Health and Human Services: Health United States 1995. 1996.

U.S. Preventive Services Task Force: Guide to Clinical Preventive Services. Williams & Wilkins, 1996.

Walsh DC: The shifting boundaries of alcohol policy. Health Aff 1990;9(2):47.

Warner KE: Cigarette taxation: Doing good by doing well. J Public Health Policy 1984;5:312.

Warner KE: Effects of the antismoking campaign: An update. Am J Public Health 1989b;79: 144.

Warner KE: Smoking and health: A 25-year perspective. Am J Public Health 1989a;79:141.

Warner KE, Goldenhar LM, McLaughlin CG: Cigarette advertising and magazine coverage of the hazards of smoking. N Engl J Med 1992;326:305.

Weinstein MC, Stason WB: Hypertension: A Policy Perspective. Harvard Univ Press, 1976.

Winslow CEA: Who killed Cock Robin? Am J Public Health 1944;34:658.

Wolff MS et al: Blood levels of organochlorine residues and risk of breast cancer. J Natl Cancer Inst 1993;85:648.

Woolf SH et al: Developing evidence-based clinical practice guidelines: Lessons learned by the US Preventive Services Task Force. Annu Rev Public Health 1996;17:511.

The Quality of Health Care

12

Each year in the United States, millions of people visit hospitals, physicians, and other care givers and receive medical care of superb quality. But that's not the whole story. Some patients' interactions with the health care system fall short.

An estimated 180,000 people die each year in the United States as a result of physician-caused injuries. Seventy percent of these deaths are a result of errors and are therefore potentially preventable (Leape, 1994). In one study, 27% of deaths in patients treated for heart attacks, strokes, and pneumonia could probably have been prevented by proper diagnosis and treatment. The preventable deaths were not primarily in older and sicker people, but rather in younger and less severely ill patients. Between one hospital and another, researchers found a 20-fold difference in mortality rates from coronary artery bypass surgery, a difference that could not be explained by variations in age of the patients or severity of the underlying illness. Mortality rates from coronary artery bypass graft (CABG) surgery, adjusted for patient age and severity of illness, varied among 18 surgeons from 2.2 to 9.3% (Dubois and Brook, 1988; Brook, 1991; Berwick, 1991). One-third of drugs prescribed may not be appropriate, and one-third of abnormal laboratory tests may not be followed up by physicians (Brook et al, 1996).

Recent studies show that African-American patients may experience an inferior quality of care compared with white patients with similar illnesses and insurance status. The likelihood of patients being harmed by medical negligence is almost three times as great in hospitals tending to serve low-income and minority patients than in hospitals with more affluent populations (Ayanian, 1994; Burstin et al, 1993a).

These and other facts demonstrate that health care in the United States suffers from uneven quality. We will first examine the factors contributing to uneven quality, and then explore what can be done to elevate all health care to the highest possible level.

THE COMPONENTS OF HIGH-QUALITY CARE

What is high-quality health care? It is health care that assists healthy people to stay healthy, cures people's acute illnesses, and allows chronically ill people to live as long and fulfilling a life as possible. What are the components of high-quality health care (Table 12–1)?

Adequate Access to Care

> Lydia and Laura were friends at a rural high school; both became pregnant. Lydia's middle class parents took her to a nearby obstetrician, while Laura, from a family on welfare, could not find a doctor who would take Medicaid. Lydia became the mother of a healthy infant, but Laura, going without prenatal care, delivered a low-birth-weight baby with severe lung problems.

Table 12–1. Components of high-quality care.

Access to care
Adequate scientific knowledge
Competent health care providers
Separation of financial and clinical decisions
Organization of health care institutions to maximize quality

To receive quality care, people must have access to care. People with reduced access to care are likely to suffer worse health outcomes, compared with those enjoying full access (see Chapter 3). Quality requires equality (Schiff et al, 1994).

Adequate Scientific Knowledge

> Brigitte Levy, a professor of family law, was started on estrogen replacement in 1960, when she reached menopause. Her doctor prescribed the hormone pills for 10 years. In 1979, she was diagnosed with invasive cancer of the uterus, which spread to her entire abdominal cavity in spite of surgical treatment and radiation. She died in 1980 at age 68, at the height of her career.

A body of knowledge must exist that informs physicians what to do for the patient's problem. If clear scientific knowledge fails to distinguish between effective and ineffective or harmful care, quality may be compromised. During the 1960s, medical science taught that estrogen replacement, without the administration of progestins, was safe. Sadly, cases of uterine cancer caused by estrogen replacement did not show up until many years later. Brigitte Levy's physician followed the standard of care for his day, but the medical profession as a whole was relying on inadequate scientific knowledge.

Between 80 and 90% of what physicians do has never been evaluated by rigorous scientific experiment (Eddy, 1993). Therapies of uncertain efficacy may cause harm and cost billions of dollars each year.

Moreover, many therapies have not been adequately tested for serious side effects, especially when such side effects may not be manifested for a decade or more. Hormone replacement by estrogen alone, as in Brigitte Levy's case, was not found to have a potentially lethal risk for many years. The possible link between widely used estrogen and progestin hormonal therapy and breast cancer is still unknown. Long-term lovastatin treatment for elevated cholesterol levels has not been in use long enough for its potential long-term adverse effects to be known.

Competent Health Care Providers

> Ceci Yu, age 77, was waking up at night with shortness of breath and wheezing. Her physician told her she had asthma and prescribed terbutaline, a bronchodilator. Two days later, Ms. Yu was admitted to the coronary care unit with a heart attack. Writing to the chief of medicine, the cardiologist charged that Ms. Yu's physician had misdiagnosed the wheezing of congestive heart failure and had treated Ms. Yu incorrectly for asthma. The cardiologist charged that the treatment may have precipitated the heart attack. The cardi-

ologist requested an investigation of the physician's competence.

The provider must have the skills to diagnose problems and choose appropriate treatments. An inadequate level of competence resulted in poor-quality care for Ms. Yu. Five to 15% of physicians are not fully competent to practice medicine, either because of inadequate medical skills, impairment caused by use of drugs or alcohol, or deficiencies resulting from mental illness. In many states, medical licensing boards have been lax in disciplining or revoking the licenses of incompetent or impaired physicians (Feinstein, 1985).

The Harvard Medical Practice study reviewed 30,000 medical records in 51 hospitals in New York State in 1984. The study found that in about 4% of hospital admissions, the patient experienced a medical injury (ie, a medical problem caused by the management of a disease rather than by the disease itself). Medical injuries can be classified as negligent or not negligent.

> Jack was given a prescription for a sulfa drug. When he took the first pill, he turned beet red, began to wheeze, and fell to the floor. His friend called 911, and Jack was treated in the emergency room for anaphylactic shock, a potentially fatal allergy. The emergency room physician learned that Jack had developed a rash the last time he took sulfa. Jack's physician had never asked Jack if he was allergic to sulfa. Jack did not realize that the prescription contained sulfa.

> Mack was prescribed a sulfa drug, following which he developed anaphylactic shock. Before writing the prescription, Mack's doctor asked whether he had a sulfa allergy. Mack had said "No."

Medical negligence is defined as failure to meet the standard of practice of an average qualified physician practicing in the same specialty. Jack's drug reaction must be considered negligence, while Mack's was not. Of the medical injuries discovered in the Harvard study, 28% were due to negligence. In those injuries that led to death, 51% involved negligence. The most common injuries were drug reactions (19%) and wound infections (14%). Eight percent of injuries involved failure to diagnose a condition, of which 75% were negligent. Seventy percent of patients suffering all forms of medical injury recovered completely in 6 months or less, but 47% of patients in whom a diagnosis was missed suffered serious disabilities (Brennan et al, 1991; Leape et al, 1991).

Negligence cannot be equated with incompetence. Any good physician may have a mental lapse, may be overtired after a long night in the intensive care unit, or may have failed to learn an important new research finding. In the view of Laffel and Berwick (1993),

> There is a fragile connection between the new knowledge generated by medical research and the care given to patients at the bedside. Physicians may not hear about or accept new findings; they may not know how or when to use them; and the health systems in which they practice may not support the implementation of new knowledge. (Laffel GL, Berwick DM: Quality health care. JAMA 1993;270:254. Copyright 1993 American Medical Association.)

Money & Quality of Care

> Nina Brown arrived at an ambulatory care clinic of a large health maintenance organization (HMO) complaining of chest pain radiating to the back. A clinic nurse described her as pale and sweaty and placed her on oxygen. The physician examined Ms. Brown, performed an EKG, which did not show clear evidence of a heart attack, diagnosed musculoskeletal pain, and sent her home. Five minutes later in the parking lot, Ms. Brown collapsed of a heart attack and was resuscitated, with severe brain damage. She died 1 week later.

> Completely healthy at age 45, Henry Fung reluctantly submitted to a treadmill exercise test at the local YMCA. The study was abnormal, and Mr. Fung, who had fee-for-service insurance, sought the advice of a cardiologist. The cardiologist knew that treadmill tests are sometimes positive in healthy people. He ordered a coronary angiogram, which was perfectly normal. Three hours after the study, a clot formed in the femoral artery at the site of the catheter insertion, and emergency surgery was required to save Mr. Fung's leg.

No one can know what motivated the HMO physician to send Ms. Brown home when a heart attack was one possible diagnosis; nor can one guess what led the fee-for-service cardiologist to perform an invasive coronary angiogram of questionable appropriateness on Mr. Fung. One factor that bears close attention is the impact of financial considerations on the quantity (and thus the quality) of medical care (Rodwin, 1993). As we noted in Chapter 4, fee-for-service reimbursement encourages physicians to perform more services, whereas capitation payment rewards those who perform fewer services. The quest for high-quality care must include a search for financially neutral clinical decision making (Schiff et al, 1994).

Over 20 years ago, John Bunker (1970) found that the United States performed twice the number of surgical procedures per capita than Great Britain did. He postulated that this difference could be accounted for by the greater number of surgeons per capita in the United States and concluded that "the method of payment appears to play an important, if unmeasured, part." Most surgeons in the United States were compensated by fee-for-service, whereas most in Great Britain were paid a salary. In his article "What puts the surge in surgery?," Harvard Medical School surgeon Francis Moore (1970) commented that Bunker's findings "add to the conviction that the American system of payment has something to do with the frequency of operations." Do excessive surgeries compromise quality of care? Dr. Moore felt that they do: "Unnecessary and meddlesome operative interventions go hand in hand with poor surgical care." A 1976 United States House of Representatives study found that in 1974, "unnecessary surgeries led to 11,900 unnecessary deaths" (Leape, 1992).

Another type of evidence linking fee-for-service reimbursement with inappropriate medical interventions is the study of cesarean sections for women with previous cesarean births. Cesarean section is the most common surgical procedure in the United States, performed in 25% of all births in 1988. The rate quadrupled during the 1970s and 1980s. Thirty-six percent were repeat cesarean sections. Vaginal birth after cesarean section (VBAC) is a safe procedure, yet in 1985, only 7% of women who had previous cesarean sections gave birth vaginally. A 1986 study showed that women giving birth in for-profit hospitals (reimbursed more for cesarean sections) had the lowest VBAC rate (5%), compared with 29% for University of California teaching hospitals. Rates of VBAC for women with private insurance (which pays more for cesarean sections) were 8%, compared with rates in the Kaiser Health Plan of 20% (where physicians do not earn more by performing cesarean sections) (Stafford, 1991). Managed care is blunting the financial incentive to perform repeat cesarean sections; already from 1985 to 1989, the VBAC rate increased from 7 to 19%, and younger obstetricians support VBAC more than older ones (Cunningham et al, 1993). Maternal mortality with cesarean section is two to four times higher than with vaginal delivery (Rothman, 1993).

The impact of reimbursement on how physicians practice is not confined to surgeons and obstetricians. In a fee-for-service for-profit ambulatory center, 15 physicians formerly paid by salary were offered bonuses that depended on the amount of income they generated for the center. A year after the bonuses were instituted, the number of patient visits increased by 12% and laboratory tests per patient visit jumped by 23% for those 15 physicians (Hemenway et al, 1990).

> It was a nice dinner, hosted by the hospital radiologist and paid for by the company manufacturing MRI scanners. After the meal came the pitch: "If you doctors invest money, we can get an MRI scanner near our hospital; if the MRI makes money, you all share in the profits." One internist explained later, "After I put in my $10,000, it was hard to resist ordering MRI scans. With headaches, back pain, and knee problems, the indications for MRIs are kind of fuzzy. You might order one or you might not. Now, I do."

During the 1980s, many doctors formed partnerships and joint ventures giving them part ownership in laboratories, MRI scanners, and outpatient surgicenters. Forty percent of practicing physicians in Florida owned services to which they referred patients. Ninety-three percent of diagnostic imaging facilities, 76% of ambulatory surgery centers, and 60% of clinical laboratories in the state were owned wholly or in part by physicians. The rates of use for MRI and CT scans were higher for physician-owned compared with non-physician–owned facilities (Mitchell and Scott, 1992). In a national study, physicians who received payment for performing x-rays and sonograms within their own offices obtained these examinations four times as often as physicians who referred the examinations to radiologists and received no reimbursement for the studies. The patients in the two groups were similar (Hillman et al, 1990). The implication is that physicians order more diagnostic tests if they profit from so doing. According to Dr. Arnold Relman,

> . . . economic incentives now play a far more important role in determining the behavior of most physicians . . . The technology explosion has provided the tools and insurance has removed the financial restraints on their use that doctor or patient may have felt in earlier times . . . In this climate, the conflict of interest that has always been inherent in the fee-for-service system takes on larger and more disturbing dimensions . . . (Relman AS: The future of medical practice. Health Aff 1983;2(2):5.)

Moving to the other side of the overtreatment–undertreatment spectrum, payment by capitation, or salaried employment by a for-profit business, may create a climate hostile to the provision of adequate services. In the 1970s, a series of HMOs called prepaid health plans (PHPs) sprang up to provide care to California Medicaid patients. The quality of care in several PHPs became a major scandal in California. At one PHP, administrators wrote a message to health care providers: "Do as little as you possibly can for the PHP patient," and charts audited by the California Health Department revealed many instances of undertreatment. The PHPs received a lump sum for each patient enrolled, meaning that the lower the cost of the services actually provided, the greater the PHP's profits (U.S. Senate, 1975).

United States House of Representatives (1988) hearings demonstrated similar problems with International Medical Centers, Inc., a Florida-based HMO caring for 130,000 Medicare patients. Many patients complained of difficulty in gaining access to services covered by Medicare. One IMC administrator brought to the attention of his superiors 130 major quality problems; he was fired.

In 1994, the state of California cited Cigna Health Plans of California for violations of state regulations, including lack of recognition of grossly abnormal laboratory tests, lack of follow-up care on post-hospital discharges, and excessive waiting periods (as long as 2 months) for appointments (Sanders, 1994). A number of probably preventable deaths have been reported of HMO patients for whom adequate care was denied for cost-saving reasons (Anders, 1996). Even in one of the nation's most highly regarded HMOs, Group Health Cooperative of Puget Sound, poor patients with chronic illnesses in the early 1980s had inferior outcomes within the HMO when compared with fee-for-service practices (Ware et al, 1986).

Most recent academic studies on managed care organizations fail to show reduced quality of care processes and outcomes when compared with traditional fee-for-service care. These studies have several limitations: They may be biased on the issue of severity of illness, they are short- and not long-term studies, and they are several years old and thus do not measure the current highly competitive marketplace with capitation-plus-bonus modes of paying physicians (Berwick, 1996).

The quantity and quality of medical care are inextricably interrelated. Too much or too little can be injurious. The research of Dr. John Wennberg (1986) has shown that similar populations in different geographic areas have widely varying rates of surgeries and days in the hospital. In these situations, someone is getting too much care or someone is getting too little. Because many clinical decisions are not based on firm scientific evidence, uncertainty pervades medicine. Medical uncertainty is fertile ground for economic influences to blossom—the tendency toward too much care under fee-for-service or too little care under capitation and other fixed reimbursements.

Health Care Institutions & Quality of Care

> The personnel cutbacks were terrible; staffing had diminished from four RNs per shift to two, with only two aides to provide assistance. Shelley Rush, RN, was 2 hours behind in administering medications and had five insulin injections to give, with complicated dosing schedules. A family member rushed to the nursing station saying, "The lady in my mother's room looks bad." Shelley ran in and found the patient comatose. She quickly checked the blood sugar, which was disastrously low at 20 mg/dL. Shelley gave 50% glucose, and the patient woke up. Then it hit her; she had injected the insulin into the wrong patient.

Health care institutions must be well organized, with an adequate, competent staff. Shelley Rush was a superb nurse, but understaffing led her to make a serious error. Studies show that hospitals with higher proportions of RNs have lower mortality rates (Fagin, 1994).

The book, *Curing Health Care,* by Berwick, Godfrey, and Roessner (1990) opens with a heartbreaking case:

> She died, but she didn't have to. The senior resident was sitting, near tears, in the drab office behind the nurses' station in the intensive care unit. It was 2:00 AM, and he had been battling for thirty-two hours to save the life of the twenty-three-year-old graduate student who had just suffered her final cardiac arrest.
>
> The resident slid a large manila envelope across the desk top. "Take a look at this," he said. "Routine screening chest x-ray, taken ten months ago. The tumor is right there, and it was curable—then. By the time the second film was taken eight months later, because she was complaining of pain, it was too late. The tumor had spread everywhere, and the odds were hopelessly against her. Everything we've done since then has really just been wishful thinking. We missed our chance. She missed her chance." Exhausted, the resident put his head in his hands and cried.
>
> Two months later, the Quality Assurance Committee completed its investigation . . . "We find the inpatient care commendable in this tragic case," concluded the brief report, "although the failure to recognize the tumor in a potentially curable stage ten months earlier was unfortunate . . ." Nowhere in this report was it written explicitly why the results of the first chest x-ray had not been translated into action. No one knew . . . The internist who had ordered that x-ray had office notes reflecting the order . . . Yet no x-ray report was found in the doctor's office folder.
>
> One year later . . . it was 2:00 AM, and the night custodian was cleaning the radiologist's office. As he moved a filing cabinet aside to sweep behind it, he glimpsed a dusty tan envelope that had been stuck between the cabinet and the wall. The envelope contained a yellow radiology report slip, and the date on the report—nearly two years earlier— convinced the custodian that this was, indeed, garbage . . . He tossed it in with the other trash, and four hours later it was incinerated along with other useless things. (Berwick DM, Godfrey AB, Roessner J: Curing Health Care. Jossey-Bass, 1990.)

This patient may have had perfect access to care for an illness whose treatment is scientifically proved; she may have seen a physician who knew how to make the diagnosis and deliver the appropriate treatment; and yet the quality of her care was disastrously deficient. Dozens of people and hundreds of processes influence the care of one person with one illness. In her case, one person—perhaps a file clerk with a near-perfect record in handling thousands of radiology reports—lost control of one report; and the physician's office had no system to monitor whether or not x-ray reports had been received. The result was the most tragic of quality failures—the unnecessary death of a young person.

How health care institutions are organized has a major impact on health care outcomes. In a study of 13 intensive care units, death rates were calculated and adjusted for severity of illness. There was a great range of adjusted death rates, with one unit showing 58% more deaths than expected, while another had 41% fewer deaths than expected. The study concluded that the organization and coordination of the physicians and nurses in the intensive care unit has a major influence on patient outcome (Knaus et al, 1986).

> Oliver Hart lived in a city with a population of 80,000. He was admitted to Primary Care Hospital with congestive heart failure caused by a defective mitral valve. He was told he needed semiurgent heart surgery to replace the valve. The cardiologist said "You can go to University Hospital 30 miles away or have the surgery done here." The cardiologist did not say that Primary Care Hospital performed only seven cardiac surgeries last year. Mr. Hart elected to remain for the procedure. During the surgery, a key piece of equipment failed, and he died on the operating table.

Quality of care must be viewed in the context of regional systems of care (see Chapter 6), not simply within each health care institution. For open heart surgery, 38% of the deaths in smaller-volume hospitals could have been averted had the procedure been done in larger-volume hospitals. Quality of care improves with the experience of those providing the care (Luft et al, 1990). Had Mr. Hart been told the relative surgical mortality rates at University Hospital, which performed 500 cardiac surgeries each year, and at Primary Care Hospital, he would have chosen to be transferred 30 miles down the road.

In the late 1980s, Dr. Donald Berwick (1989) and others realized that quality of care is not simply a question of whether or not a physician or other care giver is competent. If poorly organized, the complex systems within and among medical institutions can thwart the best efforts of professionals to deliver high-quality care.

> There are two approaches to the problem of improving quality . . . [One is] the Theory of Bad Apples, because those who subscribe to it believe that quality is best achieved by discovering bad apples and removing them from the lot . . . The Theory of Bad Apples gives rise readily to what can be called the my-apple-is-just-fine-thank-you response . . . and seeks not understanding, but escape. [The other is] the Theory of Continuous Improvement. Its postulates are simple . . . Even when people were at the root of defects, . . . the problem was generally not one of motivation or effort, but rather of poor job design, failure of leadership, or unclear purpose. Quality can be improved much more when people are assumed to be trying hard already, and are not accused of sloth. Fear of the kind engendered by the disciplinary approach poisons improvement in quality, since it inevitably leads to the loss of the chance to learn.
>
> Real improvement in quality depends . . . on continuous improvement throughout the organization through constant

effort to reduce waste, rework, and complexity. When one is clear and constant in one's purpose, when fear does not control the atmosphere (and thus the data), when learning is guided by accurate information . . . and when the hearts and talents of all workers are enlisted in the pursuit of better ways, the potential for improvement in quality is nearly boundless . . . It would be naive to counsel the total abandonment of surveillance and discipline . . . it is absolutely necessary for regulators to ferret out the truly avaricious and the dangerously incompetent. But what about the rest of us?

A test result lost, a specialist who cannot be reached, a missing requisition, a misinterpreted order, duplicate paperwork, a vanished record, a long wait for the CT scan, an unreliable on-call system—these are all-too-familiar examples of waste, rework, complexity, and error in the doctor's daily life . . . For the average doctor, quality fails when systems fail. (Berwick DM: Continuous improvement as an ideal in health care. N Engl J Med 1989;320:53. Abstracted from information appearing in *New England Journal of Medicine*.)

Dr. Berwick's analysis has led many health care institutions to embrace continuous quality improvement (CQI) as a technique for enhancing quality of care (see below).

To summarize, good quality care can be compromised at a number of steps along the way.

Angie Roth has coronary heart disease and may need CABG surgery. Here are some considerations in her case: (1) If she is uninsured and cannot get to a physician, high-quality care is impossible to obtain. (2) If clear guidelines do not exist regarding who benefits from CABG and who does not, Ms. Roth's physician may make the wrong choice. (3) Even if clear guidelines exist, if Angie Roth's physician fails to evaluate her illness correctly or sends her to a surgeon with poor operative skills, quality may suffer. (4) If indications for surgery are not clear in Ms. Roth's case but the surgeon will benefit economically from the procedure, the surgery may be inappropriately performed. (5) Even if the surgery is appropriate and performed by an excellent surgeon, faulty equipment in the operating room or a nursing staff without training to recognize complications of surgery may lead to a poor outcome.

PROPOSALS FOR IMPROVING QUALITY

Several infants at a hospital received epinephrine in error, and suffered serious medical consequences. An analysis revealed that several pharmacists had made the same mistake; the problem was caused by the identical appearance of the vitamin E and epinephrine bottles in the pharmacy. This was a system error.

An epidemic of unexpected deaths on the cardiac ward was investigated. The times of the deaths were correlated with

> personnel schedules, leading to the conclusion that one nurse was responsible. It turned out that she was administering lethal doses of digoxin to patients. This was not a system error.

Quality issues must be investigated to determine if they are system errors or problems with a particular care giver (Kritchevsky and Simmons, 1991). Whether a quality problem is caused by system failure or individual failure determines the remedy. Two simultaneous approaches are required to improve the quality of medical care in the United States: maximizing the excellence of each health care giver, and improving the function of each health care institution and each regional grouping of institutions.

Maximizing Excellence   Achieving a competent health care work force, whether physicians, nurses, pharmacists, or the many other people on whom patient care depends, requires improved high school and college education, recruitment of dedicated people into health professions, high-quality training at health science schools, thoughtful licensure examinations and reexaminations, and continuing education during professional life. In addition, four relatively new initiatives have been proposed: medical practice guidelines, peer review based on continuous quality improvement, quality report cards, and financially neutral clinical decision making.

Medical Practice Guidelines:

> Dr. Benjamin Waters was frustrated by patients who came in with urinary incontinence. He never learned about the problem in medical school, so he simply referred these patients to a urologist. In his managed care plan, Dr. Waters was known to overrefer, so he felt stuck. He could not handle the problem, yet he did not want to refer patients elsewhere. He solved his dilemma by prescribing incontinence pads and diapers, but did not feel good about it.

> Dr. Denise Drier learned about urinary incontinence in family practice residency but did not feel secure about caring for the problem. A patient brought her a brochure called *Urinary Incontinence in Adults, A Patient's Guide,* by the Agency for Health Care Policy and Research of the Department of Health and Human Services. Dr. Drier read the booklet and sent away for another publication, *Clinical Practice Guidelines on Urinary Incontinence in Adults.* She studied the material and applied it to her incontinence patients. After a few successes, she and the patients were feeling better about themselves.

For many conditions, there is a better and a worse way to make a diagnosis and prescribe treatment. Physicians may not be aware of the better way because of gaps in training, limited experience, or insufficient time or motivation to learn new techniques. For these problems, medical practice guidelines can be helpful in improving quality of care. In 1989, Congress established the Agency for Health Care Policy and Research (AHCPR) to develop practice guidelines, among other tasks. Produced by panels of experts, practice guidelines make specific recommendations to physicians on how to treat clinical conditions such as urinary incontinence or cataracts (Leape,

1990). Dozens of organizations have produced practice guidelines, and they vary in scientific reliability (Kassirer, 1993). Different guidelines on the same topic distributed by different HMOs may be confusing.

In order to develop practice guidelines, the scientific community must have data demonstrating which therapies work and which do not. Because proof of treatment efficacy is lacking in so many conditions, more research is needed to determine the outcomes (mortality and morbidity rates, improvement in symptoms) of different treatments. Outcomes research is not simple. To be definitive, research studies must be performed on a large scale, and several studies should agree before the conclusions can be widely accepted (Eddy, 1993).

Practice guidelines are not appropriate for many clinical situations. Uncertainty pervades clinical medicine, and practice guidelines are applicable only for those cases in which we enjoy "islands of knowledge in our seas of ignorance." Practice guidelines can assist but not replace clinical judgment in the quest for high-quality care (Brook, 1989).

> Pedro Urrutia, age 59, noticed mild nocturia and urinary frequency. His friend had prostate cancer, and he became concerned. The urologist said that his prostate was only slightly enlarged, his prostate-specific antigen (blood test) was normal, and surgery was not needed. Mr. Urrutia wanted surgery and found another urologist to do it.

> At age 82, James Chin noted nocturia and urinary hesitancy. He had two glasses of wine on his wife's birthday and later that night was unable to urinate. He went to the emergency room, was found to have a large prostate without nodules, and was catheterized. The urologist strongly recommended a transurethral resection of the prostate. Mr. Chin refused, thinking that the urinary retention was caused by the alcohol. Five years later, he was in good health, with his prostate intact.

Practice guidelines for benign prostatic hypertrophy (enlargement of the prostate gland) have been the topic of considerable investigation. The difficulty with creating a set of indications for surgery is that patient preferences vary markedly. Some, like Mr. Urrutia, want prostate surgery, even though it is not clearly needed; others, like Mr. Chin, have strong reasons for surgery but do not want it. Practice guidelines must take into account not only scientific data but also patient desires (Wennberg, 1990).

Do practice guidelines in themselves improve quality of care? Most studies reveal that they have been unsuccessful in influencing physicians' practices. But when guidelines are reinforced by direct feedback to physicians from colleagues who are trusted as "opinion leaders," physicians may markedly improve their clinical practice (Greco and Eisenberg, 1993).

Peer Review Based on Continuous Quality Improvement: A second component of quality improvement is peer pressure within hospitals, HMOs, and the medical community at large. Peer review is defined as the evaluation by health care practitioners of the appropriateness and quality of services performed by other practitioners, usually in the same specialty. Peer review has been a part of medicine for decades (eg, tissue committees study surgical specimens to determine whether appendectomies and hysterectomies have actually removed diseased organs; credentials committees review the qualifications of physicians for hospital staff privileges; medical society ethics committees consider potential violations of ethics). But peer review moved to center stage with the passage of the law enacting Medicare in 1965.

Medicare anointed the Joint Commission on Accreditation of Hospitals (renamed the Joint Commission on Accreditation of Healthcare Organizations, JCAHO) with the authority to terminate hospitals from the Medicare program if quality of care was found to be deficient. The JCAHO requires hospital medical staffs to set up peer review committees for the purpose of maintaining quality of care.

JCAHO traditionally used criteria of structure and process, but not outcome, to assess quality of care. Structural criteria include such factors as the cleanliness of the hospital and whether the emergency room defibrillator works properly. Criteria of process include whether medical records are dictated and signed in a timely manner, or if the credentials committee keeps minutes of its meetings. More recently, JCAHO has also paid attention to outcomes, including such measures as mortality rates for surgical procedures, proportions of deaths that are preventable, and rates of adverse drug reactions and wound infections. Outcomes are more important than, and may not always correlate with, structure and process criteria, but they are difficult to measure. Death is the most significant outcome, but it is dependent on the severity of illness, making it difficult to conclude that hospitals with higher mortality rates are inferior in quality; they may simply have sicker patients (Luce et al, 1994; Schroeder, 1987; Donabedian, 1988).

In 1972, Medicare created a new quality-monitoring structure, the Professional Standards Review Organizations, supplanted in 1982 by Peer Review Organizations (PROs). PROs were set up in each state or region to monitor hospital admissions for appropriateness and quality. With authority to deny Medicare payment to hospitals for admissions deemed unnecessary, PROs appeared to be a cost control mechanism disguised as a program to improve quality (Webber, 1988).

Peer review is less developed in outpatient settings than in hospitals. One stimulus for ambulatory peer review came with the Health Maintenance Organization Act of 1973, requiring certain HMOs to operate quality assurance programs for inpatients and outpatients. But independent physician's offices, providing the bulk of ambulatory care, have no requirement to conduct quality review.

> Angela Lopez, age 57, suffered from metastatic ovarian cancer, but was feeling well and prayed she would live 9 months more; her son was the first family member ever to attend college, and she hoped to see him graduate. It was decided to infuse chemotherapy directly into her peritoneal cavity. As the solution poured into her abdomen, she felt increasing pressure. She asked the nurse to stop the fluid. The nurse called the physician, who said not to worry. Two hours later, Ms. Lopez became short of breath and demanded that the fluid be stopped. The nurse again called the doctor, but an hour later, Ms. Lopez died. Her abdomen was tense with fluid, which pushed on her lungs and stopped circulation through her inferior vena cava. The quality assurance committee reviewed the case as a preventable death and criticized the physician for giving too much fluid and failing to respond adequately to the nurse's call. The physician replied that he was not at fault; the

nurse had not told him how sick the patient was. The case was closed.

In 1989, a hospital placed Dr. Apple on probation for performing an excessive number of bronchoscopies; the probation was lifted after 6 months. In 1991, Dr. Apple was still performing bronchoscopies on almost all of his patients with chronic obstructive pulmonary disease, a condition for which bronchoscopy is generally not indicated. Dr. Apple often failed to perform the standard noninvasive diagnostic studies such as pulmonary function tests, chest x-rays, and arterial blood gas studies. A hospital committee drew up indications for bronchoscopy, but by 1993, Dr. Apple was still not following the guidelines. His staff privileges were terminated. Dr. Apple moved to another city and applied for privileges at another hospital.

To date, peer review has not been a particularly effective tool for improving the quality of medical care.

(1) Peer review often adheres to the Theory of Bad Apples, attempting to discipline physicians (to remove them from the apple barrel) for mistakes rather than to improve their practice through education. The physician who caused Ms. Lopez's preventable death responded to peer criticism by blaming the nurse rather than learning from the mistake.

A 1990 study found that Medicare PROs failed to use positive incentives to alter practice, relying on ineffective punitive methods (Lohr, 1990). Demonstrating the ultimate effect created by fear of punishment, several hospitals were recently investigated for altering quality assurance meeting notes to hide quality problems from the JCAHO (Gottlieb, 1992); physicians have behaved similarly (Prosser, 1992). Hiding mistakes rather than correcting them is the legacy of a punitive quality assurance apparatus (Leape, 1994).

(2) In cases of repeated negligence unchanged by educational efforts (eg, Dr. Apple, who truly should have been removed from the barrel), many quality assurance committees are reluctant to act firmly.

(3) Peer reviewers frequently disagree as to whether the quality of care in particular cases is adequate or not. In a study of one state PRO, reviewers found 18% of hospital records showing inadequate quality of care, while the PRO had found only 6%. Only one of three records judged by the PRO to be below standard were felt by the study to be deficient. The study concluded that quality of care judgments by the PRO and the study reviewers agreed little more than would be expected by chance (Rubin et al, 1992). Other studies confirm that different reviewers often disagree with one another and often miss cases of substandard care (Laffel and Berwick, 1993).

(4) Recent lawsuits have made peer reviewers frightened to confront physicians because reviewers have been subject to suits. For example, Dr. Timothy Patrick, an Oregon surgeon, sued the physicians involved in peer review proceedings after his hospital privileges had been revoked for alleged poor-quality care. Dr. Patrick, claiming that the reviewing physicians used the peer review process to remove him as a com-

petitor in the medical community, won the case and collected $2.2 million in damages and attorney fees. The Patrick case has made physicians reluctant to serve on quality assurance committees or to discipline physicians practicing poor-quality care (Dolin, 1985).

Peer review could be strengthened as part of an effort to improve quality of care. Practice guidelines could become the standards upon which to measure physician performance (Brook, 1989). Berwick's concept of CQI needs to gain more widespread acceptance. Gradual improvement in the skills and judgment of all physicians will have a greater impact on quality of care than identifying and disciplining a small number of incompetent physicians. While CQI seeks to educate rather than to punish, those physicians who consistently practice an unacceptable standard of care in spite of repeated educational attempts at quality improvement should be barred from practice in order to protect the public.

Quality Report Cards: While peer review was the health care quality solution devised in the 1970s, with CQI and practice guidelines following in the 1980s, the new quality kid on the block in the 1990s is the report card. Report cards are standardized, publicly released reports on the quality of care practiced by hospitals, HMOs, medical groups, or individual physicians (Epstein, 1995).

An early report card was the Health Care Financing Administration's (HCFA's) program for publishing hospital mortality rates among Medicare patients, hospital by hospital. The report card came under intense criticism because hospitals with sicker patients naturally had higher mortality rates and looked worse in the public eye. The program was abandoned when HCFA decided—even after trying to adjust the data for severity of illness—that the data were too inaccurate to be useful (Blumenthal, 1996).

An important experiment in individual physician report cards was initiated by the New York State Department of Health in 1990. The department released data on risk-adjusted mortality rates for coronary bypass surgery performed at each hospital in the state, and in 1992 mortality rates were also published for each cardiac surgeon. Each year's list was big news, and highly controversial. The attempt to adjust mortality data for severity of illness is sophisticated enough to be recognized as the gold standard among systems of its kind; but even with this level of sophistication, the risk-adjustment methodology is limited. The problems are highlighted when one considers that in 1 year, 46% of the surgeons had moved from one half of the ranked list to the other.

Several fascinating results came of this project, which continues to function:

(1) Patients did not switch from hospitals with high mortality rates to those with lower mortality rates.

(2) Twenty-seven low-volume surgeons with risk-adjusted mortality rates 2.5 to 5 times the state average stopped performing coronary bypass surgery in New York State.

(3) In 4 years, risk-adjusted coronary artery bypass mortality dropped by 41% in New York State. Mortality for this operation has dropped in states without report cards, but not as much.

(4) Some surgeons, worried about the report cards, may have elected not to operate on the most risky patients in order to improve their report card ranking. It is possible that the reduction in surgical mortality in part resulted from denial of surgery to the sickest patients.

(5) Gaming the system, hospitals dramatically increased their reporting of coexisting medical conditions (making their patients appear sicker), thereby "upcoding" their surgeries into more risky endeavors and allowing their mortality rates to be adjusted downward.

However the New York State report card is ultimately judged, it appears to have improved the quality of care for coronary artery surgery and is being copied by other states (Green and Wintfeld, 1995; Chassin et al, 1996; Epstein, 1995).

The most important report card experiment of the late 1990s is the Health Plan Employer Data and Information Set (HEDIS). Developed by the National Committee for Quality Assurance (NCQA), a private organization controlled by large HMOs and large employers, HEDIS (version 3.0) is a list of over 70 performance indicators that can be used to evaluate HMOs. Some of the performance indicators measure patient satisfaction, access to care, utilization rates, and health plan finances; others measure quality. The quality measures include the percentage of children immunized; the percentage of enrollees of certain ages who have received cholesterol screening, Pap smears, and mammograms; the percentage of pregnant women who received prenatal care in the first trimester; the percentage of diabetics who receive retinal examinations; and the percentage of smokers for whom physicians made efforts at smoking cessation. Public report cards can be issued on HMOs listing their scores on these performance indicators.

HEDIS is a step forward in putting quality higher on the health care agenda. But HEDIS has major problems. A far less sophisticated series of measurements than the New York coronary artery bypass program, HEDIS does not risk-adjust for HMOs with sicker populations; thus, HEDIS encourages HMOs to sign up healthier people in order to look better to the public. HEDIS tends not to measure care for the seriously and chronically ill; HMOs scoring well on mammograms and Pap smears may have superior ratings in the public eye yet restrict expensive care to those who most need it. Physicians with HMO contracts are constantly being reminded to order mammograms and cholesterol tests and to send diabetics to ophthalmologists so that HMOs can score high on HEDIS measures; yet the HMO may pressure those same physicians to expedite the discharge of an elderly sick patient from the hospital. Even if an HMO does poorly on the HEDIS report card, families may be unable to leave that HMO; 48% of employees are offered only a single health plan by their employer. Moreover, a 1995 survey revealed that 97% of employers consider cost when choosing a health plan for employees, while only 29% consider quality (Epstein, 1995; Iglehart, 1996; Etheredge et al, 1996).

Financially Neutral Clinical Decision Making: For decades, most U.S. physicians have been paid on a fee-for-service basis. This type of payment gives physicians an incentive to work hard for each patient, to gain the patient's trust so that the patient will continue to come back, and, in the case of specialists, to perform timely, effective consultations and procedures for patients referred by generalist physicians so that those generalists will continue to send referrals. Fee-for-service payment has many features that improve quality of care.

The emerging payment mode, capitation, also has positive attributes. Physicians who provide excellent care will have many patients enrolled in their practices and will receive many capitation payments over many years.

However, in the increasingly business oriented health care environment, both fee-for-service and capitation payment have in some circumstances become commercialized, with potentially negative consequences for quality care.

> At their quarterly meeting, the physician partners unanimously voted to grant business manager Hy Buck a 20% raise. After all, it was Mr. Buck who had increased each physician's income by 30% in 2 years. Mr. Buck had persuaded the doctors to invest in a new MRI facility; each MRI generated $50 in profit for the ordering doctor. As an unwritten rule, each doctor ordered one MRI each day. In the second year, each physician earned $30,000 from the investment. Mr. Buck lobbied against Representative Pete Stark's legislation that would prohibit such arrangements.
>
> Mr. Buck knew how to "game" fee-for-service and capitation systems. Receptionists were instructed to allow only 10 appointments per day for patients in capitated plans, thereby freeing up as many slots as possible for fee-for-service clients. The average capitated patient, for whom the practice received $144 annually, was seen only once a year, thereby providing excellent returns from capitation contracts and allowing fee-for-service patients to be seen often. Surely, Mr. Buck was worth every cent of his $200,000 salary.

In a milieu of clinical uncertainty, financial factors can and do influence the quantity and quality of care that patients receive. The quest for quality care encompasses a search for a financial structure that does not reward over- or undertreatment and that separates physicians' personal incomes from their clinical decisions.

> Dr. Ella Justice liked her work as a general internist in a 35-member multispecialty group practice. She arrived at 8 AM to do hospital rounds and walked across the street to start her office visits at 9 AM. During her hour lunchtime, she returned to the hospital, did paperwork, or took a 2-mile walk with a colleague. She went home between 6 and 7 PM. Three nights a month and one weekend per year she was on call, which was exhausting but infrequent. Dr. Justice received a salary of $130,000 and never worried about issues related to health insurance or patient billing.

Payment by salary represents one possible escape from the payment–treatment nexus; under this arrangement, there is no direct relation between clinical decisions and physician income. Salaried physicians may face pressures that reestablish the payment–treatment linkage, however. Physicians receiving a salary are not paid more for doing extra work and thus might try to keep their appointment books light, and might choose not to hospitalize a patient or make a home visit. Doctors salaried by for-profit HMOs might be forced by management to undertreat, in order to increase HMO profits (Scovern, 1988).

Another method of minimizing the payment–treatment nexus is the traditional mode of paying general practitioners in the United Kingdom (see Chapter 14). Each physician receives a capitation payment but is rewarded with additional fees for performing preventive services and home visits. Such a balance of overtreatment and undertreatment incentives may provide a neutral financial environment.

Financially neutral clinical decision making will always be an ideal and never a reality, but laws can be passed that eliminate the worst abuses of the payment–treatment nexus. Federal laws passed in the early 1990s prohibit physicians from sending Medicare or Medicaid patients to a business providing diagnostic and treatment services if the physician has a financial interest in the business. In 1997, HCFA issued regulations limiting the bonuses that physicians can receive for reducing services to Medicare and Medicaid managed care patients. Dr. Arnold Relman (1988) has proposed three guidelines for practicing medicine in the current business-driven health care climate:

> First, salaried physicians should, whenever possible, work for a self-regulated, physician-managed professional group and not be direct employees of a business organization. This helps ensure the precedence of professional values over business imperatives that may be incompatible with the proper care of patients. Second, in the absence of a physician-managed group, individual practicing physicians should work only for nonprofit institutions committed to community service and should avoid direct employment by investor-owned businesses. Finally, regardless of the employing organization, no physician should enter into any arrangement offering rewards for withholding services or for increasing the use of services. (Relman AS: Salaried physicians and economic incentives. N Engl J Med 1988;319: 784. Abstracted from information appearing in *New England Journal of Medicine.*)

Improving Institutions   Maximizing excellence for individual health care professionals is only one ingredient in the recipe for high-quality health care. Improving institutions is the other, through CQI techniques. CQI involves the identification of concrete problems and the formation of interdisciplinary teams to gather data and propose and implement solutions to the problems.

> In LDS Hospital in Salt Lake City, variation in wound infection rates by different physicians was related to the timing of the administration of prophylactic antibiotics. Patients who received antibiotics 2 hours before surgery had the lowest infection rates. The surgery department adopted a policy that all patients receive antibiotics precisely 2 hours before surgery; the rate of postoperative wound infections dropped from 1.8% to 0.4% (Blumenthal D: Total quality management and physicians' clinical decisions. JAMA 1993;269:2775.)

Such successes only dot, but do not dominate, the health care quality landscape. CQI is hard to accomplish. In financially strapped and understaffed hospitals, finding time for administrators to organize CQI teams and for employee members of these teams to meet is a hurdle. Physicians, key players in CQI projects, often do not participate. For-profit institutions may not see CQI as affecting their bottom line. The long-term promise of CQI is its potential not only to improve quality but to reduce waste and save money as well.

CQI can bring workable systems into institutions; equally important is to bring together institutions into workable systems. To avoid the quality problems of specialty units with a low volume of procedures, each "high-tech" capability must be concentrated in a select number of facilities in each geographic region. A strong program of regional planning could eliminate the unnecessary duplication of facilities—rooted in destructive competitive arrangements between health care institutions—that undermines high-quality care. It makes no sense to apply CQI methods to upgrade the quality of a cardiac surgery unit that should be closed.

WHERE DOES MALPRACTICE REFORM FIT IN?

During a coronary angiogram, emboli traveled to the brain of Ivan Romanov, resulting in a serious stroke, with loss of use of his left arm and leg. The angiogram was appropriate and performed without any technical errors. Mr. Romanov had suffered a medical injury (an injury caused by his medical treatment), but the event was not due to negligence.

During a D&C, Judy Morrison's physician unknowingly perforated the uterus and lacerated the colon. Ms. Morrison reported severe pain, but was sent home without further evaluation. She returned 1 hour later to the emergency room with persistent pain and internal bleeding. She required a two-stage surgical repair over the following 4 months. This medical injury was found by the legal system to be negligent.

A peculiar set of institutions, called the malpractice liability system, forms an important part of U.S. health care. The goals of the malpractice system are twofold: to financially compensate people who, in the course of seeking medical care, have suffered medical injuries; and to prevent physicians and other health care personnel from negligently causing harm to their patients.

The existing malpractice system scores miserably on both counts. According to the Harvard Medical Practice Study, only 2% of patients who suffer adverse events caused by medical negligence file malpractice claims that would allow them to receive compensation, meaning that the malpractice system fails in its first goal. Moreover, the system does not deal with 98% of negligent acts performed by physicians, making it difficult to attain its second goal. Not only is the malpractice system a failure in terms of its own goals; it has serious negative side effects on medical practice (Localio et al, 1991) (Table 12–2).

(1) The system assumes that punishment, which usually involves physicians paying large amounts of money to a malpractice insurer plus enduring the overwhelming stress of a malpractice jury trial, is a reasonable method for improving the quality of medical care. Berwick's analysis of the Theory of Bad Apples suggests that fear of a lawsuit closes physicians' minds to improvement and generates an "I didn't do it" response. Malpractice litigation often discourages quality assurance; if lawyers have access to hospital committee records, physicians do not want to participate in quality assurance activities. Avoidance of malpractice suits leads doctors to deny the errors they make, even understandable nonnegligent errors. The entire atmosphere created by malpractice litigation clouds a clear analytic assessment of quality.

Table 12–2. Malpractice claims and quality of care.[1]

In 1 million hospital admissions, 37,000 patients suffer medical injuries caused by their medical management.
Of the 37,000 medical injuries, 10,212 are due to negligence. Negligence is the failure to meet the standard of
  practice of an average qualified physician practicing in the same specialty.
Of the 10,212 patients suffering medical injuries due to negligence, 204 file malpractice claims.
Of the 204 people filing malpractice claims, about 102 receive some compensation.
Thus,
Only 1% (102 of 10,212) of patients suffering a medical injury due to negligence receive any compensation for that
  injury. Ninety-nine percent receive no compensation.

Of 100 malpractice claims filed, only 17 involve cases of medical negligence. Eighty-three percent of malpractice
  claims do not involve medical negligence.
Thus,
Ninety-nine percent of patients who have been negligently harmed receive no compensation, and 83% of physicians
  who are sued for malpractice have not acted negligently. The malpractice system does not appear to be working
  for either patients or physicians.

[1] Data extracted from Brennan TA et al: Incidence of adverse events and negligence in hospitalized patients. N Engl J Med 1991;324:370; Localio AR et al: Relation between malpractice claims and adverse events due to negligence. N Engl J Med 1991;325:245; and Weiler PC, Newhouse JP, Hiatt HH: Proposal for medical liability reform. JAMA 1992;267:2355.

(2) The system is wasteful, with less than half of malpractice insurance premiums paid by physicians and other providers actually reaching patients in the form of compensation; the larger portion of malpractice money is spent on lawyers, court costs, and insurance overhead (Manuel, 1990). Recall that in the Harvard Medical Practice Study, only 28% of medical injuries actually involved negligence (Brennan et al, 1991). Many claims have no merit but create enormous waste and wreak unnecessary stress upon physicians. A recent study found that patients granted malpractice award payments had frequently received no negligent care, and patients subjected to negligent care often received no malpractice payments (Brennan et al, 1996).

(3) The system appears to generate unnecessary care, provided solely for the purpose of looking good in case of a malpractice claim. The total cost of such "defensive medicine" may approximate 2% of the nation's health expenditures.

(4) The system is based on the assumption that trial by jury is the best method of determining whether there has been negligence, and this is a highly questionable assumption.

(5) People with lower incomes generally receive smaller awards (because wages lost from a medical injury are lower) and are therefore less attractive to lawyers, who are generally paid as a percentage of the award. Accordingly, low-income patients, who suffer more medical injury, are less likely than wealthier people to file malpractice claims (Burstin et al, 1993b).

(6) Injured patients are not compensated in a timely manner. A study in New York State demonstrated that the average claim was settled about 6 years after it was filed (Garnick et al, 1991).

In summary, the malpractice system is burdened with expensive, unfounded litigation that harasses doctors who have done nothing wrong, while failing to discipline or educate most physicians committing actual medical negligence and to compensate most true victims of negligence.

A number of proposals have been made for malpractice reform. Some, which have been lumped under the heading of tort reform, simply serve to reduce a physician's malpractice insurance premiums and make little attempt to improve quality of care. More consequential proposals tackle the dual problems of compensating victims and improving quality.

> Mei Tagaloa underwent neurosurgery for compression of his spinal cord by a cervical disk. On awakening from the surgery, Mr. Tagaloa was unable to move his legs or arms at all. After 3 months of rehabilitation, he ended up as a wheelchair-bound paraplegic. He sued the neurosurgeon and his family physician. The physicians' malpractice insurer paid for lawyers to defend them. Mr. Tagaloa's lawyer used the system of contingency fees, whereby he would receive one-third of the settlement if Mr. Tagaloa won the case but would receive nothing if Mr. Tagaloa lost.
>
> After 18 months, the case went to trial; the physicians left their practices and sat in the courtroom for 3 weeks. Each physician spent many hours going over records and discussing the case with the lawyers. The family physician, who had nothing to do with the surgery, was so upset with the proceedings that he developed an ulcer. The jury found the family physician innocent and the neurosurgeon guilty of negligence. The family physician lost $8000 in income because of absence from his practice. The neurosurgeon's malpractice insurer paid $900,000 to Mr. Tagaloa, who paid $300,000 to the lawyer.

Tort Reform   A tort is a wrongful act or injury done willfully or negligently. Negligence refers to a lack of care or concern. Medical malpractice, then, fits into the larger legal field of torts. Tort reform has come to mean little more than reductions in malpractice costs for physicians. The California Medical Injury Compensation Reform Act and the Indiana Medical Malpractice Act are examples of tort reform; these acts have placed caps on damages awarded to injured parties and limits on lawyers' contingency fees. Tort reform is unfair to the patients hurt most by negligence because those who suffer the least serious injuries tend to receive compensation greater than their actual losses in medical bills and lost wages, while those with totally disabling injuries often receive awards for only a fraction of their losses. A cap on awards hurts those with the worst injuries (Saks, 1993) (Table 12–3).

Alternative Dispute Resolution   These programs would substitute mediation and arbitration for jury trials in the case of medical injury. The American Medical Association has proposed the establishment of state medical boards to settle cases. Alternatives to the jury trial could bring more compensation to injured parties by reducing legal costs, and might shift the dispute settlement to a more scientific, less emotional theater.

The Use of Practice Guidelines to Resolve Claims   A great deal of legal effort is spent in determining whether a physician named in a malpractice claim was practicing below the community standard of care. Practice guidelines could be a yardstick to judge more easily whether a physician was negligent, thereby reducing the number

Table 12–3. Malpractice reform options.

Tort reform:	Placing limits on malpractice awards paid to patients
Alternative dispute resolution:	Substituting mediation and arbitration for jury trials
Use of practice guidelines:	Improving the ability to determine whether a physician was negligent
No-fault reform:	Providing compensation to patients suffering medical injury regardless of whether the injury is due to negligence
Enterprise liability:	Making institutions (hospitals and HMOs) responsible for compensating medical injuries on a no-fault basis, thereby creating incentives for institutions to improve the quality of care provided

and cost of malpractice cases. The difficulty with this approach is that practice guidelines, which only work in straightforward medical cases, would not apply to 80% of malpractice claims, many of which involve more complex, cloudy clinical situations (Garnick et al, 1991).

No-Fault Malpractice Reform   Proposals have been made to switch compensation for medical injury from the tort system to a no-fault plan (Manuel, 1990). Under no-fault malpractice, patients suffering medical injury would receive compensation whether or not the injury was due to negligence. Without costly lawyers' fees and jury trials, waste would drop from over 50% to about 20%. A no-fault system would compensate far more people and would cost about the same as the current tort system (Johnson et al, 1992). While the no-fault approach appears superior to the tort system in compensating injured people, it plays no role in quality improvement and perhaps takes physicians "off the hook" for negligent acts.

Enterprise Liability   A relatively new idea for malpractice reform is to make health care institutions—primarily hospitals and HMOs—responsible for compensating medical injuries (Weiler et al, 1992). As with no-fault proposals, patients suffering medical injury would be compensated whether or not the injury is negligent. Enterprise liability improves upon the no-fault concept by making institutions pay more if they are the site of more medical injuries (whether caused by system failure or physician error). Institutions would pay more through experience-rated malpractice insurance premiums: Hospitals or HMOs with more claims for medical injury would have higher insurance premiums than institutions with lower rates of medical injury. Hospitals and HMOs, then, would have a financial incentive to improve the quality of their systems and of their professionals. Jury trials and towering legal fees would be averted because there would be no need to prove negligence.

CONCLUSION

In 1993, people in the United States made over 700 million visits to physicians' offices, had hundreds of millions of contacts with other health care givers, and spent over 150 million days in acute care hospitals. While quality of care provided during most of these encounters was excellent, the goal of the health care system should be to deliver high-quality care every day to every patient. This goal presents an unending challenge to each health care giver and health care institution. Physicians make hundreds of decisions each day, including which questions to ask in the patient history, which parts of the body to examine in the physical examination, which laboratory tests and x-rays to order and how urgently, which diagnoses to entertain, which treatments to offer, when to have the patient return for follow-up, and whether other physicians need to be consulted. Nurse practitioners, physician assistants, nurses, and other care givers face similar numbers of decisions. It is humanly impossible to make all these decisions correctly every day. For health care to be of high quality, mistakes should be minimized, mistakes with serious consequences should be avoided, and systems should be in place that reduce, detect, and correct errors to the greatest extent possible (Leape, 1994). Even when all decisions are technically accurate, if care givers are insensitive or fail to provide the patient with a full range of informed choices, quality is impaired.

For the clinician, each decision that influences quality of care may be simple, but the sum total of all decisions of all care givers impacting on a patient's illness makes the achievement of high-quality care elusive. To safeguard quality of care, our nation needs laws and regulations, including standards for health professional education, rules for licensure, boards with the authority to discipline clear violators, and teams to assess how a hospital or group practice is functioning. But improvement of health care quality cannot rely on regulators in Washington, D.C., in state capitals, or across town; it must come from within each institution, whether a three-physician practice, a community hospital, or a huge HMO.

The people who observe problems in quality are the people who work in the room where the problems occur. Operating room nurses know which surgeons are technically competent and which are not. Physicians in group practices who cover for one another's patients on weekends or vacations can judge each other's knowledge and judgment. Pharmacists know which doctors prescribe medications correctly and which do not. Nurses, radiology technicians, and physical therapists, among others, know which hospital departments are well organized and competently run and which need improvement. The elevation of health care quality to a higher plane requires an adequate number of well-trained people working in teams in rational administrative systems. It also requires that health care givers tell each other when something is going wrong; uncovering low quality is the first step toward achieving high quality.

REFERENCES

Anders G: Health Against Wealth. HMOs and the Breakdown of Medical Trust. Houghton Mifflin Company, 1996.

Ayanian JZ: Race, class, and the quality of medical care. JAMA 1994;271:1207.

Berwick DM: Continuous improvement as an ideal in health care. N Engl J Med 1989;320:53.

Berwick DM: The double edge of knowledge. JAMA 1991;266:841.

Berwick DM: Payment by capitation and the quality of care. N Engl J Med 1996;335:1227.

Berwick DM, Godfrey AB, Roessner J: Curing Health Care. Jossey-Bass, 1990.

Blumenthal D: Quality of care: What is it? N Engl J Med 1996;335:891.

Blumenthal D: Total quality management and physicians' clinical decisions. JAMA 1993; 269:2775.

Brennan TA, Sox CM, Burstin HR: Relation between negligent adverse events and the outcomes of medical-malpractice litigation. N Engl J Med 1996;335:1963.

Brennan TA et al: Incidence of adverse events and negligence in hospitalized patients. N Engl J Med 1991;324:370.

Brook RH: Practice guidelines and practicing medicine: Are they compatible? JAMA 1989;262:3027.

Brook RH: Quality of care: Do we care? Ann Intern Med 1991;115:486.

Brook RH, Kamberg CJ, McGlynn EA: Health system reform and quality. JAMA 1996;276:476.

Bunker J: Surgical manpower. N Engl J Med 1970;282:135.

Burstin HR et al: Do the poor sue more? JAMA 1993b;270:1697.

Burstin HR et al: The effect of hospital financial characteristics on quality of care. JAMA 1993a;270:845.

Chassin MR, Hannan EL, DeBuono BA: Benefits and hazards of reporting medical outcomes publicly. N Engl J Med 1996;334:394.

Cunningham FG et al: Williams Obstetrics, 19th ed. Appleton and Lange, 1993.

Dolin LC: Antitrust law versus peer review. N Engl J Med 1985;313:1156.

Donabedian A: The quality of care: How can it be assessed? JAMA 1988;260:1743.

Dubois RW, Brook RH: Preventable deaths: Who, how often, and why? Ann Intern Med 1988;109:582.

Eddy DM: Three battles to watch in the 1990s. JAMA 1993;270:520.

Epstein A: Performance reports on quality: Prototypes, problems, and prospects. N Engl J Med 1995;333:57.

Etheredge L, Jones SB, Lewin L: What is driving health system change? Health Aff 1996;15(4):93.

Fagin CM: Cost-effectiveness of nursing care revisited: 1981–1990. In: Health Policy and Nursing. Harrington C, Estes CL (editors). Jones & Bartlett, 1994.

Feinstein RJ: The ethics of professional regulation. N Engl J Med 1985;312:801.

Garnick DW, Hendricks AM, Brennan TA: Can practice guidelines reduce the number and costs of malpractice claims? JAMA 1991;266:2856.

Gottlieb M: Hospitals are warned not to rewrite records. New York Times, May 10, 1992.

Greco PJ, Eisenberg JM: Changing physicians' practices. N Engl J Med 1993;329:1271.

Green J, Wintfeld N: Report cards on cardiac surgeons: Assessing New York State's approach. N Engl J Med 1995;332:1229.

Hemenway D et al: Physicians' responses to financial incentives. N Engl J Med 1990;322:1059.

Hillman BJ et al: Frequency and costs of diagnostic imaging in office patients: A comparison of self-referring and radiologist-referring physicians. N Engl J Med 1990;323:1604.

Iglehart JK: The National Committee for Quality Assurance. N Engl J Med 1996;335:995.

Johnson WG et al: The economic consequences of medical injuries: Implications for a no-fault insurance plan. N Engl J Med 1992;267:2487.

Kassirer JP: The quality of care and the quality of measuring it. N Engl J Med 1993;329:1263.

Knaus WA et al: An evaluation of outcome from intensive care in major medical centers. Ann Intern Med 1986;104:410.

Kritchevsky SB, Simmons BP: Continuous quality improvement: Concepts and applications for physician care. JAMA 1991;266:1817.

Laffel GL, Berwick DM: Quality health care. JAMA 1993;270:254.

Leape LL: Error in medicine. JAMA 1994;272:1851.

Leape LL: Practice guidelines and standards: An overview. Qual Rev Bull 1990;16(2):42.

Leape LL: Unnecessary surgery. Ann Rev Public Health 1992;13:363.

Leape LL et al: The nature of adverse events in hospitalized patients. N Engl J Med 1991;324:377.

Localio AR et al: Relation between malpractice claims and adverse events due to negligence. N Engl J Med 1991;325:245.

Lohr KN (editor): Medicare: A Strategy for Quality Assurance. National Academy Press, 1990.

Luce JM, Bindman AB, Lee PR: A brief history of health care quality assessment and improvement in the United States. West J Med 1994;160:263.

Luft HS et al: Hospital Volume, Physician Volume, and Patient Outcomes: Assessing the Evidence. Health Administration Press, 1990.

Manuel BM: Professional liability: A no-fault solution. N Engl J Med 1990;322:627.

Mitchell JM, Scott E: New evidence of the prevalence and scope of physician joint ventures. JAMA 1992;268:80.

Moore F: What puts the surge in surgery? N Engl J Med 1970;282:162.

Prosser RL: Alteration of medical records submitted for medicolegal review. JAMA 1992;267:2630.

Relman AS: The future of medical practice. Health Aff 1983;2(2):5.

Relman AS: Salaried physicians and economic incentives. N Engl J Med 1988;319:784.

Rodwin MA: Medicine, Money and Morals: Physicians' Conflicts of Interest. Oxford Univ Press, 1993.

Rothman BK: Encyclopedia of Childbearing. Oryx Press, 1993.

Rubin HR et al: Watching the doctor-watchers: How well do peer review organization methods detect hospital care quality problems? JAMA 1992;267:2349.

Saks MJ: Malpractice roulette. New York Times, July 3, 1993.

Sanders E: Audit slams health group. San Francisco Examiner, Oct 2, 1994.

Schiff GD et al: A better quality alternative: Single payer national health reform. JAMA 1994;272:803.

Schroeder SA: Outcome assessment 70 years later: Are we ready? N Engl J Med 1987;316:160.

Scovern H: Hired help: A physician's experience in a for-profit staff-model HMO. N Engl J Med 1988;319:787.

Stafford RS: The impact of nonclinical factors on repeat cesarean section. JAMA 1991;265:59.

U.S. House of Representatives: 45th Report by the Committee on Government Operations, April 14, 1988. Medicare Health Maintenance Organizations: The International Medical Centers Experience. U.S. Government Printing Office, 1988.

U.S. Senate: Hearings before the Permanent Subcommittee on Investigations, Committee on Government Operations, March 13 and 14, 1975. Prepaid Health Plans. U.S. Government Printing Office, 1975.

Ware JE et al: Comparison of health outcomes at a health maintenance organization with those of fee-for-service care. Lancet 1986;1:1017.

Webber A: History and mission of quality assurance in the public sector. In: Perspectives on Quality in American Health Care. Hughes EFX (editor). McGraw-Hill Healthcare Information Center, 1988.

Weiler PC, Newhouse JP, Hiatt HH: Proposal for medical liability reform. JAMA 1992;267:2355.

Wennberg J: Which rate is right? N Engl J Med 1986:314:310.

Wennberg JE: Outcomes research, cost containment, and the fear of health care rationing. N Engl J Med 1990;323:1202.

Medical Ethics & the Rationing of Health Care

13

For those who work in the healing professions, ethical values play a special role. The specific content of medical ethics was first formulated centuries ago, based on the sayings of Hippocrates and others. The refinement of medical ethics has continued up to the present by practicing health care givers, health professional and religious organizations, and individual ethicists. As medical technology, health care financing, and the organization of health care transform themselves, so must the content of medical ethics change in order to acknowledge and guide new circumstances.

FOUR PRINCIPLES OF MEDICAL ETHICS

Over the years, participants in and observers of medical care have distilled widely shared human beliefs about healing the sick into four major ethical principles: beneficence, nonmaleficence, autonomy, and justice (Beauchamp and Childress, 1994) (Table 13–1).

Beneficence is the obligation of health care providers to help people in need.

> Dr. Rolando Bueno is a hard-working family physician practicing in a low-income neighborhood of a large city. He shows concern for his patients, and his knowledge and judgment are respected by his medical and nursing colleagues. On one occasion, he was called before the hospital quality assurance committee when one of his patients unexpectedly died; he agreed that he had made mistakes in her care and incorporated the lessons of the case into his future practice.

Dr. Bueno tries to live up to the ideal of beneficence. He does not always succeed; like all physicians, he sometimes makes clinical errors. Overall, he treats his patients to the best of his ability. The principle of beneficence in the healing professions is the obligation to help people in poor health.

Nonmaleficence is the duty of health care providers to do no harm.

> Ms. Lucy Knight suffers from insomnia and Parkinson's disease. The insomnia does not bother her, because she likes to read at night, but it irritates her husband. Mr. Knight requests his wife's physician to order strong sleeping pills for her, but the doctor declines, saying that the combination of sleeping pills and Parkinson's disease places Mrs. Knight at high risk for a serious fall.

The modern array of medical interventions has the capacity to do good or harm, or both, thereby enmeshing the principle of nonmaleficence with the principle of beneficence. In the case of Ms. Knight, the prescribing of sedatives has far more potential

Table 13–1. The four principles of medical ethics.

Beneficence:	The obligation of health care providers to help people in need
Nonmaleficence:	The duty of health care providers to do no harm
Autonomy:	The right of patients to make choices regarding their health care
Justice:	The concept of treating everyone in a fair manner

for harm than for good, particularly because Ms. Knight does not see her insomnia as a problem.

Autonomy is the right of a person to choose and follow his or her own plan of life and action.

> Mr. Winter is a frail 88-year-old found by Dr. James Washington, his family physician, to have colon cancer, which has spread to the liver. The cancer is causing no symptoms. An oncologist gives Mr. Winter the option of transfusions, parenteral nutrition, and surgery, followed by chemotherapy; or watchful waiting with palliative and hospice care when symptoms appear. Mr. Winter is terrified of hospitals and prefers to remain at home. He feels that he might live a comfortable couple of years before the cancer claims his life. After talking it over with Dr. Washington, he chooses the second option.

The principle of autonomy adds another consideration to the interrelated principles of beneficence and nonmaleficence. Would Mr. Winter enjoy a longer comfortable life by submitting himself to aggressive cancer therapy that does harm in order to do good? Or does he sense that the harm may exceed the good? The balance of risks and benefits confronts each physician on a daily basis (Eddy, 1990). But the decision cannot be made solely by a risk–benefit analysis; the patient's preference is a critical addition to the equation.

Autonomy is founded in the overall desire of most human beings to control their own destiny, to have choices in life, and to live in a society that places value on individual freedom. In medical ethics, autonomy refers to the right of competent adult patients to consent to or refuse treatment. While the physician has an obligation to respect the patient's wishes, he or she also has a duty to fully inform the patient of the probable consequences of those wishes. For children and for adults unable to make medical decisions, a parent, guardian, other family member, or surrogate decision maker named in a legal document becomes the autonomous agent on behalf of the patient.

Justice refers to the ethical concept of treating everyone in a fair manner.

> Joe, a white businessman in the suburbs, suffers crushing chest pain and within 5 minutes is taken to a nearby private emergency room, where he receives immediate thrombolytic therapy and state-of-the-art treatment for a heart attack. Five miles away, in a poor neighborhood, Josephine, an African-American woman, experiences severe chest pain, calls 911, waits 25 minutes for help to arrive, and is brought to a public hospital whose emergency department staff is attending to five other acutely ill patients. Before receiving appropriate attention, she suffers an arrhythmia and dies.

The principle of justice as applied to medical ethics is newer, more controversial, and harder to define than the principles of beneficence, nonmaleficence, and autonomy. In a general sense, people are treated justly when they receive what they deserve. It is unjust not to grant a medical degree to someone who completes medical school and passes all the necessary examinations. It is unjust to punish a person who did not commit a crime. In another meaning, justice refers to universal rights: to receive enough to eat, to be afforded shelter, to have access to basic medical care and education, and to be able to speak freely. If these rights are denied, justice has been violated. In yet another version, justice connotes equal opportunity: All people should have an equal chance to realize their human potential. Justice might be linked to the golden rule: Treat others as you would want others to treat you. While there is no clear agreement on the precise meaning of justice, most people would agree that the differential treatment of Joe and Josephine is unjust.

Distributive Justice   In exploring the concept of justice, one area of concern is the allocation of benefits and burdens in society. This realm of ethical thinking is called distributive justice, and it involves such questions as: Who receives what amount of wealth, of education, or of medical care? Who pays what amount of taxes?

The principle of justice is linked to the idea of fairness. In the arena of distributive justice, no agreement exists on what formula for allocating benefits and costs is fair. Should each person get an equal share? Should those who work harder receive more? Should the proper formula be "to each according to ability to pay," as determined by a free market? Or "to each according to need?" In allocating costs, should each person pay an equal share or should those with greater wealth pay more? Most societies construct a mixture of these allocation formulas. Unemployment benefits consider effort (having had a job) and need (having lost the job). Welfare benefits are primarily based on need. Job promotions may be based on merit. Many goods are distributed according to ability to pay. Primary education in theory (but not always in practice) is founded on the belief that everyone should receive an equal share (Beauchamp and Childress, 1994; Jonsen et al, 1992).

How is the principle of distributive justice formulated for medical care? The answer to this question must be grounded in historical trends and political debates. Throughout the history of the developed world, the concept that health care is a privilege that should be allocated according to ability to pay has competed with the idea that health care is a right and should be distributed according to need. In most developed nations, the allocation of health care according to need has become the dominant political belief, as demonstrated by the passage of universal or near-universal health insurance laws. In the United States, the failure of the 80-year battle to enact national health insurance attests to the ongoing debate between ability to pay and need as the doctrine of fairness in health care (see Chapter 15). Yet the general public, in contrast to more powerful interest groups with greater influence on the political process, for decades has endorsed the idea that basic health care should be allocated according to need. By the 1990s, this opinion had become accepted not only by most of the public, but also by many political, professional, labor, and religious organizations. For example, the President's Commission on the Study of Ethical Problems in Medicine and Biomedical and Behavioral Research (1983) affirmed society's obligation to ensure equitable access to an adequate level of health care without the imposition of excessive burdens.

If the overwhelming opinion in the developed world and in the United States holds that health care should be allocated according to need, then all people should have equal access to a reasonable level of medical care without financial barriers (ie, people should have a right to health care). In this chapter, therefore, we consider that the principle of distributive justice requires all people to equally receive a reasonable level of medical services based on medical need without regard to ability to pay.

ETHICAL DILEMMAS OLD & NEW

Ethical dilemmas (Lo, 1995) are situations in which a provider of medical care is forced to make a decision that violates one of the four principles of medical ethics in order to adhere to another of the principles. Ethical dilemmas always involve disputes in which both sides have an ethical underpinning to their position. Financial conflicts of interest on the part of physicians (see Chapters 4, 5, and 12), in contrast, pit ethical behavior against individual gain and are not ethical dilemmas.

> Anthony, a 22-year-old Jehovah's Witness, is admitted to the intensive care unit for gastrointestinal bleeding. His blood pressure is 80/60 mm Hg, and in the past 4 hours, his hematocrit has fallen from 38 to 21%. The medical resident implores Anthony to accept life-saving transfusions, but he refuses, saying that his religion teaches him that death is preferable to receiving blood products. When the blood pressure reaches 60/20 mm Hg, the desperate resident decides to give the blood while Anthony is unconscious. The attending physician vetoes the plan, saying that the patient has the right to refuse treatment, even if an avoidable death is the outcome.

In Anthony's case, the ethical dilemma is a conflict between beneficence and autonomy. Which principle has priority depends on the particular situation, and in this case, autonomy supersedes beneficence. If the patient were a child without sufficient knowledge or reasoning capability to make an informed choice, the physician would not be obligated to withhold transfusions, even if the family so demanded (Jonsen et al, 1992).

> Pedro Navarro has a lung cancer that has metastasized to his brain. No effective treatment is available, and Mr. Navarro is confused and unable to understand his medical condition. Mrs. Navarro demands that her husband undergo craniotomy to remove the tumor. The neurosurgeon refuses, arguing that the operation will do Mr. Navarro no good whatsoever and will cause him additional suffering.

The case of Mr. Navarro pits the principle of autonomy against the principle of nonmaleficence. Mr. Navarro's rightful surrogate decision maker, his wife, wants a particular course of treatment, but the neurosurgeon knows that this treatment will cause Mr. Navarro considerable harm and do him no good. In this case, nonmaleficence triumphs. Whereas patient autonomy allows the right to refuse treatment, it does not include the right to demand a harmful or ineffectual treatment.

The traditional dilemmas described in many articles and books on medical ethics feature beneficence or nonmaleficence in conflict with autonomy. In two famous ethical dilemmas, the families of Karen Ann Quinlan and Nancy Cruzan, young women with severe brain damage (persistent vegetative state), asked that physicians discontinue a respirator (in the Quinlan case) and a feeding tube (in the Cruzan case). Both cases were adjudicated in the courts. The Quinlan decision promoted the right of patients or their surrogate decision makers to withdraw treatment, even if the treatment is necessary to sustain life. The outcome of the Cruzan case placed limits on autonomy by requiring that life-supporting treatment can only be withdrawn when a patient has stated his or her wishes clearly in advance (Annas, 1993). Overall, medical ethics has moved in the direction of giving priority to the principle of autonomy over those of beneficence and nonmaleficence. For years, medical ethics has emphasized the individual doctor–patient relationship as its chief concern. In the late twentieth century, a new generation of ethical dilemmas emerged, moving beyond the individual physician–patient relationship to involve the broader society. These social–ethical problems derive from the new reality that money may not be available to pay for a reasonable level of medical services for all people.

When money and resources are bountiful, the issue of distributive justice refers to equality in medical care access and health outcomes (see Chapter 3). Is it just that some people are unable to receive needed care because they lack money and insurance? Should society provide basic health care coverage as an entitlement? Is it unjust that poor and minority people have higher mortality rates because of their socioeconomic status?

When money and resources become scarce, the issue of justice takes on a new twist. Should limits be set on treatments given people with high-cost medical needs, so that other people can receive basic services? If not, might health care consume so many resources that other social needs are sacrificed? If limits should be set, who decides these limits?

> Angela and Amy Lakeberg [actual names] were Siamese twins sharing one heart. Without surgery, they would die shortly. With surgery, Amy would die and Angela's chance of survival would be less than 1%. On August 20, 1993, a team of 18 doctors and nurses at Children's Hospital of Philadelphia performed an all-day operation to separate the twins. Amy died. The cost of the treatment was $1 million. The Indiana Medicaid program covered $700 to $1000 per day, and the hospital underwrote the balance of the costs. On June 9, 1994, Angela died; she had spent her brief life in the hospital on a respirator.

The new fiscal reality has spawned two related dilemmas.

(1) The first involves a conflict between the duty of the physician to follow the principles of beneficence and nonmaleficence and the growing sentiment that physicians should pay attention to issues of distributive justice. In the case of the Lakeberg twins, the hospital and the surgeons adhered strictly to the principle of beneficence: Even a remote chance of aiding one twin was seen as worthwhile. The hospital could have balked, arguing that its funding of the surgery would be unfairly shifted to other payers. The surgeons could have declined to operate on the grounds that the money spent on the Lakebergs could have been better used by patients with a greater chance of survival. But, the surgeons could convincingly argue, who can guarantee that the money saved would have gone to better use?

(2) The second category of social–ethical dilemma is the conflict between the individual patient's right to autonomy and society's claim to distributive justice. In the Lakeberg case, individual autonomy won out. The Lakeberg parents could have decided that spending $1 million of society's money on a less than 1% chance of saving one of two infants was excessive and could indirectly harm other patients. On the other hand, would not most parents have done what the Lakebergs did?

Physicians take up the practice of medicine with a recognition that they have a duty to help and not harm their patients. Individuals claim a right to health care and do not want others to restrict that care. Yet, the principle of distributive justice (recognizing that resources for health care are limited and should be fairly allocated among the entire population) might lead to physicians denying legitimate services or patients setting aside rightful claims to treatment.

The basis for the principle of justice is the desire shared by many human beings to live in a civilized society. To live in a state of harmony, each person must balance the concerns of the individual with the needs of the larger community. There is no right or wrong answer to the question of whether the Lakeberg surgery should have been done, but the surgery must be seen as a choice. The $1 million spent on the twins might have been spent on immunizing 10,000 children, with greater overall benefit. When health resources are scarce, the principle of justice creates ethical dilemmas that touch many people beyond those involved in an individual physician–patient relationship. Precisely because the principle of justice requires a consideration of issues broader than the physician–patient relationship, many physicians and patients have not accepted this fourth tenet of medical ethics as equal in value to beneficence, nonmaleficence, and autonomy. Nonetheless, the imperatives of cost control have thrust the topic of rationing to the forefront of health policy debate, and the very nature of rationing requires consideration of the justice principle as a central tenet of medical ethics.

WHAT IS RATIONING?

Dr. Everett Wall works in a health maintenance organization (HMO). Betty Ailes came to him with a headache and wanted an MRI scan. After a complete history and physical examination, Dr. Wall prescribed medication and denied the scan. Ms. Ailes wrote to the medical director, complaining that Dr. Wall was rationing services to her.

Perry Hiler arrives at Vacant Hospital with fever and severe cough. His chest x-ray shows an infiltrate near the hilum of the lung consistent with pneumonia or tumor. Since Mr. Hiler has no insurance, the emergency room physician sends him to the county hospital. At the time, Vacant Hospital has 35 empty beds and plenty of staff. When he recovers, Mr. Hiler calls the newspaper to complain. The next day, a headline appears: "Vacant Hospital Rations Care."

Jim Delacour is a 50-year-old man with terminal cardiomyopathy. His doctor sends him to a transplant center, where an evaluation concludes that he is an ideal candidate for a heart transplant. Because the number of transplant candidates is far larger than the supply of donor hearts available, Mr. Delacour is placed on the waiting list. After waiting 6 weeks, he dies.

When the emergency room called, Dr. Marco Intensivo's heart sank. The eight-bed intensive care unit is filled with extremely ill patients, all capable of full recovery if they survive their acute illnesses. He has worried all day about another patient needing intensive care. Here it is: a 55-year-old with a heart attack complicated by unstable arrhythmias. Which one of the nine needy cases will not get intensive care? Dr. Intensivo needs to make a decision, and fast.

The general public and the media often view rationing as a limitation of medical care such that "not all care expected to be beneficial is provided to all patients" (Aaron and Schwartz, 1984). Such a view only partially explains the concept of rationing. More precisely, rationing means a conscious policy of equitably distributing needed resources in limited supply (Reagan, 1988). Under this definition, only the last two cases presented above can be considered rationing. In the first case, Dr. Wall did not feel that the MRI was a resource needed by Betty Ailes. In the second, Vacant Hospital's refusal to care for Perry Hiler was simply a decision on the part of a private institution to place its financial well-being above a patient's health; there was no scarcity of health care resources. In the heart transplant and intensive care unit cases, in contrast, donor hearts and intensive care unit beds were, in fact, scarce. For Mr. Delacour, the scarcity was nationwide and prolonged; for Dr. Intensivo, the scarcity was within a particular hospital at a particular time. In both cases, decisions had to be made regarding the allocation of those resources.

During World War II, insufficient gasoline was available to both power the military machine and satisfy the demands of automobile owners in the United States. The government rationed gasoline, giving priority to the military, yet allowing each civilian to obtain a limited amount of fuel. In a rural area, there may be a shortage of health care providers; in an overcrowded urban public hospital, there may be an insufficient number of beds; in the transplant arena, donor organs are truly in short supply. These are cases of commodity scarcity, wherein specific items are in limited supply.

The United States is a nation with an oversupply of hospital beds and medical specialists; commodity scarcity in health care is the exception. But a different kind of health resource is becoming scarce, and that is money. Those who pay the bills are insistent that the flow of money into the health sector be restricted. Most discussions of health care rationing presume fiscal scarcity, not commodity scarcity (Morreim, 1989) (Table 13–2).

Table 13–2. Two definitions of rationing.

Popular usage of the term "rationing":
  A limitation of medical care such that not all care expected to be beneficial is provided to all patients.
Precise usage of the term "rationing":
  The limitation of resources, including money, going to medical care such that not all care expected to be beneficial is provided to all patients; and the distribution of these limited resources in a fair manner.

Rationing in medical care, then, means the limitation of resources, including money, going to medical care such that not all care expected to be beneficial is provided to all patients, and the fair distribution of these limited resources.

COMMODITY SCARCITY: THE CASE OF ORGAN TRANSPLANTS

While fiscal scarcity is the more common form of resource limitation, commodity scarcity provides an instructive example of the interaction of ethics and rationing.

> Mr. George Olds is a 76-year-old nonsmoking retired business executive with end-stage heart failure. He has good pulmonary and renal function and is not diabetic; thus, he is medically a good candidate for a heart transplant. His life expectancy without a transplant is 1 month. He has a loving family, with the resources to pay the $100,000 cost of the procedure.
>
> Mr. Matt Younger is a 46-year-old divorced man who is unemployed, having lost his job as an auto worker 3 years ago. He has a history of smoking and alcohol use. He suffers a heart attack, develops intractable heart failure, and will die within 1 month without a heart transplant. He has good pulmonary and renal function and is not diabetic, making him a good candidate for the procedure.
>
> Mr. Olds and Mr. Younger are in the same hospital, cared for by the same cardiologist, who applied for donor hearts on behalf of both patients on the same day. The cardiologist receives a call that one donor heart—histocompatible with both patients—has become available. Who should receive it?

In 1951, the first kidney transplant was performed in Massachusetts. But it was in 1967, when Dr. Christiaan Barnard sewed a living heart into the chest of a person suffering end-stage cardiac disease, that modern medicine fully entered the age of transplantation. Since that time, thousands of people have been kept alive for many years by transplantation of the kidneys, hearts, lungs, and livers of their fellow human beings. In 1996, 12,000 kidney, 2300 heart, 4000 liver, 800 lung, 1000 pancreas, and 40 heart–lung transplants were performed in the United States. The 4-year survival rate for heart transplants is 72% and for liver transplants, 71%.

Transplantation of organs is both a medical miracle and an ethical watershed. It has generated debate on such questions as these: When are people really dead (so that their organs can be harvested for use in transplantation)? What is the responsibility of the families of brain-dead people to allow their organs to be harvested? Who pays and who is paid for organ transplants? Who should receive organs that are in short supply (Jonsen, 1989)? We will focus only on the last of these issues.

As of 1996, a new patient is added to the national waiting list for organ transplants every 18 minutes, and each day, 11 people die while waiting. The number of persons on the national list increased from 16,000 in 1988 to 50,000 in 1996, yet the number of organ donors barely reaches 9,000 per year (UNOS, 1997). Even if all potential donors became actual donors, the number of organs that could be harvested each year falls far short of the required number. Transplantation presents a classic case of commodity scarcity: There is insufficient supply to meet demand. Explicit rationing, which is a system that determines who gets organs and who does not, is inevitable. For kidney transplants, the issue is less stark because live people can donate organs and because an alternative procedure, chronic dialysis, can keep renal failure patients alive indefinitely. But for heart, lung, and liver transplants, rationing is all or nothing: Those who receive organs may live, while those who do not will die.

Given the supply and demand imbalance, which potential transplant patients actually receive new organs? In the early 1980s, the major heart transplant center at Stanford University excluded people with "a history of alcoholism, job instability, antisocial behavior, or psychiatric illness," and required transplant recipients to enjoy "a stable, rewarding family and/or vocational environment." Stanford's recipients had a better than 50% chance of surviving 5 years, signifying that acceptance or rejection from the program was truly a matter of life and death. The U.S. Department of Health and Human Services was concerned about Stanford's selection criteria, which favored those middle class or wealthy people with satisfying jobs. Moreover, the $100,000 cost restricted heart transplants to those with insurance coverage or ability to pay out of pocket. Both the social and economic criteria for access to this life-saving surgery raised serious issues of distributive justice (Beauchamp and Childress, 1994).

Following the passage of the National Organ Transplantation Act of 1984, the federal government designated the United Network for Organ Sharing (UNOS) as a national system for matching donated organs and potential recipients. According to the Task Force on Organ Transplantation (1986), organ allocation should be governed by medical criteria, with the major factors being urgency of need and probability of success. The Task Force recommended that if two or more patients are equally good candidates for an organ according to the medical criteria, length of time on the waiting list is the fairest way to make the final selection.

Overall, UNOS follows these recommendations, placing potential recipients of organ transplants on its computerized waiting list. Recipients are prioritized according to a point scale based on severity of illness, time on the waiting list, and probability of a successful outcome (Childress, 1989; Hauptman and O'Connor, 1997). Problems have developed with the UNOS system; for example, people in geographic regions with more organ donors are more likely to receive liver transplants than patients with higher priority in other regions. But overall, a successful attempt has been made to allocate scarce organs on the basis of justice criteria.

Complicating the ethics of the prioritization process is the issue of ability to pay. A heart, lung, or liver transplant costs over $200,000. Transplant centers usually require recipients to pay cash in advance or show proof of insurance coverage. Currently, Medicare, some Medicaid programs, and a number of private insurers pay for needed transplants. The uninsured have little access to transplantation (Rettig, 1989; Casscells, 1986).

FISCAL SCARCITY & RESOURCE ALLOCATION

During the 1980s, technologic advances in medicine combined with the rapid rise in health care costs led to the belief that medical care rationing was upon us. The ethical issues raised by organ transplantation have thereby become generalized to all medical care. Great differences separate the case of organ transplants from that of medical care as a whole, however.

(1) Medical care in general is not a scarce resource; in many geographic areas, facilities and personnel are overabundant.

(2) Whereas a nationwide structure is in place to decide who will receive a transplant, no such structure exists for medical care as a whole.

> Dr. Ernest, who works in a for-profit HMO, wants to do her part to keep medical costs down. She prescribes low-cost ampicillin at 20 cents per capsule rather than ciprofloxacin, which is priced at $1.50 for each dose. She teaches back pain patients home exercises at no cost rather than sending them to physical therapy visits at $75 per session. At the end of each year, she enjoys calculating how many thousands of dollars she has saved, compared with one of her colleagues, who ignores costs in making medical decisions. Because of her efforts and those of other cost-conscious physicians, the HMO's pharmacy bill goes down, and HMO management is able to lay off one physical therapist, thereby raising its profit margin.

While Dr. Ernest can be praised for attempting to reduce costs without sacrificing quality, her cost savings had no impact on overall national health care expenditures. Nor were the savings used to provide more childhood immunizations or to hire a physician assistant for a nearby rural community without any health care provider. In the United States, there is no structure within which to effect a trade-off between savings in one area and benefits in another. According to analyst Joshua Wiener (1992),

> These trade-offs do not exist, because the United States does not have a fixed budget for either the Medicare and Medicaid programs or overall national health spending. Thus, it is impossible to say where the money "saved" from constraints in health spending would go. In countries that have a socially determined health budget, cuts in one area can be justified on the grounds that the money will be spent on other, higher-priority services. This closed system of funding provides a moral underpinning for resource allocation across a range of potentially unlimited demands. In the United States, it is difficult to refuse additional resources for patients, because there is no certainty that the funds will be put to better use elsewhere. (Wiener JM: Rationing in America: Overt and covert. In: Rationing America's Medical Care: The Oregon Plan and Beyond. Strosberg MA et al (editors). The Brookings Institution, 1992.)

In the United States, persuading physicians to save money on one patient in order to improve services for someone else is as illogical as telling a child to eat all the food on the plate because children in Africa are starving (Cassel, 1985).

In order for health care providers like Dr. Ernest to make their cost savings socially useful, two things are needed: a closed system of health care funding, whether governmental through a global budget or private through a network of HMOs; and a decision-making structure controlling such funding that has the responsibility to allocate budgets to health care interventions in a fair manner.

For the purposes of the following discussion, let us assume that the United States is in a position of fiscal scarcity and that a mechanism exists to fairly allocate medical care resources from one individual or population group to another. Which ethical conflicts arise between beneficence, nonmaleficence, and autonomy on the one hand and justice (equitable distribution of resources) on the other?

THE RELATIONSHIP OF RATIONING TO COST CONTROL

> Assume that Limittown, USA, has a fixed budget of $250 million for medical care in 1998. Limittown has three HMOs, each with an MRI scanner that is used only 4 hours each weekday. None of the medical facilities performs bone marrow transplantation, a procedure that can markedly prolong the lives of some leukemia patients. In 1997, Limittown spent $5 million to pay for bone marrow transplants at a university hospital 50 miles away.

> Limittown's health commissioner projects that 1998 medical care expenditures will be $5 million over budget; she must implement cost savings. She considers two choices: (1) Two of the three MRI scanners could be closed, allowing the remaining scanner's cost per procedure to be drastically reduced, or (2) Limittown could stop paying for bone marrow transplantation for leukemia patients.

Is rationing the same as cost containment? We have defined rationing in medical care as the limitation of resources, including money, going to medical care such that not all care expected to be beneficial is provided to all patients, and the fair distribution of these limited resources. While the limitation of money going to medical care is cost containment, not all cost containment reduces beneficial care to patients. In the case of Limittown, both options for saving $5 million can be considered cost containment, but only denial of coverage for bone marrow transplants requires rationing. Consolidating MRI scanning at a single facility would allow the same number of scans to be performed but at a substantially lower cost. Rationing is associated with painful cost control (reducing effective medical care), but cost containment (see Chapter 8) can be either painful or painless (not reducing effective medical care) (Table 13–3). Chapter 1 describes administrative and medical waste in the United States. The extent of such waste leads health experts to conclude that the United States may not need to ration effective medical services at this time. Brook and Lohr (1986) argue,

> The central health policy issue . . . is whether the nation will accept and act on the premise that it must ration effective medical services . . . Most of the health policy debate today focuses on how best to implement rationing and which mechanisms to use, not on whether rationing is nec-

Table 13–3. Rationing and cost control.

Not all cost control is rationing.
Painless cost control is not rationing, because no limitation is placed on medical care expected to be beneficial.
Painful cost control may require rationing because limits are placed on medical care expected to be beneficial.

essary. We believe that the correct question is whether deliberate rationing of services . . . is needed. The answer,
we contend, is "no." (Brook RH, Lohr KN: Will we need to
ration effective health care? Issues Sci Technol 1986;3(1):
68.)

The editor emeritus of the *New England Journal of Medicine,* Dr. Arnold Relman
(1990), agrees:

In a country that spends as much as we do on health care,
there should be no need to deny medically necessary services (including the best of modern technology) to anyone.
(Relman AS: Is rationing inevitable? N Engl J Med
1990;322:1809. Abstracted from information appearing in
the *New England Journal of Medicine.)*

Other health policy experts feel that explicit rationing is needed now (Eddy, 1994).
Whether or not rationing is needed today, advances in medical technology guarantee
that rationing of medically efficacious services will be necessary in the future. But to
maximize beneficence and autonomy without violating distributive justice, no rationing of beneficial services should take place until all wasteful practices are curtailed; painless cost control should precede painful cost control.

Care Provided to Profoundly Ill People

Lula Rogers is an 84-year-old diabetic woman with ampu-
tations of both legs; multiple strokes have rendered her unable to move, swallow, understand, or speak. She has been
in a nursing home for 3 years during which time her medical condition has slowly deteriorated. Ms. Rogers' son
wishes to remove her feeding tube, but her physician and
the nursing staff feel it is cruel to cause her death by malnu-
trition and dehydration. Ms. Rogers continues to live for 3
more years. Her nursing home care costs $200,000.

A hotly debated issue is the restriction of marginally effective health care provided
to the profoundly and incurably ill. Were Lula Rogers' care givers, not knowing her
wishes, right to prolong a life that had value to her? Or were they prolonging Ms.
Rogers' suffering and denying her a peaceful death? Should cost be a factor in such
decisions, or should such matters of life and death be governed by autonomy, beneficence, and nonmaleficence alone (Luce, 1990)?

About 28% of Medicare's $187 billion budget (1995) is spent on people in their
last year of life, with almost half of those funds (about $25 billion in 1995) spent in
the final 60 days (Gornick et al, 1993; Gaumer and Stavins, 1992) (Figure 13–1). It
has been estimated that in 1993, $30 billion could have been saved by reducing the
use of life-sustaining interventions for dying patients (Emanuel and Emanuel, 1994).
If there existed mechanisms to transfer these savings to more efficacious therapies for
other people, then limiting the care of the incurably ill could promote distributive justice. Does the limiting of care for profoundly and incurably ill persons necessarily in-
fringe on the principles of beneficence, nonmaleficence, and autonomy, or can these
three principles plus distributive justice be brought into unison?

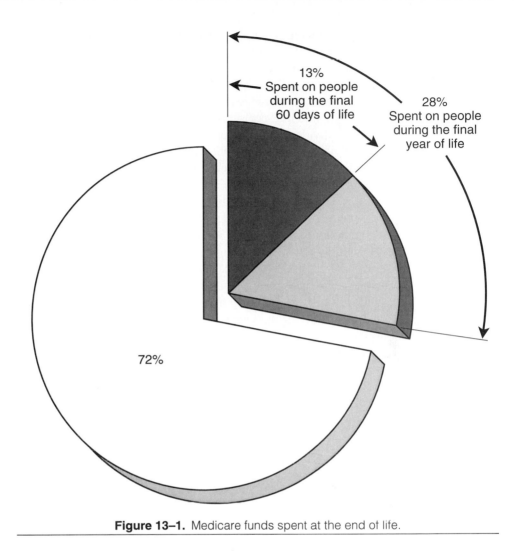

13%
Spent on people
during the final
60 days of life

28%
Spent on people
during the final
year of life

72%

Figure 13–1. Medicare funds spent at the end of life.

The precise condition of profoundly and incurably ill patients determines the ethical issues at stake (Lo, 1995). Some are people with chronic illnesses who have suffered a cardiac arrest, and the issue in these situations is whether to administer cardiopulmonary resuscitation (CPR). Some are terminally ill with cancer, AIDS, or another fatal illness, with an anticipated life span of several days or weeks. Others are people with progressive diseases who may live up to a year, but who suffer constant pain, shortness of breath, or mental anguish. In yet another category are those with severe dementia or strokes, often in nursing homes, who lie in bed year after year, communicating with no one, fed by attendants, incontinent of bowel and bladder.

The tragic human suffering of this spectrum of people in our nation is incalculable. Many of these individuals would prefer that death come sooner rather than later, and many physicians look forward to the death of these patients as a humane blessing. Yet many such patients are kept alive and receive costly medical care of little benefit and possible harm. According to Solomon et al (1993), most physicians overtreat terminally ill patients for whom there is no chance of recovery. Are care givers prolonging life or prolonging dying? In the words of George Bernard Shaw (1954), "Do not try to live forever. You will not succeed."

What are the principles under which physicians provide or withhold treatment for the profoundly and incurably ill? As a rule, autonomy is paramount. Medical therapies are often instituted or withheld based on what the patient wants. In most cases of children or adults who lack decision-making capacity, the family or a surrogate makes the decisions. Individuals are encouraged to sign living wills (which make known their preferences in the case of terminal illness) and to prepare durable power of attorney for health care documents (which name a health care decision maker should the person become incompetent). Such documents are called *advance directives* (ie, they direct physicians how to act in advance of the anticipated event). For patients with advance directives, decision making for physicians is made easier (Lo, 1995).

Does autonomy have limits? Some physicians and ethicists believe that physicians alone, without a patient's or family's consent, can decide to withhold treatment in cases of medical futility (Callahan, 1991). Such actions are ethically supported by the principles of beneficence and nonmaleficence: Treatment that has no benefit and might do harm should not be given. The difficulty with this view lies in the definition of medical futility. If a medical intervention has less than 1% chance of being successful, is it futile (Schneiderman et al, 1994)? Does "successful" mean simply alive, or does it require a reasonable level of function? If a terminal cancer patient wished to live an extra month, should all possible measures, regardless of cost, be taken to grant this wish, or would such care be futile? The 1994 court decision supporting a Virginia family's desire to keep their anencephalic (missing most of the brain and permanently unconscious) child on total life support and the 1994 decision of a Florida hospital to pay for the care of a brain-dead teenager both speak to the primacy of autonomy in current ethical thought.

> Mr. Romero, 66 years old, has incurable emphysema. For 3 weeks, he is on a respirator, an agonizing experience. Two days after going home, his breathing again becomes labored, and he returns to the hospital in a coma from severe respiratory failure. He has no close family, and his personal physician has never asked if he would choose respirator care or CPR, if that becomes necessary. The emergency room physician, after reviewing the previous hospital chart and calling Mr. Romero's physician, decides against the respirator and admits him to the hospital for comfort care.
>
> Four hours later, Mr. Romero's nurse enters the room to find him moribund, with short, agonal respirations. The personal physician had not written a DNR (do not resuscitate) order. The nurse initiates CPR. The emergency room physician appears as part of the CPR team, recognizes the patient, and calls off any further resuscitation attempts.

In this case, the emergency physician interpreted the situation as one of medical futility and withheld treatment based on beneficence and nonmaleficence, without invoking the principle of autonomy.

> Theng My's pancreatic cancer has invaded the plexus of nerves behind her stomach and is causing severe pain. Her oncologist recommends that she undergo a course of

> chemotherapy as the only hope to reduce her suffering. Though the oncologist mentions that the chance of success is only 10% while the probability of highly unpleasant nausea and vomiting is 50%, he emphasizes the chance of significant relief. Desperate, Theng My agrees to the chemotherapy. She experiences no reduction of pain and 20 days of intolerable nausea. Ms. My prays for death; her prayers are answered 1 long month later.

Oncologists in the United States sometimes offer chemotherapy for tumors that respond minimally to treatment. In the United Kingdom, chemotherapy for such tumors is infrequently provided (Aaron and Schwartz, 1984). In the United States, Theng My's situation is handled by the principle of autonomy, and she is given a choice to receive or forego chemotherapy. The physician's duty in such a case is to give Ms. My objective information on which to make her decision, without biases that might be introduced through personal preference or financial incentive. British physicians are more likely to perceive Theng My's case as one of medical futility and not even offer such therapy.

Daniel Callahan (1987), an ethicist who has written extensively on issues of aging and dying, regards death after a long, full life as a natural event rather than an evil to be battled relentlessly by medical science. For Callahan (1993), medicine's obligation is to further a good quality of life and a peaceful death while avoiding a long, tortured life's end.

> Marie is 83, and has been widowed and blind for 3 years. Active until age 80, she now sits in her chair most of the day waiting for her daughter's half-hour evening visit. She spends many hours thankful for the fulfilling life she has been given but aware that she has nothing left to accomplish. One day she falls and feels intense pain in her right hip. Though she can reach the phone, she calls no one. When her daughter arrives and calls the ambulance, Marie refuses to go. Twelve hours later, she dies peacefully of blood loss into a severely fractured hip.

Many elderly persons fear that they will be abandoned or neglected if they become critically ill, with no one caring about their fate, or that they will be excessively treated and their lives painfully extended. Death after a long, lingering illness marked by dementia and isolation in the back room of a nursing home competes as a vision of horror with that of death in an intensive care unit, a dying ever-interrupted by painful and unwanted interventions (Callahan, 1987). Marie tried to achieve a peaceful death by avoiding contact with the health care system.

RATIONING BY MEDICAL EFFECTIVENESS

We have seen that cost containment does not necessarily equal rationing and that eliminating administrative waste, medical waste, and unwanted interventions for the profoundly and incurably ill before rationing needed services best realizes the principles of beneficence and justice. If rationing of truly beneficial services is needed, however, the issues become even more difficult. If a health care system or program must compromise beneficence because of true fiscal scarcity, how can this compromise be made in a manner that yields the least harm and allocates the harm in the fairest possible way?

> Joy Fortune develops Hodgkin's disease, or cancer of the lymphatic system; she receives radiation therapy and is cured. Jessica Turner develops metastatic cancer of the ovary. She undergoes chemotherapy and dies within 8 months.

In the event of rationing, science is the best guide: The providing or withholding of care is ideally determined by the probability that the treatment will maximize benefits and minimize harm, ie, by the criterion of medical effectiveness. Radiation therapy can often cure Hodgkin's disease, but chemotherapy is unlikely to cure advanced ovarian cancer. If rationing is needed and only one of these therapies can be offered, a decision based on the criterion of medical effectiveness would allow for the treatment of Hodgkin's disease but not of metastatic ovarian cancer.

If intervention A increases person-years of reasonable-quality life more than intervention B, intervention A is more medically effective. The cost of the two interventions is not considered. Cost effectiveness adds dollars to the equation: If intervention A increases person-years of reasonable-quality life per dollar spent more than intervention B, it is more cost effective. Which is a better standard for rationing medical care: medical effectiveness or cost effectiveness?

If money were not scarce, medical effectiveness (maximizing benefit and minimizing harm) would be the ideal standard upon which to ration care (ie, the less effective the therapy, the lower its priority on the list of treatments to be offered). But if money were not scarce, we would not need to ration. It is unrealistic to pretend that costs can be ignored (Eddy, 1992).

Suppose that bone marrow transplantation saves as many person-years of life by treating advanced cancers as does penicillin by curing pneumonia. The former costs $150,000, while the latter can be obtained for $10. There is no reason to ration penicillin, as its cost is negligible, whereas to make bone marrow transplantation similarly accessible is costly. Thus, medical effectiveness is inadequate as a means of deciding which services to ration. Reality demands that costs also be factored in.

Rationing for Society as a Whole

> Mrs. Smith's breast cancer has spread to her liver and bone. She has been told that her only slim hope lies in high-dose chemotherapy with autologous bone marrow transplantation (HDC-ABMT), costing $150,000. Even with the optimistic assumption that HDC-ABMT has a 5% cure rate, screening mammography is eight times as cost-effective as HDC-ABMT in person-years of life saved.

In 1991, Dr. David Eddy (1991a) published a compelling article entitled The Individual vs Society: Is There a Conflict? Dr. Eddy poses the above case of Mrs. Smith. If medical care must be rationed, it seems logical to spend funds on mammography rather than HDC-ABMT because the former intervention is more cost effective. Dr. Eddy does not confine his analysis to cost effectiveness, however, but moves on to the ethical issues.

Each of us can be in two positions when we make judgments about the value of different health care activities. We are in one position when we are healthy, contemplating diseases we might get, and writing out checks for taxes and insurance premiums. Call this the "first position." We are in a different position when we actually have a disease, are sitting in a physician's office, and have already paid our taxes and premiums (the "second position") . . . Imagine that you are a 50-year-old woman employed by Mrs. Smith's corporation . . . [The company] is considering two options: (1) cover screening for breast cancer . . . or (2) cover HDC-ABMT . . . Now imagine you are in the first position . . . as long as you do not yet have the disease (the first position), option 1 will always deliver greater benefit at lower cost than option 2 . . . Now, let us switch you to the second position. Imagine that you already have breast cancer and have just been told that it has metastasized and is terminal . . . The value to you of the screening option has plummeted because you already have breast cancer and can no longer benefit from screening . . .

Maximizing care for individual patients attempts to maximize care for individuals when they are in the second position. Maximizing care for society expands the scope of concern to include individuals when they are in the first position. As this example illustrates, the program that delivers the most benefit for the least cost for society (option 1) is not necessarily best for the individual patient (option 2), and vice versa. But as this example also illustrates, individual patients and society are not distinct entities. Rather, they represent the different positions that each of us will be in at various times in our lives. When we serve ourselves in the second position, we can harm ourselves in the first. (Eddy DM: The individual vs society: Is there a conflict? JAMA 1991a;265:1446. Copyright 1991, American Medical Association.)

Physicians generally care for patients in Dr. Eddy's second position—when they are sick. But if the cost of treating those in the second position reduces resources available to prevent illness for the far larger number of people in the first position (who may not be seeing physicians because they feel fine), the individual principles of beneficence and autonomy are superseding the societal principle of justice. One could even say that choosing for individuals in the second position violates beneficence for those in the first position. On the other hand, if all resources go to those in the first position (eg, to cost-effective screening rather than highly technical treatment for those with life-threatening disease), injustice may be committed in the other direction by ignoring the costly needs of the very ill.

Clearly, no ideal method of rationing medical care exists. The use of cost-effectiveness as a measuring stick raises ethical problems and, because of the difficulty in determining the cost-effectiveness of different interventions, has scientific limitations (see Chapter 8). All efforts should be made to control costs painlessly before resorting to the painful limitation of effective medical care. But if rationing is inevitable, a balance must be struck among many legitimate needs: The concerns of healthy people for illness prevention, the imperative for acutely sick people to obtain diagnosis and treatment, and the obligation to provide care and comfort to those with untreatable chronic illness.

Rationing Within One Health Program: The Oregon Plan   The previous discussion of rationing medical care nationwide presumes a mechanism that redirects savings from interventions not performed toward more cost effective services. In fact, such a mechanism does not exist nationwide. Only in specific medical care programs do we find a decision-making apparatus for allocating expenditures. One example is the Oregon Health Plan.

In 1994, Oregon added 100,000 poor, uninsured Oregonians to its Medicaid program. To control costs, a prioritized list of services was developed, and the state legislature decided how many services would be covered. The prioritized list was based on how much improvement in quantity and quality of life the treatment was likely to produce. The final list contained 745 condition–treatment pairs, and the State of Oregon currently pays for items above line 578 on the list; conditions below that line are not covered. What are some of the Oregon Health Plan's ethical implications?

(1) The plan is more than a rationing proposal; its chief feature is to extend health care coverage to 100,000 more people. That aspect of the Oregon plan promotes the principle of justice.

(2) The other positive feature of the plan is its attempt to prioritize medical care services on the basis of effectiveness, which, if rationing is needed, is a reasonable method for deciding which services to eliminate.

(3) In the program's first 3 years, few if any effective services have actually been denied; in fact, poor Oregonians have enjoyed an expansion of covered services (Bodenheimer, 1997).

Other features of the Oregon plan must be viewed as negatively impacting distributive justice, or equal access to care without regard for ability to pay.

(1) If Oregon eliminated a greater number of treatments on the prioritized list, medical services would be rationed for Oregon's poor but not for anyone else.

(2) The plan targets beneficial medical services in a state with considerable medical waste. In 1988, many areas of Oregon had average hospital occupancy rates below 50%. The closing of unneeded hospital beds could have saved $50 million per year, enough to pay for some of the treatments eliminated in the plan (Fisher et al, 1992). Oregon did not exhaust its options for "painless" cost control before proceeding to potentially "painful" rationing.

Rationing Within One Institution: Intensive Care

> Ms. Wilson is a 71-year-old woman with a recently diagnosed lung cancer. Obstructing a bronchus, the tumor causes pneumonia, and Ms. Wilson is admitted to the hospital in her rural town. She deteriorates and becomes comatose, requiring a respirator. By the eighth hospital day, she is no better. On that day, Louis Ford, a previously healthy 27-year-old, is brought to the hospital with a

crushed chest and pneumothorax suffered in an automobile accident. Mr. Ford is in immediate need of a respirator. None of the six patients in the intensive care unit can be removed from respirators without dying; of the six, Ms. Wilson has the poorest prognosis. She has no family. No other respirators exist within a 50-mile radius (Jonsen, 1992). Should Ms. Wilson be removed from the respirator in favor of Mr. Ford?

Resources may be scarce throughout an entire nation or within a small hospital. *Macroallocation* refers to the amount and distribution of resources within a society, whereas *microallocation* refers to resource constraints at the level of an individual physician or institution. Macroallocation decisions may be more significant, affecting thousands or millions of people. Microallocation choices can be more acute, bringing ethical dilemmas into stark, uncompromising focus and placing issues of resource allocation squarely in the lap of practicing physicians. The microallocation choice involving Ms. Wilson incorporates all four ethical principles, which must be weighed and acted on within minutes.

(1) Beneficence: For whom? This ideal cannot be realized for both patients.

(2) Nonmaleficence: If Ms. Wilson is removed from the respirator, harm is done to her. But the price of not harming her is great for Mr. Ford.

(3) Autonomy: Withdrawal of therapy requires the consent of the patient or family, which is impossible in Ms. Wilson's case.

(4) Justice: Should resources be distributed on a first come, first served, basis or according to need?

These are tragic decisions. Many physicians would remove Ms. Wilson from the respirator and make all efforts to save Mr. Ford. The main consideration would be medical effectiveness: Ms. Wilson's chance of living more than a few months is slim, while Mr. Ford could be cured and live for many decades.

Less stark but similar decisions face physicians on a daily basis. On a busy day, which patients get more of the physician's time? In an HMO with an MRI waiting list, when should a physician call the radiologist and argue for an urgent scan, thereby pushing other people down on the waiting list? Situations involving microallocation demonstrate why, in real life, the physician is forced to balance the interests of one patient against those of another and the interests of individuals against the imperatives of society.

A BASIC LEVEL OF GUARANTEED MEDICAL BENEFITS

Don Rich is a bank executive who receives his care through a New York City HMO. He develops angina pectoris, which remains stable for over a year. An exercise treadmill test suggests mild coronary artery disease. Although this evaluation indicates that Mr. Rich's condition can be safely managed with medications, he asks his cardiologist to arrange a coronary angiogram with an angioplasty or coronary bypass if indicated. He is told that the HMO has finite resources for such procedures and limits their use to patients with unstable angina or highly abnormal treadmill tests, for whom the procedures are more efficacious. Mr. Rich flies to Texas, consults with a private cardiac surgeon, and receives a coronary angiogram at his own expense.

Most people in the United States believe that health care should be a right. But how much health care? If every person has a right to all beneficial health care, the nation may be unable to pay the bill or may be forced to limit other rights such as education or fire and police protection. One approach to this problem is to limit the health care right to a basic package of services. (In the case of Don Rich's HMO, angiography for stable angina pectoris is not within the basic package.) Any services beyond the basics can be purchased by individuals who choose to spend their own money. Under managed care, each managed care organization determines the overall benefit package, and particular services for particular patients are sometimes approved or denied in arbitrary fashion (Light, 1994).

This solution creates an ethical problem. If a service that does produce medical benefit is not included in the basic package or is denied by an HMO medical director, that service becomes available only to those who can afford it. Where should society draw the line between a basic level of care that should be equally available to all, and "more than basic" services that may be purchased according to individual ability and willingness to pay (Eddy, 1991b)? Unless the basic package covers all beneficial health services, the principle of distributive justice, that all people equally receive a reasonable level of medical services without regard to ability to pay, will be compromised.

THE ETHICS OF HEALTH CARE FINANCING

Yoshiko Takahashi's first heart attack came at age 59. It was minor, and she felt well the next day. Then came the real shock: because of her high blood pressure, her private insurance policy considers disease of the cardiovascular system a "preexisting condition" and will not cover costs for its treatment. She demands to go home to limit her hospital bill. Twelve hours later comes the second heart attack, which is severe. She is readmitted to intensive care and remains in the hospital for 8 more days. Because of persistent pain, she is a candidate for coronary angiography, which she refuses on account of the cost. When she purchased the insurance, Ms. Takahashi had not understood its terms because her English skills were poor.

Decisions by physicians encompass only one aspect of resource allocation; the payers of health care have great power in the distribution of medical care. The policies of the private insurance industry, which covers the largest number of people in the United States, raise important ethical issues. In the case of Yoshiko Takahashi, the insurance company, rather than her physicians, largely determined what kind of medical care she received.

Much private insurance is experience rated (see Chapter 2), with premiums costing more for people or groups with a higher risk of illness. Under the practice of experience rating, people who need health care the most (because they have a chronic illness) are less likely to be able to purchase affordable health insurance. Many people feel that private insurers violate the justice principle because those most in need of services have the least chance of gaining coverage for those services.

Health insurance executives, however, have a different view, believing that private health insurance is fair. An advertisement sponsored by the insurance industry argued,

> If insurance companies didn't put people into risk groups [experience rating], it would mean that low-risk people would be arbitrarily mixed in with high-risk people . . . and [low-risk people] would have to pay higher rates. That would be unfair to everyone. (Light DW: The practice and ethics of risk-rated health insurance. JAMA 1992;267:2503. Copyright 1992, American Medical Association.)

According to this notion, it is unfair to force one person or group to pay for the needs or burdens of another. An alternative view, citing the principle of distributive justice, holds that young and healthy people should pay more in health costs than they use in health services so that older and less healthy people can receive health services at a reasonable cost. Even from the perspective of one's own long-term self-interest, it may make sense to pay more for health care while young and healthy, and to pay less when age creates a greater risk of becoming sick.

A much-discussed issue involves individuals whose behavior, particularly smoking, eating unhealthy diets, and drinking alcohol in excess, is seen as contributing to their ill health.

> Jim Butts, a heavy smoker, develops emphysema and has multiple hospitalizations for respiratory failure, including many days on the respirator. Randy Schipp, a former shipyard worker, develops work-related asbestosis and has multiple hospitalizations for respiratory failure, including many days on the respirator. Should Jim pay more for health insurance than Randy?

> Gene eats a low-fat diet, exercises regularly, but has a strong family history of heart disease; he suffers a heart attack at age 44. Mac eats fast foods, does not exercise, and has a heart attack at age 44. Should Mac pay more for health care coverage than Gene?

One view holds that individuals who fall sick as a result of high-risk behavior such as smoking, substance abuse, including use of alcohol, and consumption of high-fat foods are entirely responsible for their behavior and should pay higher health insurance premiums. Opponents of this idea see it as "blaming the victim" and argue that high-risk behaviors have a complex causation that may involve genetic and environmental factors including uncontrollable addiction. They cite a number of facts to support their position. The food industry spends about $15 billion per year on television advertising; the average child sees between 15,000 and 25,000 food commercials each year, 80% for products with poor nutritional value. The tobacco industry heavily advertises to teenagers. Illegal drug use is associated with poverty, hopelessness, and easy availability of drugs. Some evidence finds a genetic predisposition to alcoholism. To the extent that individuals are not entirely at fault for their high-risk behavior, it would be unfair to charge them more for health insurance. On the other hand, it seems sensible that users of tobacco and alcohol pay through taxes on those products.

WHO ALLOCATES HEALTH CARE RESOURCES?

The predicament of limited resources has been likened to a herd of cattle grazing on a common pasture. The total grazing area may be regarded as the entirety of economic resources in the United States. A smaller pasture, the *medical commons,* comprises that portion of the grazing area dedicated to health care. The herd represents the nation's physicians, using the resources of the commons in the process of providing care to patients. Physicians, guided by medicine's moral imperative to "do everything possible for the patient," continually attempt to extend the borders of the medical commons. But communities outside the medical commons have legitimate claims to societal resources and view the herd as encroaching on resources needed for other pursuits (Hiatt, 1975; Grumbach and Bodenheimer, 1990).

Who decides the magnitude of the medical commons, that is, the resources devoted to health care? Physicians and other health care providers, whose interventions on behalf of their patients add up to the totality of medical resources used? The sum of individual consumer choices operating through a free market? Health insurance plans, watching over their particular piece of the commons? Or government, using the political process to set budgetary limits on the entire health care system?

Traditionally, physicians and patients have had a great deal to say about the size of the medical commons. In the United States, the medical commons has been an open range. The quantity and price of medical visits, hospital days, surgeries, diagnostic studies, pharmaceuticals, and other such interventions determine the total costs of medical care. This is not the case in other nations, where government health care budgets constitute a "fence" around the medical commons, setting a clear limit on the quantity of resources available. As discussed in Chapter 9, the United States may be moving toward a more fencelike approach to containing costs. Unlike in other nations, however, the U.S. approach may not have a single medical commons enclosed within a national or regional global budget. Instead, the medical commons in the United States is likely to be parcelled out into numerous subpastures, each representing an HMO or other organized health care system working within the constraints of fixed, prepaid budgets. Not all pastures will be equal in size, and the fences may have holes that allow patients to purchase additional services outside of the organized systems of care.

Ethical considerations play a role in both open and closed medical care systems. In the U.S. open range, the principles of beneficence and autonomy have the upper hand, tending toward an expanding, though not highly equitable, system. Fenced-in systems, in contrast, balance the more expansive principles of beneficence and autonomy with the demands of distributive justice in order to allocate resources within the medical commons.

As the United States moves toward a more fenced-in medical commons, decisions will be needed about who gets what. Do all 90-year-old people with multiple organ failure receive kidney dialysis that may extend their life only a few months? Are very low-birth-weight infants afforded neonatal intensive care even with a less than 5%

chance of leading a normal life? Do individual physicians, interacting with their patients, have the final say in making these decisions? Should societal bodies, such as government, commissions of interested parties, or professional associations, set the rules? Should democratic elections be held?

Ultimately, allocation issues come down to daily clinical decisions about which individual patients will receive what types of care (Lo, 1995). Physicians and other care givers may well recoil from the prospect of "bedside rationing," believing that allocative decision making unduly compromises their commitment to the principles of beneficence and autonomy. Levinsky (1984) has argued that physicians must maintain their single-mindedness in maximizing care for each patient:

> There is increasing pressure on doctors to serve two masters. Physicians in practice are being enjoined to consider society's needs as well as each patient's needs in deciding what type and amount of medical care to deliver . . . When practicing medicine, doctors cannot serve two masters. It is to the advantage both of our society and of the individuals it comprises that physicians retain their historic single-mindedness. The doctor's master must be the patient. (Levinsky, NG: The doctor's master. N Engl J Med 1984;311:1573. Abstracted from information appearing in NEJM.)

Yet, if physicians abstain from the arena of macroallocation decision making, who is to decide? Currently, these decisions are often made in a relatively arbitrary fashion by medical directors of private insurance companies and HMOs. Studies have documented that such decisions vary from plan to plan, and even within a single insurance plan, a medical director may make different decisions on different days for similar patients (Light, 1994). Some observers feel that if physicians refuse to accept two masters, then medicine will be granting microallocation decisions to HMO officials, judges, or legislatures. In this view, the physician of the twenty-first century will continue to face individual patient responsibilities, but cannot escape the obligation to balance the wishes of individual patients against the larger needs of society (Cassel, 1985; Morreim, 1989).

If physicians are to serve two masters (ie, to maintain their dedication to individual patients while at the same time responsibly managing resources), they need rules to assist them. These rules should operate at both a population and an individual level. At the population level, society should ideally decide which general treatments are to be collectively paid for through the process of universal health insurance. At the individual level, rules are needed to guide decisions about the prioritization of resources for specific patients. The workings of organ transplantation provide a model of how physicians can serve two masters: They do everything possible to procure an organ for their transplant patients, but also accept the rules of the system that attempt to allocate organs in a fair manner (Benjamin et al, 1994). A similar approach has been instituted in Canada to deal with the limited capacity for cardiac surgery. Cardiac surgeons and other physicians have cooperated in developing a formal scheme for prioritizing patients for cardiac surgery on the basis of medical urgency (Naylor, 1991).

The modern physician is caught in a global ethical dilemma. On the one hand, patients and their families expect the best that modern technology can offer, paid for through private or public insurance. The imperatives of beneficence, nonmaleficence, and autonomy rule the bedside. On the other hand, grave injustices take place on a daily basis: An uninsured young person with a curable illness is unable to pay for care, while an insured, bedridden stroke victim incurs vast medical bills during the last weeks of her ebbing life. Should not the physician at the stroke patient's bedside be concerned about both patients? However this dilemma is resolved, the principle of justice will relentlessly peek at the physician from under the bed.

REFERENCES

Aaron HJ, Schwartz WB: The Painful Prescription. The Brookings Institution, 1984.

Annas GJ: Standard of Care: The Law of American Bioethics. Oxford Univ Press, 1993.

Beauchamp TL, Childress JF: Principles of Biomedical Ethics. Oxford Univ Press, 1994.

Benjamin M, Cohen C, Grochowski E: What transplantation can teach us about health care reform. N Engl J Med 1994;330:858.

Bodenheimer T: The Oregon Health Plan: Lessons for the nation. N Engl J Med 1997;337: 651,720.

Brook RH, Lohr KN: Will we need to ration effective health care? Issues Sci Technol 1986;3(1):68.

Callahan D: Medical futility, medical necessity: The-problem-without-a-name. Hastings Center Rep 1991;21(4):30.

Callahan D: Pursuing a peaceful death. Hastings Center Rep 1993;23(4):33.

Callahan D: Setting Limits: Medical Goals in an Aging Society. Simon & Schuster, 1987.

Casscells W: Heart transplantation: Recent policy developments. N Engl J Med 1986;315: 1365.

Cassel CK: Doctors and allocation decisions: A new role in the new Medicare. J Health Polit Policy Law 1985;10:549.

Childress JF: Ethical criteria for procuring and distributing organs for transplantation. J Health Polit Policy Law 1989;4:87.

Eddy DM: Comparing benefits and harms: The balance sheet. JAMA 1990;263:2493.

Eddy DM: Cost-effectiveness analysis: A conversation with my father. JAMA 1992;267:1669.

Eddy DM: The individual vs society: Is there a conflict? JAMA 1991a;265:1446.

Eddy DM: Rationing resources while improving quality. JAMA 1994;272:817.

Eddy DM: What care is "essential?" What services are "basic?" JAMA 1991b;265:782.

Emanuel EJ, Emanuel LL: The economics of dying. N Engl J Med 1994;330:540.

Fisher ES, Welch HG, Wennberg JE: Prioritizing Oregon's hospital resources. JAMA 1992;267:1925.

Gaumer GL, Stavins J: Medicare use in the last 90 days of life. Health Serv Res 1992;26:725.

Gornick M, McMillan A, Lubitz J: A longitudinal perspective on patterns of Medicare payments. Health Aff 1993;12(2):140.

Grumbach K, Bodenheimer T: Reins or fences: A physician's view of cost containment. Health Aff 1990;9(4):120.

Hauptman PJ, O'Connor KJ: Procurement and allocation of solid organs for transplantation. N Engl J Med 1997;336:422.

Hiatt HH: Protecting the medical commons: Who is responsible? N Engl J Med 1975:293:235.

Jonsen AR: Ethical issues in organ transplantation. In: Medical Ethics. Veatch RM (editor). Jones & Bartlett, 1989.

Jonsen AR, Siegler M, Winslade WJ: Clinical Ethics. McGraw-Hill, 1992.

Levinsky, NG: The doctor's master. N Engl J Med 1984;311:1573.

Light DW: Life, death, and the insurance companies. N Engl J Med 1994;330:498.

Light DW: The practice and ethics of risk-rated health insurance. JAMA 1992;267:2503.

Lo B: Resolving Ethical Dilemmas. Williams and Wilkins, 1995.

Luce JM: Ethical principles in critical care. JAMA 1990;263:696.

Morreim EH: Fiscal scarcity and the inevitability of bedside budget balancing. Arch Intern Med 1989;149:1012.

Naylor CD: A different view of queues in Ontario. Health Aff 1991;10(3):110.

President's Commission on the Study of Ethical Problems in Medicine and Biomedical and Behavioral Research: Securing Access to Health Care. U.S. Government Printing Office, 1983.

Reagan MD: Health care rationing: What does it mean? N Engl J Med 1988;319:1149.

Relman AS: Is rationing inevitable? N Engl J Med 1990;322:1809.

Rettig RA: The politics of organ transplantation: A parable of our time. J Health Polit Policy Law 1989;14:191.

Schneiderman LJ, Faber-Langendoen K, Jecker NS: Beyond futility to an ethic of care. Am J Med 1994;96:110.

Shaw GB: The Doctor's Dilemma. Penguin Books, 1954.

Solomon MZ et al: Decisions near the end of life: Professional views on life-sustaining treatments. Am J Public Health 1993;83:14.

Task Force on Organ Transplantation: Issues and Recommendations. U.S. Department of Health and Human Services, 1986.

UNOS: Facts and statistics. www.unos.org. June 1997.

Wiener JM: Rationing in America: Overt and covert. In: Rationing America's Medical Care: The Oregon Plan and Beyond. Strosberg MA et al (editors). The Brookings Institution, 1992.

Health Care in Three Nations

14

The financing and organization of medical care throughout the developed world spans a broad spectrum (Roemer, 1993). In most countries, the great bulk of medical care is financed or delivered (or both) in the public sector; in others, like the United States, most people both pay for and receive their care through private institutions.

In this chapter, we describe the health care systems of three nations: Germany, Canada, and the United Kingdom (UK). These nations reside at quite different points on the international spectrum. Their diversity assists in illuminating the search for a suitable health care system for the United States.

Recall from Chapter 2 the four varieties of health care financing: out-of-pocket payments, individual private insurance, employment-based private insurance, and government financing. Germany, Canada, and the UK use the first two modes of payment to a minimal degree. Germany finances medical care through government-mandated, employment-based private insurance, though German private insurance is a world apart from that found in the United States. Canada and the UK are essentially government-financed systems. Regarding the delivery of medical care, the German and Canadian systems are predominantly private, while the UK's is largely public.

Although these three nations demonstrate great differences in their manner of financing and organizing medical care, in one respect they are identical. They all provide universal health care coverage, thereby guaranteeing to their populations financial access to medical services.

GERMANY

Health Insurance

> Hans Deutsch is a bank teller living in Germany (formerly in West Germany). He and his family receive health insurance through a sickness fund that insures other employees and their families at his bank and at other workplaces in his city. When Hans went to work at the bank, he was required by law to join the sickness fund selected by his employer.
>
> The bank contributes 6% of Hans's salary to the sickness fund; an additional 6% is withheld from Hans's paycheck and sent to the fund. Hans's sickness fund collects the same 12% employer–employee contribution for all its members. Some bank employees were grumbling 2 years ago because the sickness fund raised the rate from 11% to 12%. But Hans feels relatively lucky. He has friends in other sickness funds whose contribution rate is 16%, half from employer and half from employee.

Germany was the first nation to enact compulsory health insurance legislation. Its pioneer law of 1883 required certain employers and employees to make payments to existing voluntary sickness funds, which would pay for the covered employees' medical care. Initially, only industrial wage earners with incomes less than $500 per year were included; the eligible population was extended in later years.

About 90% of Germans now receive their health insurance through the mandatory sickness funds (Figure 14–1). Most people belong to the same fund throughout their lives, although switching does take place. Several categories of sickness funds exist. Forty percent of people (mostly blue collar workers and their families) belong to funds organized by geographic area; 27% (for the most part the families of white collar workers) are in nationally based "substitute" funds; 12% are employees or dependents of employees who work in 700 companies that have their own sickness funds; and another 12% are in funds covering all workers in a particular craft.

The sickness funds are nonprofit, closely regulated entities that lie somewhere between the private and public sectors. The funds collect money from their members and their members' employers and pay for the care of their members. About 1000 sickness funds exist in Germany. The funds are not allowed to exclude people due to illness, or to raise contribution rates according to age or medical condition, ie, they may not use experience rating. The funds are required to cover a broad range of benefits, including hospital and physician services, prescription drugs, and dental, preventive, and maternity care. There are no deductibles and copayments are minimal (Iglehart, 1991).

> Hans's father, Peter Deutsch, is retired from his job as a machinist in a steel plant. When he worked, his family received health insurance through a sickness fund set up for employees of the steel company. The fund was run by a board, half of whose members represented employees and the other half the employer. On retirement, Peter's family continued its coverage through the same sickness fund, with no change in benefits. The sickness fund continues to pay about 60% of his family's health care costs (subsidized by the contributions of active workers and the employer), with 40% paid from Peter's retirement pension fund.

> Hans has a cousin, Georg, who formerly worked for a gas station in Hans's city but is now unemployed. Georg remained in his sickness fund after losing his job. His contribution to the fund is paid by the government.

> Hans's best friend at the bank was diagnosed with lymphoma and became permanently disabled and unable to work. He remained in the sickness fund, with his contribution paid by the government.

Upon retiring from or losing a job, people and their families retain membership in their sickness funds. Health insurance in Germany, as in the United States, is employment based; but German health insurance, unlike in the United States, must continue to cover its members whether or not they change jobs or stop working for any reason.

> Hans's Uncle Karl is an assistant vice-president at the bank. Because he earns over $40,000 per year, he is not required to join a sickness fund, but can opt to purchase private health insurance. If he chooses private insurance, he will not be able to enter a sickness fund in the future. Most

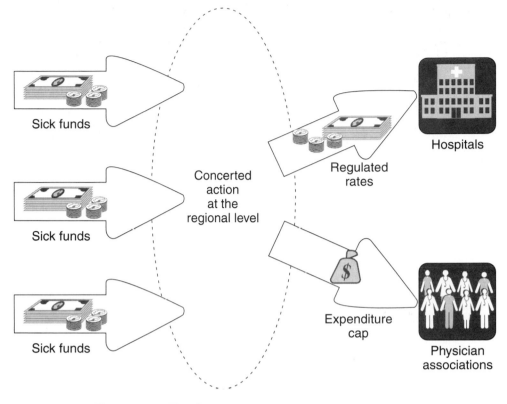

Figure 14–1. The German national health insurance system.

higher-paid employees choose a sickness fund; they are not required to join the fund selected by the employer for lower paid workers, but can join one of 15 national "substitute" funds.

Eight percent of Germans, all with incomes over $40,000, choose private insurance. Private insurers pay substantially higher fees to physicians than do the sickness funds, often allowing their policyholders to receive preferential treatment when seeing a physician (Iglehart, 1991). In summary, in Germany, 90% of the populace belongs to the mandatory sickness fund system, 8% opt for private insurance, 2% receive medical services as members of the armed forces or police, and less than 0.2% (all of whom are wealthy) have no coverage (Saltman, 1988; Files and Murray, 1995).

Germany finances health care through a merged social insurance and public assistance structure (see Chapters 2, 10, and 15 for discussion of these concepts), such that no distinctions are made between employed people who contribute to their health insurance, and unemployed people, whose contribution is made by the government. Germany's social insurance concept is slightly different from that of Medicare in the United States: The employer and employee payments in Germany go to quasi-public sickness funds rather than to the government.

Germany's method of financing tends to be regressive. Hans Deutsch contributes 6% of his paycheck to his sickness fund, but other employees contribute as little as

4% or as much as 8% (U.S. General Accounting Office, 1991). The higher the average wage level of a sickness fund's members, the lower the percentage of payroll needed to cover medical expenses. Thus, lower-wage employees tend to pay a greater proportion of their wages for health care than higher-wage employees. An appreciation of the growing inequity in payroll contributions prompted recent reforms in health care financing in Germany. In 1994, Germany instituted a method to reduce disparities in the rate of health care payroll taxes among different sick funds. Under this new system, sick funds that have enrollees with higher incomes and lower health needs must refund a portion of their payroll revenues to a national pool. The government then distributes money from this risk pool to sick funds with poorer and sicker enrollees. Since implementation of this program, the differential in payroll contribution rates across sick funds has diminished, with rates falling somewhat for lower-income populations and rising for higher-income groups (Files and Murray, 1995).

Medical Care

> Hans Deutsch develops chest pain while walking, and it worries him. He does not have a physician, and a friend recommends a general practitioner (GP), Dr. Helmut Arzt. Because Hans is free to see any ambulatory care physician he chooses, he indeed visits Dr. Arzt, who diagnoses angina pectoris—coronary artery disease. Dr. Arzt prescribes some medications and a low-fat diet, but the pain persists. One morning, Hans awakens with severe, suffocating chest pain. He calls Dr. Arzt, who orders an ambulance to take Hans to a nearby hospital. Hans is admitted for a heart attack, and is cared for by Dr. Edgar Hertz, a cardiologist. Dr. Arzt does not visit Hans in the hospital. Upon discharge, Dr. Hertz sends a report to Dr. Arzt, who then resumes Hans's medical care. Hans never receives a bill.

German medicine maintains a strict separation of ambulatory care physicians and hospital-based physicians. Most ambulatory care physicians are prohibited from treating patients in hospitals, and most hospital-based physicians do not have private offices for treating outpatients. People often have their own primary care physician (PCP), but have traditionally been allowed to make appointments to see ambulatory care specialists without referral from the primary care doctor. This practice is now changing, with specialty visits increasingly requiring a referral from a PCP. Fifty-five percent of Germany's physicians are generalists, compared with only 35% in the United States. The German system tends to use the dispersed model of medical care organization characteristic of the United States (see Chapter 6), with little coordination between ambulatory care physicians and hospitals (Light and Schuller, 1986).

Paying Doctors & Hospitals

> Dr. Arzt was used to billing his regional association of physicians and receiving a fee for each patient visit and for each procedure done during the visit. In 1986, he was shocked to find that spending caps had been placed on the total ambulatory physician budget. If in the first quarter of the year, the physicians in his regional association billed for

more patient services than expected, each fee would be proportionately reduced during the next quarter. If the volume of services continued to increase, fees would drop again in the third and fourth quarters of the year. Dr. Arzt discussed the situation with his friend, Dr. Hertz, but Dr. Hertz, as a hospital physician, received a salary and was not affected by the spending cap.

Ambulatory care physicians are required to join their regional physicians' association. Rather than paying physicians directly, sickness funds pay a global sum each year to the physicians' association in their region, which in turn pays physicians on the basis of a detailed fee schedule. Since 1986, physicians' associations, in an attempt to stay within their global budgets, have reduced fees on a quarterly basis if the volume of services delivered by their physicians was too high (U.S. General Accounting Office, 1991). Sickness funds pay hospitals on a basis similar to the diagnosis-related groups used in the U.S. Medicare program. Included within this payment is the salary of hospital-based physicians.

Cost Control   Between 1965 and 1975, West German health care costs flew out of control, rising from 5.1% to 7.8% of the gross domestic product (Schieber and Poullier, 1989). As a remedy, the government intervened by passing the 1977 Cost Containment Act. This law imposed a number of fiscal restrictions and created a body called Concerted Action, made up of representatives of the nation's health providers, sickness funds, employers, unions, and different levels of government. Concerted Action is convened twice each year, and every spring it sets guidelines for physician fees, hospital rates, and the prices of pharmaceuticals and other supplies. Based on these guidelines, negotiations are conducted at state, regional, and local levels between the sickness funds in a region, the regional physicians' association, and the hospitals to set physician fees and hospital rates that reflect Concerted Action guidelines. Since 1986, not only have physician fees been controlled, but, as described in the above vignette about Dr. Arzt, the total amount of money flowing to physicians has been capped (U.S. General Accounting Office, 1991). As a result of these efforts, Germany's health expenditures as a percentage of the gross domestic product actually fell between 1985 and 1991, from 8.7% to 8.5% (Schieber et al, 1993).

Germany's cost control troubles, however, are not over. In 1991, health care costs had a new upward surge, paving the way for a 1993 cost control law restricting the growth of sickness fund budgets. By 1996, this measure had failed to stem rising costs, and the German government is seeking new cost containment measures (Jackson, 1997). As in every nation, the German cost control story has no ending.

CANADA

Health Insurance

The Maple family owns a small grocery store in Outer Snowshoe, a tiny Canadian town. Grandfather Maple has a heart condition for which he sees Dr. Rebecca North, his family physician, regularly; the rest of the family is healthy and goes to Dr. North for minor problems and preventive care, including children's immunizations. Neither as employers nor as health consumers do the Maples worry about health insurance. They receive a plastic card from their provincial government and show the card when they visit Dr. North.

The Maples do worry about taxes. The federal personal income tax, the 1991 goods and services tax, and the various provincial taxes take almost 40% of the family's income. But the Maples would never let anyone take away their health insurance system.

In 1947, the province of Saskatchewan initiated the first publicly financed universal hospital insurance program in North America. Other provinces followed suit, and in 1957, the Canadian government passed the Hospital Insurance Act, which was fully implemented by 1961. Hospital, but not physician, services were covered. In 1963, Saskatchewan again took the lead and enacted a medical insurance plan for physician services. The Canadian federal government passed universal medical insurance in 1966; the program was fully operational by 1971 (Taylor, 1990).

Canada has a tax-financed, public, single-payer health care system. In each Canadian province, the single payer is the provincial government (Figure 14–2). During the 1970s, federal taxes financed 50% of health services, but since the 1980s, the provinces have had to pay medical costs increasing above the gross national product's growth rate. From 1980 to 1990, the contribution of the federal government to national health expenditures dropped from 45% to 37% (Iglehart, 1990). Provincial taxes vary in type from province to province and include income taxes, payroll taxes, and sales taxes. Two provinces, British Columbia and Alberta, charge a compulsory health care premium to finance a small portion of their health budgets.

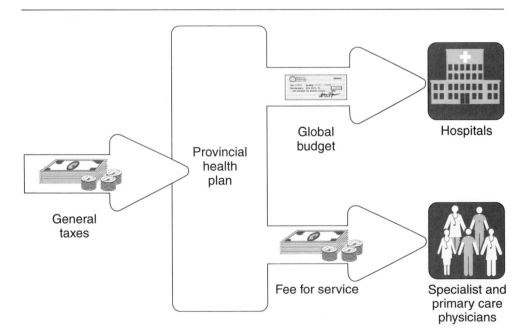

Figure 14–2. The Canadian National Health insurance system.

Canada, unlike Germany, has severed the link between employment and health insurance. Wealthy or poor, employed or jobless, retired or under age 18, every Canadian receives the same health insurance, financed in the same way. No Canadian would even imagine that leaving, changing, retiring from, or losing a job has anything to do with health insurance. In Canada, no distinction is made between the two public financing mechanisms of social insurance (in which only those who contribute receive benefits) and public assistance (in which people receive benefits based on need rather than on having contributed). Everyone contributes through the tax structure and everyone receives benefits.

The benefits provided by Canadian provinces are broad, including unlimited hospital, physician, and ancillary services. Not all provinces pay for outpatient prescription drugs, and long-term care benefits vary from province to province.

The Canadian health care system is unique in its prohibition of private health insurance for coverage of services included in the provincial health plans. Hospitals and physicians that receive payments from the provincial health plans are not allowed to bill private insurers for such services, thereby avoiding the preferential treatment of privately insured patients that occurs in many health care systems. A small number of upper-income Canadians purchase health insurance policies for the few gaps in provincial health plan coverage or for such amenities as private hospital rooms.

Medical Care

> Grandfather Maple wakes up one morning with a feeling of palpitations in his chest. He calls Dr. North, who tells him to come right over. An electrocardiogram reveals rapid atrial fibrillation, an abnormal heart rhythm. Because Mr. Maple is tolerating the rapid rhythm, Dr. North treats him with digoxin in the office, tells him to return the next day, and writes out a referral slip to see Dr. Jonathan Hartwell, the cardiologist in a nearby small city.

> Dr. Hartwell arranges a stress echocardiogram at the local hospital to evaluate Mr. Maple's arrhythmia, finds severe coronary ischemia, and explains to Mr. Maple that his coronary arteries are narrowed. He recommends a coronary angiogram and possible coronary artery bypass surgery. Because Mr. Maple's condition is not urgent, Dr. Hartwell arranges for his patient to be placed on the waiting list at the University Hospital in the provincial capital 50 miles away. One month later, Mr. Maple awakens at 2 AM in a cold sweat, gasping for breath. His daughter calls Dr. North, who urgently sends for an ambulance to transport Mr. Maple to the University Hospital. There, Mr. Maple is admitted to the coronary care unit, his condition is stabilized, and he undergoes emergency coronary artery bypass surgery the next day. Ten days later, Mr. Maple returns home, complaining of pain in his incision but otherwise feeling well.

Fifty-five percent of Canadian physicians are general GPs or family practitioners who act as gatekeepers to the medical care delivery system. Canadians have free choice of physician. As a rule, Canadians see their GP for routine medical problems and visit specialists only through referral by the GP. Specialists are allowed to see patients without referrals, but only receive the higher specialist fee if they include the referral slip in their billing; for that reason, most specialists will not see patients without a referral. Because 55% of Canadian physicians are GPs or family practitioners (contrasted with the United States, where only 35% of physicians are generalists), primary care services are in ample supply, except in remote rural areas. Elderly Canadians receive 17% more physician services than the elderly in the United States (Welch et al, 1996). Unlike the European model of separation between ambulatory and hospital physicians, Canadian family physicians are allowed to care for their patients in hospitals, although they tend to perform less inpatient work than U.S. family physicians.

Because of the close scientific interchange between Canada and the United States, the practice of Canadian medicine is similar to that in the United States; the differences lie in the financing system and the far greater use of PCPs as gatekeepers. The treatment of Mr. Maple's heart condition is not significantly different from what would occur in the United States, with two exceptions:

(1) High-technology procedures such as cardiac surgery and MRI scans are regionalized in a limited number of facilities and performed less frequently than in the United States (Grumbach et al, 1995; Anderson et al, 1993; Katz et al, 1996a); and

(2) There are waiting lists for some specialized elective procedures. The average patient scheduled for a knee-replacement operation in Ontario in the late 1980s waited 8 weeks, compared with a 3-week wait for the average patient in the United States (Coyte et al, 1994). On the other hand, patients diagnosed with leukemia in Canada did not wait longer to receive bone marrow transplantation than patients in the United States with the same condition (Silberman et al, 1994).

Although Canadians may in some instances wait longer for operations than do insured people in the United States, Canada's universal insurance program has created a fairer system for distributing health services. Studies of the United States and Canada have compared how receipt of a variety of services, ranging from cardiac surgery to mental health care, may vary according to income in the two nations. These studies indicate that while in the United States, people with higher incomes tend to use more services, no similar differential according to income exists in Canada for most services studied. In some cases, lower-income groups in Canada are the *most* likely to receive health services such as cardiac surgery, a pattern that corresponds to the higher burden of disease among lower-income groups (Anderson et al, 1993; Katz et al, 1996b; Katz et al, 1997).

Paying Doctors & Hospitals

For Dr. Rebecca North, collecting fees is a simple matter. Each week she sends a computer disk to the provincial government, listing the patients she saw and the services she provided. Within a month, she is paid in full, according to a fee schedule. Dr. North wishes the fees were higher, but loves the simplicity of the billing process. Her staff spends 2 hours per week on billing, compared with the 30 hours of staff time her friend, Dr. South, in Michigan, needs for billing purposes.

> Dr. North is less happy about the global budget approach used to pay hospitals. She often begs the hospital administrator to hire more physical therapists, to speed up the reporting of laboratory results, and to institute a program of diabetic teaching. The administrator responds that he receives a fixed payment from the provincial government each year, and there is no extra money.

Physicians in Canada—GPs and specialists—are paid on a fee-for-service basis, with fee levels negotiated between provincial governments and provincial medical associations (Figure 14–2). Previously, physicians were allowed to bill patients in addition to billing the government; this practice was prohibited in 1984 (Lomas et al, 1989). Canadian hospitals, most of which are private nonprofit institutions, negotiate a global budget with the provincial government each year. Hospitals have no need to prepare the itemized patient bills that are so administratively costly in the United States. Hospitals must receive approval from their provincial health plan for new capital projects such as the purchase of expensive new technology or the construction of new facilities.

Cost Control   The Canadian system has attracted the interest of many people in the United States because, in contrast to the United States, the Canadians have found a way to deliver comprehensive care to their entire population at far less cost. In 1970, the year before Canada's single-payer system was fully in place, Canada and the United States spent approximately the same proportion of their gross domestic products on health care—7.2% and 7.4%, respectively. By 1991, Canada's health expenditures had risen to 10% of the gross domestic product, compared with 13.2% for the United States. Since 1991, Canada's health care costs have actually declined, compared with continued cost increases in the United States. In 1995, Canada spent 9.6% of its gross domestic product on health care; the United States spent 14.2%. The 1995 per capita cost of health care in the United States was 80% higher than the per capita cost in Canada (OECD, 1997).

Notably, as discussed in Chapter 9, the differences in cost between the United States and Canada are not a result of Canadians receiving fewer services overall. In fact, Canadians on the average spend more days in the hospital and see physicians more often than people in the United States. Lower costs in Canada are primarily accounted for by three items: (1) administrative costs, which are 300% greater in the United States per capita; (2) cost per patient day in hospitals, which reflects a greater intensity of service in the United States; and (3) physician fees, which are much higher in the United States (Evans et al, 1989; Fuchs and Hahn, 1990; Woolhandler and Himmelstein, 1991).

Viewed from its southern border, Canada appears to be doing well in containing health care costs, but within Canada, costs are seen as a serious problem. After all, aside from the United States, Canada has one of the most expensive health care systems in the world. Health expenditures account for about one-third of provincial budgets. Rising taxes and governmental budget deficits are attributable in part to health care inflation. Some Canadian analysts feel that the fee-for-service method of paying physicians is a major impetus to health cost inflation (Evans, 1990; Rachlis and Kushner, 1989). As a remedy for its inflation problem, all provinces have put into effect caps on physician payments similar to those used in Germany (Barer et al, 1996).

THE UNITED KINGDOM

Health Insurance

> Roderick Pound owns a small bicycle repair shop in the north of England; he lives with his wife and two children. His sister Jennifer is a lawyer in Scotland. Roderick's younger brother is a student at Oxford, and their widowed mother, a retired saleswoman, lives in London. Their cousin Anne is totally and permanently disabled from a tragic automobile accident. A distant relative, who became a U.S. citizen 15 years before, recently arrived to help care for Anne.

> Simply by virtue of existing on the soil of the U.K.—whether employed, retired, disabled, or a foreign visitor—each of the Pound family members is entitled to receive tax-supported medical care through the National Health Service (NHS)

In 1911, Great Britain established a system of health insurance similar to that of Germany. About half the population was covered, and the insurance arrangements were highly complex, with contributions flowing to "friendly societies," trade union and employer funds, commercial insurers, and county insurance committees. In 1942, the world's most renowned treatise on social insurance was published by Sir William Beveridge. The Beveridge Report proposed that Britain's diverse and complex social insurance and public assistance programs, including retirement, disability and unemployment benefits, welfare payments, and medical care, be financed and administered in a simple and uniform system. One part of Beveridge's vision was the creation of a national health service for the entire population. In 1948, the NHS began (Saltman, 1988; Klein, 1983; Sidel and Sidel, 1983).

Eight-two percent of NHS funding comes from taxes, 13% from employer–employee contributions similar to social security payments in the United States, and 4% from user charges (Maynard and Bloor, 1996). As in Canada, the UK completely delinks health insurance from employment, and no distinction exists between social insurance and public assistance financing. Unlike Canada, the UK allows private insurance companies to sell health insurance for services also covered by the NHS. A number of affluent people purchase private insurance in order to receive preferential treatment, "hopping over" the queues for services present in parts of the NHS (Lister, 1988). Some employers offer such supplemental insurance as a perk. Naturally, the 11% of the population with private insurance are also paying taxes to support the NHS (Figure 14–3).

Medical Care

> Dr. Timothy Broadman is an English GP, whose list of patients numbers 1750. Included on his list is Roderick Pound and his family. One day, Roderick's son broke his leg playing soccer; he was brought to the NHS district hospital by ambulance and treated by Dr. Pettibone, the hospital orthopedist, without ever seeing Dr. Broadman.

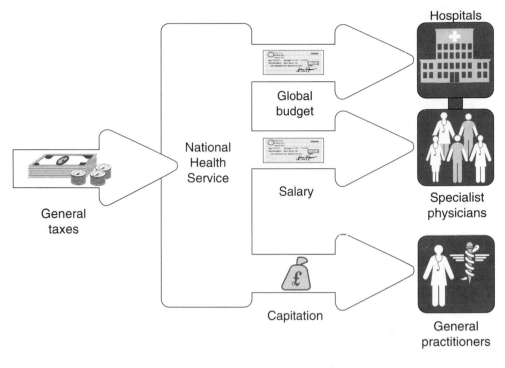

Figure 14–3. The British National Health Service: traditional model.

Roderick's mother has severe degenerative arthritis of the hip, which Dr. Broadman cares for. A year ago, Dr. Broadman sent her to Dr. Pettibone to be evaluated for a hip replacement. Because this was not an emergency, Mrs. Pound required a referral from Dr. Broadman to see Dr. Pettibone. The orthopedist examined and x-rayed her hip and agreed that she needed a hip replacement, but not on an urgent basis. Mrs. Pound has been on the waiting list for her surgery for over 6 months. Mrs. Pound has a wealthy friend with private health insurance who got her hip replacement within 3 weeks from Dr. Pettibone, who has a private practice in addition to his employment with the NHS.

Prior to the NHS, most primary medical care was delivered through GPs. The NHS maintained this tradition and formalized a gatekeeper system by which specialty and hospital services (except in emergencies) are available only by referral from a GP. Every person in the UK who wants to use the NHS must be enrolled on the list of a GP. There is free choice of GP (unless the GP's list of patients is full), and people can (but rarely do) switch from one GP's list to another (Saltman, 1988; Hiatt, 1987; Grumbach and Fry, 1993).

Whereas the creation of the NHS in 1948 left primary care essentially unchanged, it revolutionized Britain's hospital sector. As in the United States, hospitals had mainly been private nonprofit institutions or were run by local government; most of these hospitals were nationalized and arranged into administrative regions. Because the NHS unified the UK's hospitals under the national government, it was possible to institute a true regionalized plan (see Chapter 6).

Patient flow in a regionalized system tends to go from GP (primary care for common illnesses) to local hospital (secondary care for more serious illnesses) to regional or national teaching hospital (tertiary care for complex illnesses). Traditionally, most specialists have had their offices in hospitals. As in Germany, GPs do not provide care in hospitals. GPs have a tradition of working closely with social service agencies in the community, and home care is highly developed in the UK (Sidel and Sidel, 1983).

Paying Doctors & Hospitals

> Dr. Timothy Broadman does not think much about money when he goes to his surgery (office) each morning. He receives a payment from the NHS to cover part of the cost of running his office, and every month he receives a capitation payment for each of the 1750 patients on his list. Because he cannot influence the number of people on his list, there isn't much he can do to change his income. Recently, 10% of his income has been coming from extra fees he receives when he gives vaccinations to the kids and does Pap smears, family planning, and other preventive care. He also gets extra payment for making home visits after hours. There is no particular reason for money to be on Dr. Broadman's mind when he cares for his patients.

Since early in the twentieth century, the major method of payment for British GPs has been capitation (see Chapter 4). This mode of payment did not change when the NHS took over in 1948. The NHS did add some fee-for-service payments as an encouragement to provide certain preventive services and home visits during nights and weekends. Consultants (specialists) are salaried employees of the NHS, though some consultants are allowed to see privately insured patients on the side, whom they bill fee-for-service.

Cost Control   Health expenditures in the UK accounted for 5.9% of the gross domestic product in 1985 and 6.9% in 1995. In 1995, UK per capita health spending was only 34% of the U.S. figure (OECD, 1997).

Two major factors allow the UK to keep its health care costs low: the power of the governmental single payer to limit budgets and the mode of reimbursement of physicians. While Canada also has a single payer of health services, it pays most physicians fee-for-service and only recently has moved toward physician expenditure caps (like Germany) in an attempt to control the inflationary tendencies of fee-for-service reimbursement. The UK, in contrast, relies chiefly on capitation and salary to pay physicians; payment can more easily be controlled by limiting increases in capitation payments and salaries. Moreover, because consultants (specialists) in the UK are NHS employees, the NHS can and does tightly restrict the number of consultant slots, including those for surgeons. As a result, queues have developed for nonemergency consultant visits, and the rates of some forms of surgery such as gallbladder operations are half those in the United States and Canada (Hiatt, 1987). Overall, the UK controls costs by controlling the supply of personnel and facilities and the budget for medical resources.

Critics both within and outside the UK suggest that health care costs are controlled too tightly (Lister, 1988; Aaron and Schwartz, 1984). In the 1980s, the Thatcher government strictly limited the rate of growth of the NHS budget. In the late 1980s, underpaid nurses were leaving employment at the rate of 30,000 per year. Even with hospital beds, operating theatres, and surgeons available, the shortage of skilled nurses caused increases in queues. For the first time, the overwhelming public support for the NHS was beginning to erode (Lister, 1988).

Related to the low level of health expenditures, the UK is often viewed as a nation that rations certain kinds of health care. In fact, primary and preventive care are not rationed, and average waiting times to see a GP are probably shorter than primary care appointment delays in many parts of the United States. Even some high-technology services (eg, radiation therapy for cancer and bone marrow transplantation) are performed at the same rates as in the United States. But waiting times to see consultants for nonurgent problems, elective hospital admissions, and such elective surgeries as hip replacement and cataract removal, may be substantial (though 90% of elective waits are under 3 months) (Hiatt, 1987; Potter and Porter, 1989). Renal dialysis is performed far less often in the UK than in the United States, especially for people over 60 years of age, a practice that has been criticized by U.S. observers (Aaron and Schwartz, 1984). Overall, a striking characteristic of British medicine is its economy. British physicians simply do less of nearly everything—perform fewer surgeries, prescribe fewer medications, and order fewer x-rays; they are more skeptical of new technologies than U.S. physicians (Payer, 1988).

The single-payer form of health care system, as the UK exemplifies, is capable of keeping health expenditures down. However, not all single-payer health care systems have low per capita costs: Canada's per capita expenditures are relatively high. In part, the UK dedicates less to health care because of its poor economy. As a general rule, nations such as the UK, with a low gross domestic product per capita, spend a smaller portion of that gross domestic product on health care (Schieber et al, 1993).

Recent Reforms of the NHS

> Dr. Broadman attended a lecture given by Dr. Cornelius Merchant, a GP from a 10-physician group practice across town. Dr. Merchant explained that his practice has chosen to become a fund-holding practice, meaning that the NHS gives the group practice funds from which the GPs must pay for outpatient specialty referrals, diagnostic tests, prescription drugs, and some hospital expenses. The physicians can contract with whichever specialists, laboratories, or hospitals give them the best service. Dr. Merchant explained that his practice had contracted with a hospital 30 miles away for orthopedic care, to reduce patient waiting times.

In 1990, the British government, led by Prime Minister Margaret Thatcher, enacted major changes in the NHS (Light and May, 1993) (Figure 14–4). These reforms were intended to address problems such as waiting times for elective surgery. The reforms introduced market incentives and competition to produce greater efficiency in the delivery of services within existing funding levels. Two types of "internal markets" were established within the NHS, one aimed at hospitals and the other at GP practices. Hospitals are no longer assured global budgets under the NHS, but must now market their services to local NHS district health authorities that act as purchasers of hospital services for the populations in their district. District authorities may negoti-

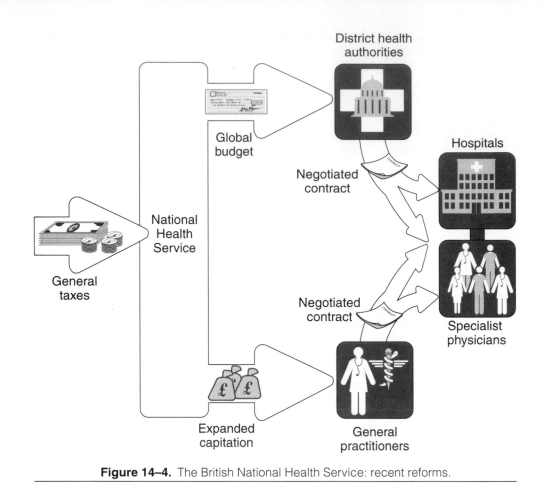

Figure 14–4. The British National Health Service: recent reforms.

ate contracts with different hospitals in an attempt to obtain the best quality of care at the best price. Hospitals are expected to improve their responsiveness to patients, eg, by reducing waiting times for consultations and procedures, or risk losing contracts.

The second internal market centers on GP practices. The key feature in the restructuring of GP practices is the option for GP "fund-holding." In the traditional NHS arrangement, services such as specialist consultations, physical therapy, and pharmaceuticals are covered under the budgets of district health authorities that are responsible for the entire population in a region. Under fund-holding, portions of these budgets are transferred from the district health authority to a GP group. The fund-holding GP group uses this budget to purchase ancillary and elective referral services for the group's panel of enrolled patients. GPs negotiate contracts with specialists and other providers for services for their enrolled patients, with terms of these contracts including items such as the timeliness of appointments.

As in the case of the hospital competitive market, the goal is to make hospital administrators and hospital-based consultants more responsive to GPs (and the patients of GPs) in order to be awarded contracts from GPs. Although fund-holding might appear to resemble some of the managed care capitation arrangements that place U.S. PCPs at financial risk for referral and hospital services (see Chapters 4 and 5), there is an "ocean" of difference between UK fund-holding and U.S.–style capitation. Most important, fund-holding is a risk-free (and profit-free) proposition for PCPs in the UK. If a fund-holding GP group generates referral and ancillary costs that exceed the fund-holding allotment, the district health authority supplements the budget rather than forcing GPs to pay for deficits out of their own income. Conversely, surpluses in fund-holding budgets may not be used to increase physicians' personal income; surpluses must be invested in expanded services or improvements in practice facilities (Maxwell, 1996).

The reforms have their strengths and weaknesses. On the positive side, they promote primary and preventive care, and could—by instilling some competition—improve the services provided by specialists and hospitals. The time spent on waiting lists for elective admissions and surgeries has fallen sharply, though the number of people on waiting lists has risen (Klein, 1995). On the negative pole, the internal markets are already producing more administrative costs and more managers; it has been reported that 50,000 nursing jobs have disappeared since 1990 while the number of managers has grown by 20,000 (Whitney, 1996). Physicians are more preoccupied with budgets and financial incentives. Non–fund-holding GPs are concerned that their patients may become "second-class citizens" and receive less preferential treatment from specialists than patients from fund-holding practices. Most problematic, fund-holding GP practices have the incentive to maximize healthy persons on their lists and see few chronically ill patients, whose high use of diagnostic, specialty, pharmacy, and hospital services deplete the fund-holders' budgets (Maxwell, 1996).

In 1997, the election of a Labour government has created uncertainty about the future direction of the NHS. On the one hand, the new government has suggested that it will dismantle the internal market. On the other hand, the dynamics of the internal market could further evolve, merging many small GP offices into larger primary care centers with salaried physicians (Groves, 1997).

CONCLUSION

Key issues in evaluating and comparing health care systems are access to care, level of health expenditures, public satisfaction with health care, and the overall quality of care as expressed by the health of the population. We have seen that Germany, Canada, and the UK provide universal financial access to health care through government-run or government-mandated programs. We have also seen that these three nations have controlled health care costs more successfully than has the United States (see Tables 14–1 and 14–2), though all three continue to face challenges in containing their spending.

Table 14–1. Total health expenditures as a percentage of gross domestic product (GDP) 1960–1995.

	1960	1970	1980	1985	1990	1995
Germany	4.7	5.5	7.9	8.7	8.3	10.4
United Kingdom	3.9	4.5	5.8	6.0	6.2	6.9
Canada	5.5	7.2	7.4	8.5	9.5	9.6
United States	5.2	7.4	9.2	10.5	12.2	14.2

Sources: Schieber GJ and Poullier JP, 1987; Schieber GJ, Poullier JP and Greenwald LM, 1993; OECD, 1997.

Table 14–2. Per capita health spending in U.S. dollars, 1985–1995.

	1985	1995
Germany	$1175	2134
United Kingdom	685	1246
Canada	1244	2049
United States	1711	3701

Source: OECD, 1997.

In a 1990 survey of 10 nations, Canada ranked first in public satisfaction with the health care system, West Germany ranked third, the UK ranked eighth, and the United States came in last (Blendon et al, 1990). In a 1991 survey of practicing physicians in three nations, 23% of U.S. respondents felt that the health care system works well and 77% felt that fundamental changes are needed. Thirty-three percent of Canadian and 48% of West German physicians felt that their systems work well (Blendon et al, 1993). In 1994, public satisfaction with the health care system in Canada and Germany was less than in 1990, but still higher than the level in the United States (Blendon et al, 1995).

Cross-national comparisons of health care quality are treacherous and tend to confuse the impacts of socioeconomic factors and of medical care on the health status of the population. But such comparisons can convey crude impressions of whether a health care system is functioning at a reasonable level of quality. From Table 14–3, it is clear that the United States has an infant mortality rate higher than that of Germany, Canada, and the UK, with the German rate the lowest. Canada has the highest male and female life expectancy rates at birth. The life expectancy rate at age 60 is believed by some observers to measure the impact of medical care, especially its more "high-tech" component, more than it measures underlying socioeconomic influences; by this standard, Canada and the United States have the highest scores (OECD, 1997).

Just as epidemiologic studies often derive their most profound insights from comparisons of different populations (see Chapter 11), so can research into health services reveal volumes from the experience of other nations. As the United States confronts its dual health care problems of access and cost, it must look across its borders and overseas to nations who have been more successful in solving those problems.

Table 14–3. Health outcome measures, 1995.

	Infant mortality*	Life expectancy at birth		Life expectancy at age 60	
		Men	Women	Men	Women
Germany	5.3	73.0	79.5	18.1	22.5
United Kingdom	6.2	74.3	79.7	18.3	22.4
Canada	6.3	75.3	81.3	19.9	24.3
United States	8.0	72.5	79.2	18.9	22.9

* per 1000 live births
Source: OECD, 1997.

REFERENCES

Aaron HJ, Schwartz WB: The Painful Prescription: Rationing Hospital Care. The Brookings Institution, 1984.

Anderson GM et al: Use of coronary artery bypass surgery in the United States and Canada. JAMA 1993;269:1661.

Barer ML, Lomas J, Sanmartin C: Re-minding our Ps and Qs: Medical cost controls in Canada. Health Aff 1996;15(2):216.

Blendon RJ et al: Physicians' perspectives on caring for patients in the United States, Canada, and West Germany. N Engl J Med 1993;328:1011.

Blendon RJ et al: Satisfaction with health systems in ten nations. Health Aff 1990;9(2):185.

Blendon RJ et al: Who has the best health care system? A second look. Health Aff 1995;14(4):220.

Coyte PC et al: Waiting times for knee-replacement surgery in the United States and Ontario. N Engl J Med 1994;331:1068.

Evans RG: Tension, compression, and shear: Directions, stresses, and outcomes of health care cost control. J Health Polit Policy Law 1990;15:101.

Evans RG et al: Controlling health expenditures: The Canadian reality. N Engl J Med 1989;320:571.

Files A, Murray M: German risk structure compensation: Enhancing equity and effectiveness. Inquiry 1995:32:300.

Fuchs VR, Hahn JS: How does Canada do it? N Engl J Med 1990;323:884.

Groves T: Primary care: Opportunities and threats. What the changes mean. BMJ 1997;314:436.

Grumbach K, Fry J: Managing primary care in the United States and in the United Kingdom. N Engl J Med 1993;328:940.

Grumbach K et al: Regionalization of cardiac surgery in the United States and Canada. JAMA 1995;274:1282.

Hiatt HH: America's Health in the Balance. Harper & Row, 1987.

Iglehart JK: Canada's health care system faces its problems. N Engl J Med 1990;322:562.

Iglehart JK: Germany's health care system. N Engl J Med 1991;324:503, 1750.

Jackson JL: The German health system. Arch Intern Med 1997;157:155.

Katz SJ et al: Comparing use of diagnostic tests in Canadian and US hospitals. Med Care 1996a;34:117.

Katz SJ et al: Mental health care use, morbidity, and socioeconomic status in the United States and Ontario. Inquiry 1997;34:38.

Katz SJ et al: Physician use in Ontario and the United States: The impact of socioeconomic status and health status. Am J Public Health 1996b;86:520.

Klein R: Big bang health care reform: Does it work? The case of Britain's 1991 National Health Service reforms. Milbank Mem Fund Q 1995;73:299.

Klein R: The Politics of the National Health Service. Longman Group Limited, 1983.

Light DW, May A: Britain's Health System: From Welfare State to Managed Markets. Faulkner and Gray, 1993.

Light DW, Schuller A: Political Values and Health Care: The German Experience. MIT Press, 1986.

Lister J: Prospects for the National Health Service. N Engl J Med 1988;318:1473.

Lomas J et al: Paying physicians in Canada: minding our Ps and Qs. Health Aff 1989;8(1):80.

Maxwell JG: Changes in Britain's health care. JAMA 1996;275:189.

Maynard A, Bloor K: Introducing a market to the United Kingdom's National Health Service. N Engl J Med 1996;334:604.

OECD: Health Data 97. Organization for Economic Cooperation and Development, 1997.

Payer L: Medicine and Culture. Henry Holt, 1988.

Potter C, Porter J: American perceptions of the British National Health Service: Five myths. J Health Polit Policy Law 1989;14:341.

Rachlis M, Kushner C: Second Opinion: What's Wrong with Canada's Health Care System and How to Fix It. Collins, 1989.

Roemer MI: National Health Systems of the World, Vols 1 and 2. Oxford Univ Press, 1993.

Saltman RB (editor): The International Handbook of Health-Care Systems. Greenwood Press, 1988.

Schieber GJ, Poullier JP: International health care expenditure trends: 1987. Health Aff 1989;8(3):169.

Schieber GJ, Poullier JP, Greenwald LM: Health spending, delivery, and outcomes in OECD countries. Health Aff 1993;12(2):120.

Sidel VW, Sidel R: A Healthy State. Pantheon Books, 1983.

Silberman G et al: Availability and appropriateness of allogenic bone marrow transplantation for chronic myeloid leukemia in 10 countries. N Engl J Med 1994;331:1063.

Taylor MG: Insuring National Health Care. The Canadian Experience. Univ of North Carolina Press, 1990.

U.S. General Accounting Office: Health Care Spending Control: The Experience of France, Germany, and Japan. 1991.

Welch WP et al: A detailed comparison of physician services for the elderly in the United States and Canada. JAMA 1996;275:1410.

Whitney CR: Rising health costs threaten generous benefits in Europe. New York Times, Aug 6, 1996.

Woolhandler S, Himmelstein DU: The deteriorating administrative efficiency of the U.S. health care system. N Engl J Med 1991;324:1253.

National Health Insurance

15

For 80 years, reformers in the United States have argued for the passage of a national health insurance program, a government guarantee that every person is insured for basic health care. Yet, in 1997, the United States remained the only industrialized Western nation lacking such a guarantee.

The subject of national health insurance has seen five periods of intense legislative activity, alternating with times of political inattention. From 1912 to 1919, 1946 to 1949, 1963 to 1965, 1970 to 1974, and 1991 to 1994, it was the topic of major national debate. In 1916, 1949, 1974, and 1994, national health insurance was defeated and temporarily consigned to the nation's back burner. Guaranteed health coverage for two groups—the elderly and some of the poor—was enacted in 1965 through Medicare and Medicaid; and health insurance for some low-income children was legislated in 1997. While the specific phrase "national health insurance" has been replaced by the general 1990s term "health care reform," the central issue is unchanged: how to provide health insurance to all residents of the United States.

National health insurance means the guarantee of health insurance for all the nation's residents. The principal goal of any national health insurance proposal is to arrange universal health care financing. The issues of how physicians and hospitals are paid, how health care is organized, and how costs are controlled are not necessarily included in a national health insurance plan. Nonetheless, because of the close relationship among health care financing, provider reimbursement, organization of health care, and cost containment, many national health insurance proposals do concern themselves with those topics. However, the essence of any national health insurance plan is its mode of financing health care.

The controversies that erupt over universal health care coverage become simpler to understand if one returns to the four basic modes of health care financing outlined in Chapter 2: out-of-pocket payment, individual private insurance, employment-based private insurance, and government financing. There is general agreement that out-of-pocket payment does not work as a sole financing method for costly contemporary health care. National health insurance involves the replacement of out-of-pocket payments by one, or a mixture, of the other three financing modes.

Under government-financed national health insurance plans, funds are collected by a government or quasi-governmental fund, which in turn pays hospitals, physicians, health maintenance organizations (HMOs), and other health care providers. Under private individual or employment-based national health insurance, funds are collected by private insurance companies or HMOs, which then pay providers of care.

Historically, health care financing began with out-of-pocket payment and progressed through individual private insurance, then employment-based insurance, and finally government financing (for Medicare and Medicaid). In the history of U.S. national health insurance, the chronologic sequence is reversed. Early attempts at national health insurance legislation proposed government programs; private employment-based national health insurance was not seriously entertained until 1971, and individually purchased universal coverage was not suggested until the 1980s (Table 15–1).

Table 15–1. Attempts to legislate national health insurance.

1912–1919:	American Association for Labor Legislation
1946–1949:	Wagner-Murray-Dingell bill supported by President Truman
1963–1965:	Medicare and Medicaid passed as a first step toward national health insurance
1970–1974:	Kennedy and Nixon proposals
1991–1994:	A variety of proposals introduced, including President Clinton's plan

Following this historical progression, we shall first discuss government-financed national health insurance, followed by private employment-based and then individually purchased universal coverage.

GOVERNMENT-FINANCED NATIONAL HEALTH INSURANCE

The American Association for Labor Legislation Plan   In the early 1900s, 25–40% of people who became sick did not receive any medical care. In 1915, the American Association for Labor Legislation (AALL) published a national health insurance proposal to provide medical care, sick pay, and funeral expenses to lower-paid workers—earning less than $1200 a year—and to their dependents. The program would be run by states rather than the federal government, and would be financed by a payroll tax–like contribution from employers and employees, perhaps with an additional contribution from state governments. Payments would go to regional funds (not private insurance companies) under extensive government control. The funds would pay physicians and hospitals. Thus, the first national health insurance proposal in the United States—because the money was collected by quasi-public funds—can be considered a government-financed program (Starr, 1982; Myers, 1970).

> In 1910, Edgar Peoples worked as a clerk for Standard Oil, earning $800 a year. He lived with his wife and three sons. Under the AALL proposal, Standard Oil and Mr. Peoples would each pay $13 per year into the regional health insurance fund, with the state government contributing $6. The total of $32 (4% of wages) would cover the Peoples family.

The AALL's road to national health insurance followed the example of European nations, which often began their programs with lower-paid workers and gradually extended coverage to other groups in the population. Key to the financing of national health insurance was its compulsory nature and its coverage of large segments of the population; mandatory payments were to be made on behalf of every eligible person, thereby ensuring sufficient funds in the program to pay for that proportion of people who fell sick.

The AALL proposal initially had the support of the American Medical Association (AMA) leadership, and major initiatives to pass the program took place in several states. However, the AMA reversed its position and the conservative branch of labor, the American Federation of Labor, along with business interests, opposed the plan (Starr, 1982). The first attempt at national health insurance failed.

The Wagner–Murray–Dingell Bill   In 1943, Democratic Senators Robert Wagner of New York, and James Murray of Montana, and Representative John Dingell of Michigan, introduced a national health insurance bill into Congress. The Wagner–

Murray-Dingell bill was organized as an expansion of the social security system that had been enacted in 1935. Employer and employee contributions to cover physician and hospital care would be paid to the federal social insurance trust fund, which would in turn pay health providers.

> In the 1940s, Edgar Peoples' daughter Elena worked in a General Motors plant manufacturing trucks to be used in World War II. Elena earned $3500 per year. Under the 1943 Wagner–Murray–Dingell bill, General Motors would pay 6% of her wages up to $3000 into the social insurance trust fund for retirement, disability, unemployment, and health insurance. An identical 6% would be taken out of Elena's check for the same purpose. One-fourth of this total amount ($90) would be dedicated to the health insurance portion of social security. If Elena or her children became sick, the social insurance trust fund would reimburse their doctor and hospital.

> Edgar Peoples, in his 70s, would also receive health insurance under the Wagner–Murray–Dingell bill, because he was a social security beneficiary.

> Elena's younger brother, Marvin, was permanently disabled and unable to work. Under the Wagner–Murray–Dingell bill, he would not have received government health insurance, unless his state added unemployed people to the program.

As discussed in Chapter 2, government-financed health insurance can be divided into two categories. Under the social insurance model, only those who have paid into the program, usually through social security contributions, are eligible for the program's benefits. Under the public assistance (welfare) model, eligibility is based on a means test; those below a certain income may receive assistance. In the welfare model, those who benefit may not necessarily contribute, and those who do contribute (usually through taxes) may not benefit (Bodenheimer and Grumbach, 1992). The Wagner–Murray–Dingell bill, like the AALL proposal, was a social insurance proposal. Working people and their dependents were eligible because they made social security contributions, and retired people receiving social security benefits were eligible because they paid into social security prior to their retirement. The permanently unemployed were not eligible and were required to seek charity care at public hospitals or to have their care paid for by a state welfare program.

In 1945, President Harry S. Truman, in embracing the general principles of the Wagner–Murray–Dingell legislation, became the first U.S. president to strongly support national health insurance. After Truman's surprise election in 1948, the AMA organized a massive and expensive campaign to defeat the Wagner–Murray–Dingell bill. The AMA succeeded, and in 1950, national health insurance returned to obscurity (Starr, 1982; Poen, 1979).

Medicare & Medicaid   In the late 1950s, less than 15% of the elderly had health insurance (see Chapter 2), and a strong social movement clamored for the federal government to come up with a solution. The Medicare law of 1965 took the Wagner–Murray–Dingell approach to national health insurance and narrowed it to coverage of people over 65 years of age. Medicare was financed through social security contributions, federal income taxes, and individual premiums. Congress also enacted the Medicaid program in 1965, a public assistance or "welfare" model of government insurance that covered a portion of the low-income population. Medicaid was paid for by general federal and state taxes.

> In 1966, at age 66, Elena Peoples was automatically enrolled in the federal government's Medicare Part A hospital insurance plan, and she chose to sign up for the Medicare Part B physician insurance plan by paying a $3 monthly premium to the Social Security Administration. Elena's son, Tom, and Tom's employer helped to finance Medicare Part A; each paid 0.5% of wages (up to a wage level of $6600 per year) into a Medicare trust fund within the social security system. Elena's Part B coverage was financed in part by federal income taxes and in part by Elena's monthly premiums. In case of illness, Medicare would pay for most of Elena's hospital and physician bills.
>
> Elena's disabled younger brother, Marvin, age 60, was too young to qualify for Medicare in 1966. Marvin instead became a recipient of Medicaid, the federal–state program for certain groups of low-income people. When Marvin required medical care, the state Medicaid program paid the hospital, physician, and pharmacy, and a substantial portion of the state's costs were picked up by the federal government.

Medicare is a social insurance program, requiring individuals or families to have made social security contributions to gain eligibility to the plan. Medicaid, in contrast, is a public assistance program that does not require recipients to make contributions but is financed from general tax revenues. Because of the rapid increase in Medicare costs, the social security contribution has risen substantially. In 1966, Medicare took 1% of wages, up to a $6600 wage level (0.5% each from employer and employee); in 1997, the payments had risen to 2.9% of all wages. The Part B premium has jumped from $3 per month in 1966 to $43.80 per month in 1997.

The 1970 Kennedy Bill & the Single-Payer Plan of the 1990s   Many people felt that Medicare and Medicaid were a first step toward national health insurance. European nations started their national health insurance programs by covering a portion of the population and later extending coverage to more and more people. Medicare and Medicaid seemed to fit into that tradition. Shortly after Medicare and Medicaid became law, the labor movement, Senator Edward Kennedy of Massachusetts, and Representative Martha Griffiths of Michigan drafted legislation to cover the entire population through a national health insurance program. The 1970 Kennedy–Griffiths Health Security Act followed in the footsteps of the Wagner–Murray–Dingell bill, calling for a single federally operated health insurance system that would replace all public and private health insurance plans (Somers, 1971).

> Under the Kennedy-Griffiths 1970 Health Security Program, Tom Peoples, who worked for Great Books, a small book publisher, would continue to see his family physician as before. Rather than receiving payment from Tom's private insurance company, his physician would be paid by the federal government, perhaps through a regional intermedi-

ary. Tom's employer would no longer make a social security contribution to Medicare (which would be folded into
the Health Security Program) and would instead make a
larger contribution of 3% of wages up to a wage level of
$15,000 for each employee. Tom's employee contribution
was set at 1% up to a wage level of $15,000. These social
insurance contributions would pay for about 60% of the
program; federal income taxes would pay for the other
40%.

Tom's Uncle Marvin, on Medicaid since 1966, would be included in the Health Security Program, as would all residents of the United States. Medicaid would be phased out
as a separate public assistance program.

The Kennedy–Griffiths Health Security Act went one step further than the AALL
and Wagner–Murray–Dingell proposals: It combined the social insurance and public
assistance approaches into one unified program. In part because of the staunch opposition of the AMA and the private insurance industry, the Health Security Program
went the way of its predecessors: political defeat.

In 1989, the latest incarnation of government-financed national health insurance
resurfaced. The plan came to be known as the "single-payer" program, because it
would establish a single government fund within each state to pay hospitals, physicians, and other health care providers, replacing the current multipayer system of private insurance companies and HMOs (Himmelstein and Woolhandler, 1989). Several
versions of the single-payer plan were introduced into Congress in the early 1990s,
each bringing the entire population together into one health care financing system,
merging the social insurance and public assistance approaches (Table 15–2).

EMPLOYMENT-BASED NATIONAL HEALTH INSURANCE

In response to Democratic Senator Edward Kennedy's introduction of the 1970
Health Security Act, President Richard M. Nixon, a Republican, countered with a
plan of his own, the nation's first employment-based, privately administered national
health insurance proposal (Somers, 1971). For 3 years, the Nixon and Kennedy approaches competed in the congressional battleground; however, because most of the
population was covered under private insurance, Medicare, or Medicaid, there was
relatively little public pressure on Congress. In 1974, the momentum for national
health insurance collapsed, not to be seriously revived until the 1990s.

Table 15–2. Categories of national health insurance plans.

1. Government-financed health insurance plans	Money is collected through taxes or premiums by a public or quasi-public fund that reimburses health care providers.
2. Employer-mandated private health insurance plans	The government requires employers to pay for all or part of private health insurance policies for their employees.
3. Individual-mandated private health insurance plans	The government requires individuals to purchase private health insurance, with subsidies for low-income people.
4. Mixed plans	Government-financed insurance for the elderly and the poor, employer-mandated private insurance for the employed and their dependents, individual-mandated private insurance for people without employment.

The essence of the Nixon proposal was the employer mandate, under which the federal government requires (or mandates) employers to purchase private health insurance for their employees.

> Tom Peoples' cousin Blanche was a receptionist in a physician's office in 1971. The doctor did not provide health insurance to his employees. Under Nixon's 1971 plan, Blanche's employer would be required to pay 75% of the private health insurance premium for his employees; the employees would pay the other 25%.

> Blanche's boyfriend, Al, had been laid off from his job in 1970 and was receiving unemployment benefits. He had no health insurance. Under Nixon's proposal, the federal government would pay a portion of Al's health insurance premium.

No longer was national health insurance equated with government financing. Employer mandate plans preserve and expand the role of the private health insurance industry, while government-financed plans reduce or eliminate private health insurance. Thus, the Nixon proposal changed the entire political landscape of national health insurance, moving it toward the private sector. In later years, Senator Kennedy embraced the employer mandate approach himself, fearing that the opposition of the insurance industry and organized medicine would kill any attempt to legislate government-financed national health insurance.

During the 1980s and 1990s, the number of people in the United States without any health insurance rose from 25 to 40 million (see Chapter 3). About three-quarters of the uninsured were employed or were dependents of employed persons. The rapidly rising cost of health insurance premiums made insurance unaffordable for many businesses.

In response to this crisis in health care access, President Bill Clinton submitted legislation to Congress in 1993 calling for universal health insurance through an employer mandate. Like the proposal introduced by President Nixon, the essence of the Clinton plan was the requirement that employers pay for most of their employees' private insurance premiums (Starr and Zelman, 1993).

A variation on the employer mandate type of national health insurance is the voluntary approach. Rather than requiring employers to purchase health insurance for employees, employers are given incentives such as tax credits to cover employees voluntarily. The attempt of some states to implement the voluntary approach, however, has failed to reduce significantly the numbers of uninsured workers.

Another voluntary innovation is the Medical Savings Account (MSA) proposal, backed by the AMA, conservative Republicans, and non-managed care private insurers. MSAs can be offered by employers as an alternative to other coverage. For example, an employer may pay a modest premium for a family insurance policy with a $4000 per year deductible and place $1800 per year in the family's MSA. The family must pay the first $4000 of medical expenses each year and can use the money in the MSA to help make these payments. Families using no health services may keep the money for future years or spend it on a new TV or a summer vacation. The supporters of MSAs wish to make them tax deductible if the money is used for medical expenses. MSA proponents contend that patients would exercise greater restraint in their health care expenditures if they could financially benefit from seeking less health care. The Health Insurance Portability and Accountability Act of 1996 includes a pilot program allowing tax-deductible MSAs for some employees.

Because families with MSAs must pay for medical expenses below the deductible, their incentive is to skimp on preventive services. Healthy people would tend to choose MSAs because they could keep the money, whereas people with chronic illnesses would be unlikely to choose MSAs because the funds in the MSA would not cover their medical expenses below the deductible. If millions of healthy HMO enrollees switched to MSAs, leaving HMOs with a sicker and costlier population, HMOs would be forced to raise their premiums by an estimated 60% (Thorpe, 1995). MSAs divide the population into low-risk and high-risk pools; low-risk people no longer would subsidize high-risk people, and the latter would see an unprecedented increase in their health insurance costs. Since the great majority of health care expenses are concentrated in a small number of acutely or chronically ill people, the incentive created by MSAs for families to restrain health care services would have little impact on the nation's health care costs.

Individually Purchased National Health Insurance   In 1989, a new species of national health insurance appeared, sponsored by the conservative Heritage Foundation. In contrast to the government-financed or employer mandate approaches, the Heritage Foundation called for an individual mandate. Just as many states require motor vehicle drivers to purchase automobile insurance, the Heritage plan called for the federal government to require (or mandate) all U.S. residents to purchase individual health insurance policies. Tax credits would be made available on a sliding scale to individuals and families too poor to afford health insurance premiums (Butler, 1991). In 1993, Republican Senator John Chafee of Vermont introduced a bill based on the principle of an individual mandate.

> Tom Peoples received health insurance through his employer, Great Books. Under the Chafee plan, Tom would be legally required to purchase health insurance for his family. Great Books would be obligated to offer a health plan to Tom and his coworkers but would not be required to contribute anything to the premium. If Tom purchased private health insurance for his family at a cost of $4000 per year, he would receive a tax credit of $800 (ie, he would pay $800 less in income taxes). Tom's Uncle Marvin, formerly on Medicaid, would be given a voucher to purchase a private health insurance policy.

In 1993, the individual mandate approach was not confined to the conservative pole of the political spectrum. President Clinton's plan included an employer mandate for employed people and their families and an individual mandate (with subsidies for lower-income families) for people without jobs.

SECONDARY FEATURES OF NATIONAL HEALTH INSURANCE PLANS

The primary distinction among national health insurance approaches is the mode of financing: government versus employment-based versus individual-based health insurance. A plan may contain a mixture of these modes; eg, the 1993 Clinton plan merged government financing (Medicaid and Medicare) for the poor and the elderly, an employer mandate for working people, and an individual mandate for those without jobs who are ineligible for Medicare or Medicaid. However, complex a national health insurance plan may be, it can always be broken down into one or more of these three financing modes.

The complexity of national health insurance plans frequently stems from their secondary characteristics, ie, those features of the plan that modify or add to the basic financing mechanism (see Table 15–3). What are some of these secondary features?

Benefit Package

> Elena Peoples is a beneficiary of Medicare Parts A and B, which cover her for most hospital and physician services but not for outpatient medications or long-term care. Elena's brother Marvin receives Medicaid, which pays for most hospital and physician services plus many outpatient medications and long-term care.

An important feature of any health plan is its benefit package. Most national health insurance proposals cover hospital care, physician visits, laboratory, x-rays, physical and occupational therapy, inpatient pharmacy, and other services usually emphasizing acute care. Outpatient medications and long-term care are often not included, and mental health services may be covered with a restricted number of visits per year. Chiropractic care and acupuncture may or may not be part of the package. In the past, many private insurance plans and Medicare failed to cover routine preventive care, but most HMOs and most national health insurance proposals now include clinical preventive services.

Patient Cost Sharing

> In 1972, Tom Peoples turned on his television and caught a debate between advocates of the Kennedy and Nixon national health insurance plans. One big difference between the plans attracted his attention. Under the Nixon plan, he would pay 25% of his insurance premium, the entire cost of the first 2 days of the hospital bill, a $100 deductible for each family member on doctor bills, and 25% coinsurance on all medical bills up to $5000 in a year. In contrast, the Kennedy plan would take about 1% of Tom's wages in a

Table 15–3. Features of national health insurance plans.

Primary feature	
How the plan is financed:	Government, employer mandate, or individual mandate?
Secondary features	
Benefit package:	Which services are covered?
Patient cost sharing:	Does the plan require deductibles or copayments, or both?
Effect on existing programs:	Do Medicare, Medicaid, and private insurance arrangements continue in their current form?
Cost containment:	Are cost controls introduced, and, if so, what type of controls (see Chapter 9)?

social security tax but charge Tom no deductibles or coinsurance payments when he needed care.

Patient cost sharing involves payments made by patients at the time of receiving medical care services. It is sometimes broadened to include that portion of health insurance premiums paid by the employee rather than by the employer. Naturally, the breadth of the benefit package influences the amount of patient cost sharing: The more services not covered, the more patients must pay out of pocket. Many plans impose patient cost sharing requirements on covered services, usually in the form of deductibles (a lump sum each year), coinsurance payments (a percentage of the cost of the service), or copayments (a fixed fee, eg, $5 or $10 per visit or per prescription). In general, proposals based on individual mandates, such as the Heritage Foundation plan, impose large cost-sharing requirements, eg, a $5000-per-year deductible; government-financed plans tend to reduce patient cost sharing.

Effects on Medicare, Medicaid, & Private Insurance

As a senior citizen in 1993, Elena Peoples always worried about her Medicare plan. There was so much talk about cutting this and cutting that out of Medicare. In the publications she received from senior citizen organizations, Elena read that some plans, like the single-payer plan, would eliminate Medicare and Medicaid, making them part of a single universal health care system. Other plans would keep Medicare separate. President Clinton's plan was somewhere in between, with the option for states to fold Medicare into purchasing cooperatives. She did not know which she preferred, but was worried about any possible change.

Any national health insurance program must interact with existing health care programs, whether Medicare, Medicaid, or private insurance plans. Single-payer proposals make the most far-reaching changes: Medicare, Medicaid, and private insurance are eliminated in their current form and are melded into the single insurance program. Individual mandates would have a major impact on private insurance: By moving from employment-based insurance (the dominant current financing mode) toward individually mandated insurance, major disruptions would take place in the health insurance market. Medicare and Medicaid would be less affected. Employer mandates, which extend rather than supplant employment-based coverage, tend to have the least effect on existing dollar flow in the health care system. Depending on the benefit package required under an employer mandate plan, however, employees receiving rich benefits could lose some of their coverage.

Cost Containment

Tom Peoples' son Chris was doing a report for his 1994 high school civics class; health care costs was his topic. Confused by the rhetoric, he talked to his dad one night. "I remember a debate back in 1972," offered Tom. "It was the Nixon people against Ted Kennedy's people. The Nixon folks said there were only two ways to keep costs down: Make people pay more out of pocket, and pay doctors to keep you healthy through those things called HMOs. The

Kennedy people said that wouldn't work. You needed to slap a budget on the whole health care system and make the patients, doctors, and hospitals live within that budget, because that's all the money there's going to be."

"That sounds just like what they're saying in 1994," ventured Chris. "The HMO advocates say that if people have to pay more for their health insurance premiums, they'll choose cheaper plans. And with a big coinsurance, they'll go to the doctor less. The cheapest health plans will be HMOs that stop paying doctors more for doing more tests and more surgeries. Health plans will compete by offering cheaper premiums than other plans and the costs will go down. They call it 'managed competition.' "

"Sounds like a modern version of the Nixon philosophy," interjected Tom. "But does anyone nowadays say what Kennedy was saying?"

"You bet," said Chris. "The single-payer people argue that managed competition has never been tried anywhere and we need a global budget to control health care costs. But the managed competition folks say a global budget means rationing and government bureaucracy. I don't know what I think."

By increasing people's access to medical care, national health insurance has the capacity to cause a rapid increase in national health expenditures, as did Medicare and Medicaid (see Chapter 2). By the 1990s, policymakers recognized that an increase in access must be balanced with measures to control costs.

Different national health insurance proposals have vastly disparate methods of containing costs. Individual- and employment-based proposals tend to use patient cost sharing and managed competition as their chief cost control mechanisms (see Chapter 9). In contrast, government-financed plans look more to global budgeting to keep expenditures down. Single-payer plans, which concentrate health care funds in a single public insurer, can more easily establish a global budgeting approach than can plans with multiple private insurers.

WHICH NATIONAL HEALTH INSURANCE PLAN IS BEST?

Historically, in the United States, the government-financed road to national health insurance—now called the single-payer proposal—is the oldest and most traveled of the three approaches. Advocates of government financing cite its universality: Everyone is insured in the same plan simply by virtue of being a U.S. resident. Its simplicity creates a potential cost saving: The 20–25% of health expenditures spent on administration could be reduced, thus making available funds to extend health insurance to the uninsured. Employers would be relieved of the burden of providing health insurance to their employees. Employees would regain free choice of physician, choice that is being lost as employers are increasingly choosing which health plans (and therefore which physicians) are available to their work force. Health insurance would be delinked from jobs, so that people changing jobs or losing a job would not be forced to change or lose their health coverage. Single-payer advocates, citing the experience of other nations, argue that cost control only works when all health care moneys are channeled through a single mechanism with the capacity to set budgets. While opponents accuse the government-financed approach as an invitation to bureaucracy, single-payer advocates point out that private insurers have average administrative costs of 14%, far higher than government programs such as Medicare, with its 2% administrative overhead (Burner et al, 1992). A cost control advantage intrinsic to tax-financed systems in which a public agency serves as the single payer for health care is the administrative efficiency of collecting and dispensing revenues under this arrangement.

Single-payer detractors charge that one single government payer would have too much power over people's health choices, dictating to physicians and patients which treatments they can receive and which they cannot, resulting in waiting lines and the rationing of care. Opponents also state that the shift in health care financing from private payments (out-of-pocket, individual insurance, and employment-based insurance) to taxes would be unacceptable in an antitax society (Blendon et al, 1994). Moreover, the United States has a long history of politicians and government agencies being overly influenced by wealthy private interests, and this has contributed to making the public mistrustful of the government.

The employer mandate approach—requiring all employers to pay for the health insurance of their employees—is seen by its supporters as the only way to raise enough funds to insure the uninsured without massive tax increases (though employer mandates have been called hidden taxes). Because most people under age 65 now receive their health insurance through the workplace, it may be less disruptive to extend this process rather than change it.

The conservative advocates of individual-based insurance and the liberal supporters of single-payer plans both criticize employer mandate plans, saying that forcing small businesses—many of whom do not insure their employees—to shoulder the fiscal burden of insuring the uninsured is inequitable and economically disastrous; rather than purchasing health insurance for their employees, many small businesses may simply lay off workers, thereby pitting health insurance against jobs. Moreover, because millions of people change their jobs in a given year, job-linked health insurance is administratively cumbersome and insecure for employees, whose health security is tied to their job. Finally, critics point out that under the employer mandate approach, "Your boss, not your family, chooses your doctor;" changes in the health plans offered by employers often force employees and their families to change physicians, who may not belong to the health plans being offered.

Advocates of the individual mandate assert that their approach would free employers of the obligation to provide health insurance, and would grant individuals a stable source of health insurance whether they are employed, change jobs, or become disabled. There would be no need either to burden small businesses with new expenses and thereby disrupt job growth, or to raise taxes substantially. While opponents argue that low-income families would be unable to afford the mandatory purchase of health insurance, supporters claim that income-related tax credits are a fair and effective method to assist such families (Butler, 1991).

The individual mandate approach is criticized as inefficient, with each family having to purchase its own health insurance. The awarding of tax credits would require a cumbersome means-testing apparatus. To enforce a requirement that every person buy coverage would be even more difficult for health insurance than for automobile insurance. Moreover, to reduce the price of their premiums, many families would purchase low-cost, high-deductible coverage with a scanty benefit package (called by some "bare-bones insurance"), thereby leaving lower-income families with potentially unaffordable out-of-pocket costs.

Regrettably, the national health insurance debate will not be decided by logic or rational persuasion. In 1994, most observers predicted that Congress, with the leadership of President Clinton, would legislate some form of national health insurance or would at least take a major step toward universal coverage. No legislation was passed. The public was besieged with, and confused by, slick and often inaccurate television advertisements produced by such powerful interest groups as the Health Insurance Association of America. Special-interest groups spent over $100 million to influence the outcome of the legislation (Skocpol, 1995).

Health care is a trillion dollar business, and those dollars represent income or profits for health insurers, HMOs, hospitals, nursing homes, pharmaceutical manufacturers, physicians, and other health care givers. At the same time, these billions represent costs for powerful business interests that pay a portion of their employees' health insurance. Every stake-holder in the health care economy has a keen interest in preserving or bettering their financial position. In the money-driven political environment in the United States, powerful interest groups will play a major role in shaping any future national health insurance program.

To overcome the moneyed interest groups would require an electorate mobilized in support of a particular national health insurance plan. Such an electorate does not exist in the United States. While three-quarters of the public in recent polls expresses a desire for universal health insurance coverage, less than half the people surveyed are willing to pay more taxes to finance universal coverage, and only half think that business should be required to pay for their employees' health insurance. Less than one-quarter of the public trusts the federal government to do the right thing (Blendon et al, 1994). The strength of the public's antitax and antigovernment sentiments erodes support for the overall concept of national health insurance.

The concept of national health insurance rests on the belief that everyone should contribute to finance health care and everyone should benefit. People who pay more than they benefit are likely to benefit more than they pay 10 years down the road when they face an expensive health problem. The achievement of national health insurance in the United States may depend on the development of such community-minded attitudes.

REFERENCES

Blendon RJ et al: The American public and the critical choices for health system reform. JAMA 1994:271:1539.

Bodenheimer T, Grumbach K: Financing universal health insurance: Taxes, premiums, and the lessons of social insurance. J Health Polit Policy Law 1992;17:439.

Burner ST, Waldo DR, McKusick DR: National health expenditures projections through 2030. Health Care Fin Rev 1992;14(1):1.

Butler SM: A tax reform strategy to deal with the uninsured. JAMA 1991;265:2541.

Himmelstein DU, Woolhandler S: Writing Committee of Physicians for a National Health Program: A national health program for the United States: A physicians' proposal. N Engl J Med 1989;320:102.

Myers RJ: Medicare. Richard D. Irwin, 1970.

Poen MM: Harry S. Truman Versus the Medical Lobby. Univ Missouri Press, 1979.

Skocpol T: The rise and resounding demise of the Clinton plan. Health Aff 1995;14(1):66.

Somers AR: Health Care in Transition: Directions for the Future. Hospital Research and Educational Trust, 1971.

Starr P: The Social Transformation of American Medicine. Basic Books, 1982.

Starr P, Zelman WA: A bridge to compromise: competition under a budget. Health Aff 1993; 12(Suppl):7.

Thorpe KE: Medical savings accounts: Design and policy issues. Health Aff 1995;14(3):254.

The Ascendance of Managed Care 16

The book's introduction describes the paradigm shift in health care in the United States; managed care has become the overarching concept within which many details can be understood. Managed care expresses a power shift whereby those who pay for medical care services have acquired the authority to make decisions formerly reserved for those who provide the care. How did managed care achieve its ascendance? How has it changed medical practice?

THE FOUR MAJOR ACTORS

The health care sector of the nation's economy is a trillion dollar system that finances, organizes, and provides health care services for the people of the United States. Four major actors can be found on this stage (Table 16–1).

(1) *The payers* supply the funds. These include individual health care consumers, businesses that pay for the health insurance of their employees, and the government, which pays for care through public programs such as Medicare and Medicaid. In fact, all payers of health care are ultimately individuals, because individuals finance businesses by purchasing their products and fund the government by paying taxes. Nonetheless, businesses and the government assume special importance as the nation's *organized* payers of health care.

(2) *The insurers* receive money from the payers and reimburse the providers. Traditional insurers take money from payers (individuals or businesses), assume risk, and pay providers when policyholders require medical care. Yet, some insurers are the same as payers; the government can be viewed as insurer or payer in the Medicare and Medicaid programs, and businesses that self-insure their employees can similarly occupy both roles.

(3) *The providers,* including hospitals, physicians, nurses, nurse practitioners, physician assistants, other care givers, nursing homes, home care agencies, and pharmacies, actually provide the care. While HMOs are generally insurers, some are also providers, owning hospitals and employing physicians.

(4) *The suppliers* are the pharmaceutical and medical supply industries, which manufacture equipment, supplies, and medications used by providers to treat patients.

Insurers, providers, and suppliers make up the health care industry. Each dollar spent on health care represents an expense to the payers and a gain to the health care industry. In the past, payers viewed this expense as an investment, money spent to improve the health of the population and thereby the economic and social vitality of the nation. But more recently, payers have been reluctant to continue to pour dollars into the health care industry. A fundamental conflict has intensified between the pay-

Table 16–1. The four major actors.

Payers
   Individuals
   Business
   Government
Insurers
   Blue Cross and Blue Shield
   Commercial insurance companies
   Health maintenance organizations
Providers
   Hospitals
   Nursing homes
   Home care agencies
   Pharmacies
   Physicians
   Other care givers
Suppliers
   Pharmaceutical companies
   Medical supply companies

ers and the health care industry: The payers wish to reduce, and the health care industry to increase, the number of dollars spent on health care. We will now explore the changing relationships among payers, insurers, and providers (leaving out the suppliers) in a historical progression.

THE YEARS 1945 to 1970: THE PROVIDER–INSURER PACT

Until recently, independent hospitals and small private practices of office-based physicians populated the U.S. health delivery system (see Chapter 7). Some large institutions existed that combined hospital and physician care (eg, the Kaiser–Permanente system, the Mayo Clinic, and urban medical school complexes), but these were the exception (Starr, 1982). Competition among health care providers was minimal because most geographic areas did not have an excess of facilities and personnel. The health care financing system included hundreds of private insurance companies, joined by the governmental Medicare and Medicaid programs enacted in 1965. The United States had a relatively dispersed health care industry.

> Bert Neighbor was a 63-year-old man who developed abdominal pain in 1962. Because he was well insured under Blue Cross, his physician placed him in Metropolitan Hospital for diagnostic studies. On the sixth hospital day, a colon cancer was surgically removed. On the fifteenth day, Mr. Neighbor went home. The hospital sent its $1200 bill to Blue Cross, which paid the hospital for its total costs in caring for Mr. Neighbor. In calculating Mr. Neighbor's bill, Metropolitan Hospital included a small part of the cost of the 80-bed new building under construction.
>
> At a subsequent meeting of the Blue Cross board of directors, the hospital administrator (also a Blue Cross director) was asked whether it was reasonable to include the cost of

capital improvements when preparing a bill. Other Blue Cross directors, also hospital administrators with construction plans, argued that it was proper, and the matter was dropped. In the same meeting, the directors voted a 34% increase in Blue Cross premiums. Sixteen years later, a study revealed that the metropolitan area had 300 excess hospital beds, with hospital occupancy down from 82 to 60% over the past decade.

A defining characteristic of the health care industry was an alliance of insurers and providers of care. This provider–insurer pact was cemented with the creation of Blue Cross and Blue Shield, the nation's largest health insurance system for half a century (see Chapter 2). Blue Cross was formed by the American Hospital Association, and Blue Shield was run by state medical societies affiliated with the American Medical Association. Thus, in the case of the Blues, the provider–insurer relationship was more than a political alliance; it involved legal control of insurers by providers. As in the example of Metropolitan Hospital, the providers set generous rules of reimbursement, and the Blues made the payments without asking too many questions (Law, 1974). Commercial insurers usually played by the reimbursement rules already formulated by the physicians, hospitals, and Blues, paying for medical services without asking providers to justify their prices or the reasons for the services (Weiss, 1992).

By the 1960s, the power of the provider–insurer pact was so great that the hospitals and Blue Cross virtually wrote the reimbursement provisions of Medicare and Medicaid, guaranteeing that doctors and hospitals would be paid with the same bountiful formulas used for private patients. The providers even set up a payment apparatus to shield them from the government: Under Medicare and many state Medicaid programs, the government paid fiscal intermediaries (in most cases, Blue Cross or Blue Shield), who in turn reimbursed doctors and hospitals for treating Medicare and Medicaid patients (Law, 1974). With relatively open-ended reimbursement policies, the costs of health care inflated at a rapid pace.

With some exceptions, the payers were relatively apathetic about the amount of money pouring into the health care industry. Millions of individual consumers hardly noticed the cost increases because their medical bills appeared to be paid by their employers. Moreover, individual consumers were seldom organized and thus incapable of exerting much clout. The government became a major payer only in 1965; as a latecomer to the triad of payers, it was not a major actor during the 1945 to 1970 period.

The disinterest of the chief organized payer (ie, business) stemmed from two sources: the healthy economy and the tax subsidy for health insurance. From 1945 through 1970, U.S. business controlled domestic and foreign markets with little foreign competition. Labor unions in certain industries had successfully gained generous wages and fringe benefits, and business could afford these costs because profits were high and world economic growth was robust (Kennedy, 1987; Kuttner, 1980). The cost of health insurance for employees was a tiny fraction of total business expenses. Moreover, payments by business for employee health insurance were considered a tax-deductible business expense, thereby cushioning any economic drain on business (Reinhardt, 1993). For these reasons, increasing costs generated by the providers and reimbursed by the insurers were passed on to business, which, with few complaints, paid higher and higher premiums for employees' health insurance and thereby underwrote the expanding health care system. No countervailing forces "put the brakes" on the enthusiasm that united providers and the public in support of a medical industry that strived to translate the proliferation of biomedical breakthroughs into an improvement in people's lives.

THE 1970s: TENSIONS DEVELOP

> Jerry Neighbor, Bert Neighbor's son, developed abdominal pain in 1978. Because Blue Cross no longer paid for in-hospital diagnostic testing, his doctor ordered outpatient x-ray studies. When colon cancer was discovered, Jerry Neighbor was admitted to Metropolitan Hospital on the morning of his surgery. His total hospital stay was 9 days, 6 days shorter than his father's stay in 1962. Since 1962, medical care costs had risen by about 10% per year. Blue Cross paid Metropolitan Hospital $460 for each of the 9 days Jerry Neighbor spent in the hospital, for a total cost of $4140. The Blue Cross board of directors, which in 1977 included for the first time more business than hospital representatives, submitted a formal proposal to the regional health planning agency to reduce the number of hospital beds in the region, in order to keep hospital costs down. The planning agency board had a majority of hospital and physician representatives, and they voted the proposal down.

In the early 1970s, two developments took place that fundamentally changed the economy of the United States. The world entered a prolonged recession, with rates of economic growth of industrialized nations falling markedly from the levels of the 1960s (Thurow, 1992). At the same time, the United States fell from its postwar position of economic dominance, as Western Europe and Japan gobbled up markets (not only abroad but in the United States itself) formerly controlled by U.S. companies. The U.S. share of world industrial production was dropping, from 60% in 1950 to 30% in 1980. In the early 1970s, the profits of U.S. companies had dropped far below their previous levels (Castells, 1980). Except for a few years during the mid 1980s, inflation or unemployment plagued the United States from 1970 to the early 1990s.

The new economic reality has been a critical motor of change in the health care system. With less money in their respective pockets, individual health care consumers, business, and government gradually became concerned with the accelerating flow of dollars into the health care industry. The payers also became concerned that more health care dollars did not appear to be buying better health. Prominent business-oriented journals published major critiques of the health care industry and its rising costs (Bergthold, 1990). A new concern for community and preventive medicine, which seemed underemphasized in relation to specialty and hospital care, spread within the health professions. As a result of these influences, payers became more critical of the health care industry, thereby producing tensions within the industry itself.

During the 1970s, the effects on the health care system produced by the payers' change in attitude were in their infancy. Faced with Blue Cross premium increases of 25 to 50% in a single year, angry Blue Cross subscribers protested at state hearings in eastern and midwestern states, and challenged hospital control over Blue Cross boards (Law, 1974; Health Policy Advisory Center, 1971). Some state governments began to regulate hospital construction, and a few states initiated hospital rate regulation. The federal government established a network of health planning agencies, attempting to slow down hospital growth. Peer review was established to monitor the appropriateness of physician services under Medicare. The payers, then, took on an additional role as health care regulators. But the health care industry resisted these attempts of payers to control health care costs through regulation. Medical inflation continued at a rate far above that of inflation in the general economy (Starr, 1982).

Nonetheless, these early initiatives from the payers made an impact on the provider–insurer pact. As pressure mounted on insurers not to increase premiums, insurers demanded that services be provided at lower cost. Blue Cross, widely criticized as playing the role of a middleman that passed increased hospital costs on to a helpless public, legally separated from the American Hospital Association in 1972 (Law, 1974). State medical societies were forced to relinquish some of their control over Blue Shield plans. Conflicts erupted between providers and insurers as the latter imposed utilization review procedures to reduce the length of hospital stays. Hospitals, which had hitherto purchased the newest diagnostic and surgical technology desired by physicians on their medical staffs, began to deny such requests because insurers questioned the need for such equipment and would no longer guarantee its reimbursement. Moreover, the glut of hospital beds and specialty physicians, which had been produced by the attractive reimbursements of the 1960s and the influence of the biomedical model on medical education (see Chapter 6), turned on itself as half-empty hospitals and half-busy surgeons began to compete with one another for patients. Strains were showing within the provider–insurer pact.

By the late 1970s, the deepening of the economic crisis created a nationwide tax revolt; as a result, governments attempted to reduce spending on such programs as health care (Kuttner, 1980). But major change was still awaiting the arrival of the most powerful payer: business.

THE 1980s: THE REVOLT OF THE PAYERS

> In 1989, Ryan Neighbor, Jerry Neighbor's brother, became concerned when he noticed blood in his stools; he decided to see a physician. Six months earlier, his company had increased the annual health insurance deductible to $1000, which could be avoided by joining one of the health maintenance organizations (HMOs) offered by the company. Ryan Neighbor opted for the Blue Cross HMO, but his family physician was not involved in that HMO, and Mr. Neighbor had to pick another physician from the HMO's list. The physician diagnosed colon cancer; Ryan Neighbor was not allowed to see the surgeon who had operated on his brother, but was sent to a Blue Cross HMO surgeon. While Mr. Neighbor respected Metropolitan Hospital, his surgery was scheduled at Crosstown Hospital; Blue Cross had refused to sign a contract with Metropolitan when the hospital failed to negotiate down from its $1800 per diem rate. Ryan Neighbor's entire Crosstown Hospital stay was 5 days, and the HMO paid the hospital $7500, based on its $1500 per diem contract.

By 1980, U.S. business had entered an era of austerity, with wage reductions and plant relocations to low-wage areas of the nation and the globe (Bluestone and Harrison, 1982). But business had not yet confronted the impact of health care costs. A 1981 survey of corporate executives reported that companies were not strongly motivated to do much about their health care costs, and concluded that business was unlikely to be a major force for health care system reform (Sapolsky et al, 1981).

The late 1980s produced a severe shock: The cost of employer-sponsored health plans jumped 18.6% in 1988 and 20.4% in 1989 (Cantor et al, 1991). Between 1976 and 1988, the percentage of total payroll spent on health benefits almost doubled, from 5 to 9.7% (Bergthold, 1991). In another development, many large corporations began to self-insure. Rather than paying money to insurance companies to cover their employees, employers increasingly took on the health insurance function themselves and used insurance companies only for claims processing and related administrative tasks. In 1991, 40% of employees receiving employer-sponsored health benefits were in self-insured plans (Sullivan et al, 1992). Self-insurance placed employers at risk for health care expenditures and forced them to pay more attention to the health care issue. These three developments (ie, a troubled economy, rising health care costs, and self-insurance) catapulted big business into the center of the health policy debate, with cost control as its rallying cry. Business, the major private payer of health care, became the motor driving unprecedented change in the health care landscape (Bergthold, 1990).

Employers pursued their cost control goals through two major avenues:

(1) As U.S. business was losing domestic and foreign markets, pressure mounted to cut the costs of production by reducing wages and benefits, one of which was health insurance for employees. In the late 1980s, employers began to shift their costs onto employees through increases in employee deductible and coinsurance payments (Sullivan et al, 1992).

(2) Business threw its clout behind managed care, particularly HMOs, as a cost control device, thereby allying with those insurers owning HMOs (Harris, 1992). By shifting from fee-for-service to capitated reimbursement, managed care could transfer a portion of the health expenditure risk from payers and insurers to providers (see Chapter 4).

Individual health care consumers, in their role as payers, also showed some clout during the late 1980s. Because employers were shifting health care payments to employees, labor unions began to complain bitterly about health care costs, and major strikes took place over the issue of health care benefits. Over 70% of people polled in a 1992 Louis Harris survey favored serious health care cost controls (Smith et al, 1992). The growing tendency of private health insurers to reduce their risks by dramatic premium increases and policy cancellations for policyholders with chronic illnesses created a series of horror stories in the media that turned health insurance companies into highly unpopular institutions.

During the 1980s, the government was facing the tax revolt and budget deficits, and it took measures designed to slow the rising costs of Medicare and Medicaid, with limited success. The 1983 Medicare Prospective Payment System (diagnosis-related groups [DRGs]) did somewhat reduce the rate of increase of Medicare hospital costs, but outpatient Medicare costs and costs borne by private payers escalated in response (Califano, 1986). In 1989, Medicare physician payments were brought under tighter control, resulting in Medicare physician expenditures growing at only 5.3% per year from 1991 to 1993, compared with 11.3% per year from 1984 to 1991 (Davis and Burner, 1995). Numerous states scaled back their Medicaid programs, but because of the economic recession and the growing crisis of uninsurance (see Chapter 3), the federal government was forced to expand Medicaid eligibility, and Medicaid costs rose faster than ever before. Governments began to experiment with managed care for Medicare and Medicaid as a cost control device.

The most significant development of the 1980s was the growth of selective contracting. Payers and insurers had usually reimbursed any and all physicians and hospitals. Under selective contracting, payers and insurers choose which providers they will pay and which they will not. In 1982, for example, California passed a law bringing selective contracting to the state's Medicaid program and to private health insurance plans. The law was passed because large California corporations formed a political coalition to challenge physician and hospital interests and because insurers deserted their former provider allies and joined the payers (Bergthold, 1990). The message of selective contracting was clear: Payers and insurers will do business only with providers who keep costs down. This development, especially when linked with capitation payments that placed providers at risk, changed the entire dynamic within the health care industry. For patients, it meant that, like Ryan Neighbor, they had lost free choice of physician because employers could require employees to change health plans and therefore physicians. For the health care industry, selective contracting meant fierce competition for contracts and the crumbling of the provider–insurer pact.

As a result of the payers' revolt, managed care became a burgeoning movement in U.S. health care. By 1990, 95% of insured employees were enrolled in some form of managed care plan, including fee-for-service plans with utilization management, preferred provider organizations (PPOs), and HMOs. Thirty-nine million people were enrolled in HMOs, up from 9 million in 1980. The growth of managed care plans, especially HMOs, competing against one another for contracts with business and the government, changed the entire political topography of U.S. health care (Table 16–2).

THE 1990s: THE BREAKUP OF THE PROVIDER–INSURER PACT

> In 1994, Pamela Neighbor, Ryan's cousin, developed constipation. Earlier that year, her law firm had switched from Blue Cross HMO to Apple a Day HMO because the premiums were lower; all employees of the firm were forced to change their physicians. Apple a Day contracted only with Crosstown Hospital, whose rates were lower than those of Metropolitan, resulting in Metropolitan losing patients and closing its doors. Ms. Neighbor's new physician diagnosed colon cancer and arranged for her admission to Crosstown Hospital for surgery. The physician's office was across the street from the now-closed Metropolitan Hospital, and she did not see her patients at Crosstown Hospital. Instead, she transferred the care of her hospitalized patients to a salaried inpatient physician called a hospitalist, who cared for Ms. Neighbor during her 4-day hospital stay. Apple a Day paid Crosstown Hospital $6000, $1500 per diem.

Table 16–2. Historical overview of U.S. health care.

1945–1970: Provider–insurer pact
  Independent hospitals and small private practices
  Many private insurers
  Providers tended to dominate the insurers, especially in Blue Cross and Blue Shield
  Payers (individuals, businesses, and, after 1965, government) had relatively little power
  Reimbursements for providers were generous
The 1970s: Tensions develop
  Payers (especially government) become concerned about costs of health care
  Under pressure from payers, insurers begin to question generous reimbursements of providers
The 1980s: Revolt of the payers
  Payers (business joining government) become very concerned with rising health care costs
  Attempts are made to reduce health cost inflation through Medicare DRGs, fee schedules, capitated HMOs, and
    selective contracting
The 1990s: Breakup of the provider–insurer pact
  Spurred by the payers, selective contracting spreads widely as a mechanism to reduce costs
  Price competition is introduced
  Large integrated health networks are formed
  Large physician groups emerge
  Insurance companies dominate many managed care markets
  For-profit institutions increase in importance
  Insurers gain increasing power over providers, creating conflict and ending the provider–insurer pact

During the 1990s, every metropolitan area in the United States, and many smaller cities and towns, experienced major upheavals of their medical care landscape. The myriad small physician offices and independent hospitals were replaced, to greater or lesser degrees in different regions of the country, by large managed care plans contracting with a shrinking number of hospitals and with medical groups that encompassed most of the community's physicians. In the most mature managed care markets, three or four health care networks are competing for those patients with private insurance, Medicare, or Medicaid. Hospitals and physicians not affiliated with one of the networks are likely to close their doors. Several major trends that will determine the trajectory of health care in the next century are apparent.

Selective Contracting   Many employers offer their employees one or several managed care plans with which they have contracts and will not pay noncontracted physicians or hospitals. Under such a system, large payers amass countervailing power to discipline providers whose costs inflate too rapidly. Within a few years, many metropolitan areas will see most of their populations enrolled in whichever HMO plans are able to get contracts with large payers.

Selective contracting has a tendency to disorganize rather than organize medical care patterns. Physicians may be forced to admit patients from one HMO to one hospital and those from another HMO to a different hospital. Laboratory, x-ray, and specialist services close to a primary care physician's office (PCP) may not be covered under contracts with that physician's patients' HMO, forcing referrals to be made across town. In one highly publicized case with a tragic outcome, the parents of a 6-month-old infant with bacterial meningitis were told by their HMO to drive the child almost 40 miles to a hospital that had a contract with that HMO, passing several high-quality hospitals along the way (Anders, 1996).

Price Competition   Selective contracting has brought price competition to the health care sector for the first time. In the past, hospitals competed with one another for patients, but the competition was not based on price. Rather, each hospital bought the most modern equipment and technology to attract physicians; it was up to the physicians to provide the patients. Rather than reducing costs, this kind of "medical arms race" competition increased costs. With the advent of selective contracting, HMOs (rather than physicians) provide the patients. Hospitals without HMO contracts can find themselves empty, and HMO contracts come to hospitals that can offer lower prices than other hospitals in the region. The health care system is moving toward price competition driven by the large business and government payers.

Mergers and Acquisitions   Health care providers and HMOs have responded to selective contracting with an unprecedented wave of mergers and acquisitions. With 40% of the nation's hospital beds empty on the average day, and with hospital use decreasing under managed care, a third of the nation's 5500 hospitals are predicted to close (Johnsson, 1993). To survive, hospitals are joining forces by merging or affiliating with one another. In 1994 alone, 10% of the nation's hospitals were involved in merger or acquisition activity. In 1994 and 1995, 375 for-profit hospitals were acquired by another investor-owned hospital chain. The largest hospital chain, Columbia/HCA, grew from 94 hospitals in early 1994 to over 340 by the end of 1995. By 1994, 61% of all acute general hospitals were involved in multihospital systems (Zelman, 1996; Kuttner, 1996).

Not only hospitals but also insurance companies and HMOs are merging. In 1952, 150 Blue Cross and Blue Shield plans spanned the nation; in 1993 only 69 were left, and the number will drop to 40 in the future. By the end of the 1990s, 70 to 80% of Blues subscribers are likely to be in HMOs (Albertson, 1993). While the number of HMO enrollees grows, the number of HMOs is declining. In 1991, the largest 20 HMOs had 33% of total HMO enrollment; by 1994, that percentage had jumped to 57%. Large HMOs are buying up smaller ones and are merging with one another. Aetna, previously the nation's tenth largest HMO, acquired U.S. HealthCare, the fifth largest, in 1996. United HealthCare acquired MetraHealth, thereby becoming the nation's largest managed care organization, with over 14 million members (Zelman, 1996). PacifiCare and FHP, two of the top 10 HMOs, recently merged, as did Health-Net and Foundation Health.

The Emergence of Large Physician Groups   In 1965, 10% of physicians practiced in groups; by 1991, that figure had risen to one-third. The average group has grown from 6.3 physicians in 1969 to 11.5 in 1991 (Clements, 1992). Between 1991 and 1995, the number of group practices increased by 20%, and the number of groups with over 100 physicians grew by 26% (Zelman, 1996). Physicians in solo practice and small groups are being excluded from managed care networks in favor of physicians in large group practices (Stevens, 1993).

Two types of groups are available for physicians to join. One is the hospital-centered group, which may involve entire medical staffs. Many hospitals have assisted physicians in creating groups to obtain managed care contracts. With occupancy rates low, hospitals want to "lock in" physicians, so they will admit patients exclusively to their beds. The difficulty with these hospital-based groups is that they perpetuate the excess number of specialists and hospital patient-days rather than moving toward a more competitive, lower-cost primary care and outpatient orientation.

The alternative to hospital-based physician groups is large investor-owned groups. Worried doctors across the country are selling their practices to such practice management companies as Caremark, Pacific Physician Services, Phycor Inc., Mullikin, and Kelsey-Seybold, in order to obtain managed care contracts. These for-profit companies are engaged in a process of merger and consolidation similar to that taking place among hospitals and HMOs. For example, MedPartners acquired Mullikin Medical Enterprises in 1995, creating the nation's largest multispecialty physician management company; in 1996, MedPartners/Mullikin bought Caremark, creating a mega-group with contracts covering 1.5 million patients. In California, large integrated medical groups are contracting with HMOs and assuming risk for HMO patients (see Chapter 5); these groups have prospered by sharing in the cost savings generated from marked reductions in hospital utilization (Robinson and Casalino, 1995).

The Growth of For-Profit Institutions   The pharmaceutical and medical equipment functions of the health care system have always been carried out by for-profit companies. But health care delivery has traditionally been nonprofit. This situation is changing. The 1970s saw rapid growth of corporate-owned proprietary (for-profit) hospital chains; in 1980, about 20% of the nation's private general hospitals were owned or managed by for-profit companies such as Humana and Hospital Corporation of America (Relman, 1980). During the 1990s, the for-profit hospital environment was altered by the hegemony of Columbia/HCA, but most for-profit acquisitions were of other for-profit hospitals; about three-fourths of hospitals continue to be nonprofit, private, or public. However, from 1993 through 1996, over 100 nonprofit hospitals have been taken over by for-profit chains. Moreover, the influence of for-profit hospitals is greater than their numbers. In order to compete with for-profits, some nonprofit hospitals are acting more and more like their for-profit competitors, primarily concerned with market share and net income rather than community service. For-profit hospitals provide less charity care, treat fewer Medicaid patients, and have higher administrative costs than nonprofit hospitals (Kuttner, 1996; Woolhandler and Himmelstein, 1997). Columbia/HCA has been under a federal criminal investigation examining whether it is illegal for Columbia to give physicians monetary incentives to admit patients to their hospitals. Columbia is also suspected of defrauding Medicare by overbilling for services performed (Eichenwald, 1997).

Seventy-seven percent of nursing homes and 50% of home health care organizations are for-profit organizations. Many diagnostic laboratories are run by for-profit companies. Ambulatory surgery centers, urgent care clinics (irreverently called "docs-in-the-box"), and large physician groups have proliferated, many run by investor-owned companies (Relman, 1991).

Because of the availability of federal funds for nonprofit HMO development, most HMOs prior to the 1980s were nonprofit. By the early 1980s, most governmental prohibitions against for-profit HMOs had been lifted, and federal funds were no longer available for nonprofit HMOs. For-profit companies had greater access to capital, and began to proliferate in the HMO arena. During the 1980s, many nonprofit HMOs converted to for-profit status (Langwell, 1990). For example, Blue Cross of California set up a for-profit subsidiary to run its large California Care HMO. HealthNet, California's second largest HMO, converted from nonprofit to for-profit status. In all, since 1983, 28 of California's HMOs have converted to for-profit status. One hundred percent of HMOs newly formed in 1990 were for-profit, compared with about 40% of new HMOs formed prior to 1981 (Marion Merrell Dow, 1990). As a result, 67% of HMOs in 1994 were for-profit.

Nine of the 10 largest HMOs in 1994 were for-profit companies (Zelman, 1996). Some for-profit HMO executives have been paid enormous compensation packages. In 1994, Dan Crowley, chief executive of Foundation Health, had a $19 million pay package. The founder and chairman of Oxford Health Plans, Steve Wiggins, collected options on Oxford stock between 1992 and 1994 that were valued at $35 million. When Qual-Med became a publicly traded for-profit HMO in 1991, CEO Dr. Malik Hasan's fortune climbed to $67 million. U.S. Healthcare's CEO Leonard Abramson negotiated the receipt of $967 million in cash and stocks plus a corporate jet as part of that company's purchase by Aetna. Around the time of that sale, U.S. Healthcare was spending only 68% of its funds on medical care, with the remainder going for administration, profits, and executive compensation (Anders, 1996).

In 1992, Dr. Arnold Relman, editor-in-chief emeritus of the *New England Journal of Medicine,* estimated that 35–40% of all health care services and facilities were owned by for-profit businesses (Relman, 1992). If the trend continues toward large integrated networks controlled by for-profit HMOs, for-profit hospital chains, and for-profit physician management corporations, most health care services may be under the control of for-profit companies by the year 2000.

Entrepreneurialism in medicine will inevitably create conflicts between the physician's professional commitment to patient welfare and the corporate manager's fiduciary responsibility to earn money for investors and stockholders. The new forms of for-profit medicine have similarities and differences with traditional financial arrangements in health care. Fee-for-service physicians have often acted as profit maximizers. Private nonprofit institutions have engaged in profit-seeking behavior; for example, some nonprofit Blue Cross plans have granted excessive salaries and "perks" for their high-level officials (Light, 1994), and nonprofit hospitals are often motivated by income generation more than community need (Relman, 1991). Whether conducted by for-profit corporations, private nonprofit institutions, or individual professionals, decisions based on the profit motive often conflict with behavior solely motivated by service to the patient (see Chapter 12) (Rodwin, 1993). These are the similarities between investor-run medical organizations and traditional physician-run or nonprofit structures. The chief difference lies in the fact that the traditional arrangements tended to retain excess income largely within the health care sector, where it might be used to purchase improved equipment or provide new services. In contrast, investor-owned for-profit health institutions distribute profits to their investors, who are less likely to contribute to health care sector improvement. The commitment of physicians and other care givers to the ethical principles of beneficence, nonmaleficence, patient autonomy, and distributive justice will be tested on a daily basis in the increasingly profit dominated environment of modern medicine.

The Demise of the Provider–Insurer Pact Selective contracting gives payers a great deal of power because they can deny contracts with insurers and providers who fail to keep costs down. The heightened power of the payers has led to a new relationship between insurers and providers.

(1) Staff and group model HMOs and vertically integrated health networks (see Chapter 7) merge insurers and providers into one organization; in these cases, insurers have become providers.

(2) Within both staff/group model HMOs and IPA/network HMOs, and within vertically and virtually integrated health networks, the insurers play the role of managers, while the true providers (ie, hospitals and physicians) are the direct producers of medical services. Conflict tends to develop between insurers and providers over who gets how much money. A lower physician capitation payment or hospital per diem rate (see Chapter 4) means more money for health plan administrators and stockholders and less for providers. Although on the one hand insurers are more tightly connected to providers, at the same time insurers and providers are more antagonistic than ever before. Rather than a provider–insurer pact dominated by providers, the health care industry is moving toward an insurer–provider relationship dominated by insurers.

Numerous rifts have appeared in the health care industry. HMOs and insurers compete with one another to obtain contracts with business and government. The Health Insurance Association of America, for years the powerful organization of commercial health insurance companies, has fractured, with several large insurers (CIGNA, Aetna, and Metropolitan Life) leaving the organization in 1992. The large commercial companies and the Blues (with managed care networks) have split with the small insurers and hope to take away the portion of the commercial health insurance market controlled by more than 1000 smaller insurance firms (Weiss, 1992). Hospitals and physicians fight with insurers for higher fees and less interference in medical practice. Large insurer-run HMOs have abruptly terminated contracts with physician groups, thereby taking away many of the physicians' patients and forcing the patients to go to other physicians (Meyer, 1994). Hospitals compete with each other for entry into emerging integrated networks and for physicians who can bring them patients. Large physician groups and physician management companies battle to swallow up more and more independent medical offices. Hospitals, PCPs, and specialists argue over what proportion of the capitation payment each will receive. Health care consumers are protesting reduced access to services provided by managed care organizations while managed care executives earn millions of dollars in compensation and stock options (Bodenheimer, 1996).

THE OPTIONS FOR HEALTH CARE PROFESSIONALS

From 1945 through 1970, developments in U.S. health care were dominated by a mutuality of interests between insurers and providers, who forged a pact that facilitated a flow of funds from the payers of care to the insurers, providers, and suppliers. These monies were stimulated by, and helped to further, the postwar flourishing of scientific progress in the field of medicine. In the 1970s and 1980s, the deterioration of the economy clashed with the imperatives of biotechnologic development and the public's desire for the most advanced diagnosis and treatment. The major payers (business and government) attempted to slow the torrent of money pouring into health care. The tensions thereby placed upon insurers and providers caused a fracturing of their alliance, opening the health care sector to unprecedented political and economic change. As the payers limited which insurers and providers would receive payments, competition intensified within the health care industry, with the big (ie, large insurers, large hospitals, and large physician groups) gaining ascendancy over the small.

As the twenty-first century begins, the landscape of the health care system will have been fundamentally altered. The multiplicity of independent hospitals and physician offices will have given way to a small number of large integrated health care organizations and networks. What do these changes portend for physicians, nurses, and other health care professionals?

> Susan is in her final year of family practice residency in a large university hospital program. Starting in September 1999, she is visited by a parade of recruiters from the four health plans that care for 85% of the people in her metropolitan area and from plans in nearby cities. She is determined to work in a small setting with two of her fellow residents. They are denied bank loans to start their own practice; the loan officer tells them they would have no patients to see. Susan finally accepts a job at a large health plan that seems to have well-trained physicians, gives her the opportunity to work closely with nurse practitioners and physician assistants from high-quality training programs, and offers her good vacation and maternity benefits.

> In 1999, Luisa is one of the few anesthesiology residents finishing the program in a large hospital; most of her medical school classmates chose primary care careers because of the greater number of employment opportunities. Luisa is so busy in the operating room that she does not have much time to worry about her career. When she finishes the program, she takes a 6-month rest and then starts looking for work. After 2 months, she takes an evening job at an urgent care center in one of the large local health plans. In the first year, she does not even enter the operating room, which is disappointing, but she enjoys the variety of clinical problems she encounters. Meanwhile, she submits applications to several health plans for anesthesia positions.

> In nursing school, Felicia is excited about intensive care unit nursing, and upon graduation is hired to work in the university hospital's intensive care unit. After 3 years, she becomes tired of the long hours and high level of intensity. She is irritated about teaching each new wave of medical residents everything she knows, only to have them order her around even though their knowledge is less than hers. Felicia becomes a home health care nurse, and finds that her clinical training in the intensive care unit has given her the skills to care for patients without much help from their physicians. She talks to her friend, who worked in labor and delivery and went on to become a certified nurse–midwife. Even though she enjoys her work in home care nursing, Felicia decides to return to school and become a nurse practitioner.

Until very recently in the United States, most graduates of physician training programs faced abundant practice opportunities in the specialty of their choice. The ascendance of managed care may be dramatically changing practice opportunities, especially for specialists.

Between 1965 and 1992, the growth in the number of practicing physicians outpaced growth of the overall population by almost 75%. In 1965, there were 115 practicing physicians for every 100,000 people in the nation. By 1992, that number had risen to 190 per 100,000 (Council on Graduate Medical Education, 1996). In 1965, the ratio of specialists to generalists in the United States was 1:1. In 1992, the ratio was 2:1. (See Figure 16–1). Much of this expansion was fueled by federal dollars to support residency training programs.

Nearly two decades ago, policy analysts warned that the United States was producing too many specialist physicians and called for public regulation to curb further growth (Graduate Medical Education National Advisory Committee, 1981). These analysts argued that continued expansion of physician supply would add considerable costs to the system without necessarily enhancing patients' access to appropriate care or overall health. Most nations allow public agencies to regulate the number of training positions in exchange for public subsidy of the costs of medical training. In the United States, however, attempts to exact these types of regulations have been repeatedly rejected.

In the absence of explicit public regulation, the "invisible hand" of the market may now be imposing limitations on practice opportunities. HMOs tend to staff their organizations with a level of specialists per enrollee that is far lower than the level of specialists per population in the nation as a whole. Estimates suggest that if the United

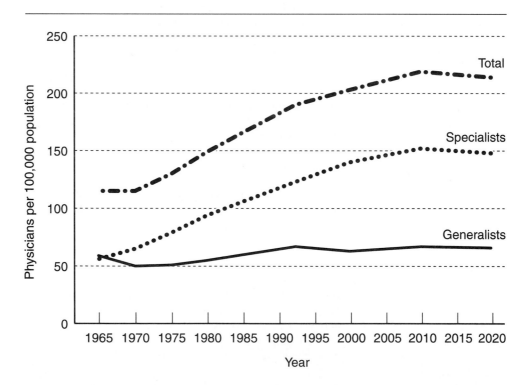

Figure 16–1. Supply of practicing physicians in the United States. Note: Data beyond 1992 are estimated projections based on continuation of 1992 training and retirement patterns. Source: Council on Graduate Medical Education. Patient care physician supply and requirements: testing COGME recommendations. United States Department of Health and Human Services, 1996 (HRSA-P-DM 95-3).

States completely converted to managed care, the nation would have 40% more specialists than required by HMO staffing patterns (Council on Graduate Medical Education, 1996).

Through direct employment of physicians and selective contracting, managed care organizations now wield considerable power over physicians' ability to find and maintain gainful practice. A physician without managed care contracts risks becoming a physician without patients. Whether the "invisible hand" of the market will operate with such harshness that it will actually produce a significant amount of unemployment and underemployment among physicians remains to be determined. Some practicing physicians are experiencing denials of contract applications or termination of existing contracts. Some physicians graduating from specialty training programs in the mid-1990s may be facing difficulties finding an acceptable practice placement. However, it is unlikely that the public will tolerate major unemployment among physicians at a time when millions of Americans continue to go without access to basic care. More likely, young physicians will not have the unlimited choice of specialty and practice location that was afforded their predecessors. Medical students will need to weigh considerations of existing supply when selecting a specialty for residency training, and residency graduates may have to settle for practice in less "desirable" regions and settings.

Managed care is also having a major impact on the nursing profession. In the 1980s, a consensus existed that the United States faced a shortage of nurses. By the mid-1990s, nurses—like physicians—began hearing warnings of an oversupply brought on by the upheavals of managed care. Registered nurses (RNs) represent the single largest profession in health care. In 1992, the country had 2.2 million licensed registered nurses, 83% of whom were actively working in health care fields. The supply of registered nurses per capita in the United States more than doubled between 1960 and 1992 (Coffman et al, 1998). Two-thirds of registered nurses are employed by hospitals.

Managed care has profoundly reduced the amount of care delivered in hospitals, a trend with major ramifications for nursing. Patients are discharged home much sooner, and many procedures formerly performed only on an inpatient basis are now done as "come-and-go" surgery. Moreover, many hospitals have responded to the cost containment pressures of managed care by "re-engineering" hospital staffing (Gordon, 1997). One method of economizing has been to replace more highly trained, highly paid nurses with lower-paid nurse's aides (often referred to as "unlicensed assistive personnel"). Nurses and physicians are extremely concerned about the impact of these changes on patient care.

Two things are clear about the future of nursing. First, more nurses will be employed outside the hospital, in settings such as home care, public health nursing, and ambulatory care clinics. Second, reforms will be needed in the educational preparation of registered nurses. Fewer than 40% of nurses in the United States have a bachelor's degree (Coffman et al, 1998). The majority of registered nurses trained in "diploma" or "associate degree" programs that required less extensive educational preparation. As nurses care for hospitalized patients with greater complexity and acuity of illness and assume greater responsibility for patient care in other settings, training programs will need to adjust to meet the higher level of clinical demands. Nurses may also find more opportunities to pursue advanced training to practice as nurse practitioners in a health care system desiring a wider variety of primary care practitioners.

Within the new structures of medical care lies the opportunity for solving the stubborn social problems of health care access and health care costs. On the other hand, dangers lurk as the traditional model of professional control over health care is replaced with corporate forms of organization. These changes will have profound effects on both patients and their care givers. The next and final chapter explores the tensions inherent in the emerging health care system.

REFERENCES

Albertson D: Blues plans seek links to improve competitive edge. Phys Fin News, Sept 15, 1993.

Anders G: Health Against Wealth: HMOs and the Breakdown of Medical Trust. Houghton Mifflin Company, 1996.

Bergthold L: The fat kid on the seesaw: American business and health care cost containment, 1970–1990. Ann Rev Public Health 1991;12:157.

Bergthold L: Purchasing Power in Health. Rutgers Univ Press, 1990.

Bluestone B, Harrison B: The Deindustrialization of America. Basic Books, 1982.

Bodenheimer T: The HMO backlash: Righteous or reactionary? N Engl J Med 1996;335: 1601.

Califano JA: America's Health Care Revolution. Random House, 1986.

Cantor JC et al: Business leaders' views on American health care. Health Aff 1991;10(1):98.

Castells M: The Economic Crisis and American Society. Princeton Univ Press, 1980.

Clements B: Group practice: A profile. Am Med News, Sept 7, 1992.

Coffman J et al: Overview of trends in the nursing workforce and nursing education. In: O'Neil EH, Coffman J (editors): Seven Strategies for the Future of Nursing. Jossey-Bass, 1998.

Council on Graduate Medical Education: Patient care physician supply and requirements: Testing COGME recommendations. United States Department of Health and Human Services, 1996 (HRSA-P-DM 95-3).

Davis MH, Burner ST: Three decades of Medicare: What the numbers tell us. Health Aff 1995;14(4):231.

Eichenwald K: A makeover may change more than Columbia. New York Times, Aug 8, 1997.

Gordon S: Life Support: Three Nurses on the Front Lines. Little, Brown and Company, 1997.

Graduate Medical Education National Advisory Committee (GMENAC): Summary report of the GMENAC. United States Department of Health and Human Services, 1981 (HRA-81-651).

Harris N: Managed care is right course, employers say. Bus Health 1992;10(8):32.

Health Policy Advisory Center: The American Health Empire. Vintage Books, 1971.

Johnsson J: PHOs, friends or foes? Am Med News, Aug 9, 1993.

Kennedy P: The Rise and Fall of the Great Powers. Random House, 1987.

Kuttner R: Columbia/HCA and the resurgence of the for-profit hospital business. N Engl J Med 1996;335:362,446.

Kuttner R: Revolt of the Haves. Simon & Schuster, 1980.

Langwell KM: Structure and performance of health maintenance organizations. Health Care Fin Rev 1990;12(1):71.

Law SA: Blue Cross: What Went Wrong? Yale Univ Press, 1974.

Light DW: Life, death, and the insurance companies. N Engl J Med 1994;330:498.

Marion Merrell Dow, Inc: Managed Care Digest, HMO Edition, 1990.

Meyer H: Insurance giants bet on managed care. Am Med News, Feb 7, 1994.

Reinhardt UE: Reorganizing the financial flows in U.S. health care. Health Aff 1993; 12(Suppl):172.

Relman AS: The choices for healthcare reform. Pennsylvania Blue Shield Institute, 1992.

Relman AS: The new medical-industrial complex. N Engl J Med 1980;303:963.

Relman AS: Shattuck lecture: The health care industry: Where is it taking us? N Engl J Med 1991;325:854.

Robinson JC, Casalino LP: The growth of medical groups paid through capitation in California. N Engl J Med 1995;333:1684.

Rodwin MA: Medicine, Money, and Morals: Physicians' Conflicts of Interest. Oxford Univ Press, 1993.

Sapolsky HM et al: Corporate attitudes toward health care costs. Milbank Mem Fund Q 1981; 59(4):561.

Smith MD et al: Taking the public's pulse on health system reform. Health Aff 1992; 11(2):125.

Starr P: The Social Transformation of American Medicine. Basic Books, 1982.

Stevens S: Health plans seen favoring groups over solo doctors. Phys Fin News, May 15, 1993.

Sullivan CB et al: Employer-sponsored health insurance in 1991. Health Aff 1992;11(4):172.

Thurow L: Head to Head: The Coming Economic Battle Among Japan, Europe, and America. William Morrow, 1992.

Weiss LD: No Benefit: Crisis in America's Health Insurance Industry. Westview Press, 1992.

Woolhandler S, Himmelstein DU: Costs of care and administration at for-profit and other hospitals in the United States. N Engl J Med 1997;336:769.

Zelman WA: The Changing Health Care Marketplace. Jossey-Bass, 1996.

Conclusion: Tensions & Challenges   17

The perfect health care system is like perfect health—a noble aspiration but one that is impossible to attain. In the preceding chapters, we have discussed many fundamental issues and principles involved in formulating health care policy. A recurrent theme has been the notion that "magic bullets" are hard to come by. As stated in Chapter 2, policies tend to evolve in a process of solution-creating-new-problem-requiring-new-solution. Policy changes may offer a degree of relief for a pressing problem, such as inadequate access to care, but frequently also give rise to various side effects, such as stimulating health care cost inflation.

All health care systems face the same challenges: improving health, controlling costs, prioritizing allocation of resources, enhancing the quality of care, and distributing services fairly. These challenges require the management of various tensions that pull at the health care system (O'Neil and Seifer, 1995). The goal of health policy is to find the points of equilibrium producing the optimal system of health care (Table 17–1).

Dr. Madeleine Longview is chief resident in critical care medicine and supervises the intensive care unit of a large municipal hospital. It's 5:30 AM, and the intensive care unit team has finally stabilized the condition of a 15-year-old admitted the prior evening with gunshot wounds to the abdomen and chest. Dr. Longview sits by the nursing desk and surveys the other patients in the unit: a 91-year-old woman admitted from a nursing home with sepsis from a urinary tract infection, a 50-year-old man with shock lung due to drugs ingested in a suicide attempt, and a 32-year-old woman with lupus erythematosus who is rejecting her second kidney transplant. Dr. Longview feels personally responsible for the care of every one of these patients. She tells herself that she will do her best to help each of them survive.

As Dr. Longview gazes out the windows of the intensive care unit, the apartment houses surrounding the hospital take shape in the breaking dawn. She wonders: Which block will be the scene of the next drive-by shooting or episode of spouse abuse? Which window shade hides a homebound elder lying on the floor dehydrated and unable to move, waiting for someone to find him and bring him to the emergency room? Which one of the unvaccinated kids in the neighborhood will one day be rushed into the unit limp with meningitis? In which room is someone lighting up the first cigarette of the day? Dr. Longview somehow feels responsible for all those patients-to-be, as well as for the patients lying in the hospital beds around her. After these sleepless nights on duty, the doubts about the value of all the work she does in the intensive care unit creep into her thoughts. She has visions of shutting down the unit and

Table 17–1. Major tensions in health care.[1]

Health of the individual patient	Health of the population
Tertiary care	Primary care
Acute care	Chronic and preventive care
Cost unawareness in medical practice	Cost awareness
Unlimited expectations for care	Affordability of care
Individual physician	Organized health care team
Professional management	Corporate management
Market competition	Government regulation
Inequity in distribution	Fair distribution

[1] Adapted from O'Neil and Seifer, 1995.

> putting all the money to work hiring public health nurses in the community, or maybe just paying for a better grammar school in the neighborhood. But then, what would happen to the patients needing her care right now?

One of the most basic tensions affecting physicians and other care givers is the tension between caring for the individual patient and caring for the larger community or population. Many of the most important decisions to be made in health policy—decisions such as allocating health care resources, addressing the social context of health and illness, and augmenting activities in prevention and public health—depend on broadening the practitioner's view to encompass the population health perspective. The challenge for physicians and other clinicians will be to make room for this broader perspective while preserving the ethical duty to care for the individual patients under their charge.

Like Dr. Longview, the health care system as a whole will continue to struggle over finding the proper balance between the provision of acute care services and preventive and chronic care services, as well as striking the right balance between the levels of tertiary and primary care. Few observers would encourage Dr. Longview to succumb to her despair, close all the intensive care units, and expel all the critical care subspecialists from the health care system. Yet, most would agree that health care in the United States has drifted too far away from the primary care end of the tertiary care–primary care axis.

> Dr. Tom Ransom has performed what he believes to be a reasonably thorough workup for Zed's abdominal pain and decreased appetite, including a detailed history and physical examination, upper gastrointestinal x-ray series, and abdominal ultrasound test—all of which were normal. When Dr. Ransom tells Zed that they will have to work together to manage Zed's symptoms, Zed tells Dr. Ransom that he wants one more test, an abdominal CT scan. Zed says that he had a cousin with similar symptoms who was eventually diagnosed with advanced-stage lymphoma after complaining of pain for over a year.
>
> Dr. Ransom feels in a quandary. He believes it extremely unlikely that Zed has serious pathologic changes in his abdomen that will be detected on CT scan. He could order the scan, but then there's the issue of the cost. He can't recall

whether Zed is covered by a fee-for-service plan or by one of the health maintenance organizations (HMOs) that pays on a capitated basis and puts Dr. Ransom at financial risk for all radiologic tests ordered. He starts to ask Zed about his coverage, but feels a pang of guilt that he should allow these economic considerations to intrude into his clinical judgment.

The desire (and in many instances, expectation) of patients to receive all potentially beneficial care, and the unwillingness of these same individuals in their role as purchasers to spend unlimited amounts to finance health care, creates a strain for all care givers and systems of care. Physicians increasingly are being called upon to incorporate considerations of costs when making clinical decisions. Debate will continue about the best ways to encourage physicians to be more accountable for the costs of care in a manner that is socially responsible and does not unduly intrude on the physician's ability to serve the individual patient. Is it necessary to use payment methods that place physicians at individual financial risk for their treatment decisions in order to control costs? Are more global methods available to induce physicians and other care givers to practice in a more cost-conscious manner? If Zed does not get a CT scan, does that constitute painless or painful cost control?

On the eve of his retirement, Dr. Melvin Steadman reminisces with his son, Dr. Kevin Steadman. The elder Dr. Steadman has practiced as a solo pediatrician for over 40 years in the same town. The only boss he has known in his professional life has been himself. He has served as president of the local medical society, helped spearhead efforts to build a special children's wing of the local hospital, and antagonized several of his colleagues when he pushed for a change in hospital policy that required physicians to attend extra continuing medical education courses in order to maintain their hospital privileges. Mel swore that he'd never retire; but he also swore that he'd never let the insurance companies "tell me how to practice medicine." He has refused to sign any managed care contracts. Facing a dwindling supply of patients, Mel has decided to call it quits.

His son Kevin is also a pediatrician, working as a staff physician for a large for-profit HMO that recently opened up an office in town. Kevin remembers the many nights when his father didn't get home from work until after he had gone to bed. Kevin's work hours are more regular at the HMO, and he is on call for only one weekend every 2 months. He considers his father's approach to medicine old-fashioned in many ways—excessively paternalistic toward patients and irrationally scornful of the pediatric nurse practitioners that work with Kevin. He does, however, envy his father's professional independence. Just this week, the HMO refused to authorize a bone marrow transplant for one of Kevin's patients with a rare blood disorder. The HMO also just notified Kevin that he would have to divide his time between his current office and a new site that would soon open in a suburban mall. His schedule will be limited to 10-minute drop-in appointments at the new site, rather than the continuity style of practice that allows him to get to know his patients over time.

A system of health care formerly managed according to a professional model by independent practitioners is being pulled toward a corporate model of care featuring large organizations managed by administrators. As the role of commercial, for-profit entities expands, traditional responsibilities toward patients and local communities are vying with new obligations to shareholders. Power relationships are changing, with insurance companies and organized purchasers challenging the dominance of the medical profession. A shift toward multidisciplinary group practice may provide more opportunity for health professionals to work collegially and implement new approaches to quality improvement to elevate the competence of all health care providers. At the same time, a competitive, for-profit health care environment may induce physicians to compromise their humanity and turn toward the "homo economicus," basing clinical decisions in part on monetary considerations.

> Aurora can't wait any longer in the crowded county hospital emergency room. She's already been there for 6 hours, and the doctor hasn't seen her yet. Her lower abdomen still hurts, but she figures she'll just have to put up with it for a few more days. She really doesn't have much choice. Poor and uninsured, where else could she go? Aurora has two young children at home who need to be put to bed. In half an hour, their father has to get to his night job as a security officer. As she enters her apartment, she collapses, the pregnancy in her fallopian tube having ruptured, producing internal hemorrhage. Her husband frantically dials 911, praying that his wife won't die.

Perhaps no tension within the U.S. health care system is as far from reaching a point of satisfactory equilibrium as the achievement of a basic level of fairness in the distribution of health care services and the burden of paying for those services. Despite 2 years of intense debate on health care reform following the 1992 presidential election, more people in the country are uninsured in 1997 than in 1994, with prospects dim for attainment of universal insurance coverage in this century. Due to persistent financial barriers, more patients will go without early detection of potentially curable cancers, more patients with chronic diseases will be hospitalized because of lack of timely outpatient care, more hypertensive patients will forego the medications that might avert the occurrence of strokes and kidney failure, and more babies will be born prematurely and spend their first weeks of life in a neonatal intensive care unit. The poor will continue to pay a greater proportion of their income for health care than do more affluent families, and catastrophic health care costs will ravage countless middle class families.

People providing and receiving care in the United States must work together to achieve a brighter future for the nation's health care system. Changing the future will require that people look beyond their immediate self-interest to view the common good of a health care system that is accessible, affordable, and of high quality for all. A heightened level of public discourse will be needed, with a populace that is better informed and more actively engaged in shaping the future of their health care system. Abstract concepts in health policy will need to be discussed and debated in a manner that connects with the daily realities experienced by patients and care givers. The attitudes and actions of physicians and other health professionals will play a major role in determining the future of health care in the United States. With leadership and foresight among the community of health professionals, our nation may yet achieve a system that allows the most honorable features of the healing professions to flourish.

REFERENCE

O'Neil E, Seifer S: Health care reform and medical education: Forces towards generalism. Acad Med 1995;70:337.

Questions and Discussion Topics

18

CHAPTER 2: PAYING FOR HEALTH CARE

1. What are the four modes of financing health care? Describe each.

2. Describe regressive, proportional, and progressive financing. Explain how each of the following is regressive, proportional, or progressive: out-of-pocket payments, experience-rated individual private insurance, community-rated individual private insurance, health insurance purchased 100% by the employer (assuming that employees actually pay for health insurance as explained in the text), and the federal income tax.

3. Harvey, who has worked all his life for General Electric, reaches 65. He does not retire. Is he eligible for Medicare Part A? Part B? Six months later, his wife, who has never worked, reaches 65. Is she eligible for Medicare Part A? Part B? How are Parts A and B paid for?

4. Hubert has received social security disability for 24 months because he has AIDS. Is he eligible for Medicare?

5. Rena developed chronic renal failure and started renal dialysis 2 weeks ago. She feels fine and is working. Is she eligible for Medicare?

6. Heidi, age 72, on Medicare Part A and B without Medicaid or a Medigap policy, is hospitalized for a stroke complicated by a deep vein thrombosis of the leg and a pulmonary embolus. She is in the acute hospital for 70 days, is cared for by a family practitioner and a neurologist. She improves somewhat, and is then transferred to the skilled nursing facility (SNF) for rehabilitation. She remains in the SNF for 30 days, is still severely disabled and unable to go home. She is sent to a nursing home for custodial care, where she stays for 3 months. Surprisingly, she improves, and goes home, where she receives skilled physical therapy services from a home care agency and also has a homemaker come in for 4 hours a day to buy food, cook, and clean the house. She is on three prescription medications at home. What does Heidi pay and what does Medicare pay? Acute hospital? SNF? Nursing home? Home care? Physicians? Prescriptions while in hospital? Prescriptions while at home?

Discussion Topics

1. Discuss your experiences with health insurance that was provided through a job. How did you obtain the insurance? Did you pay part of the premium? Were there deductibles or copayments? How many choices of plans did you have? What happened if you left your job?

2. Divide into two groups: one insurance company selling community-rated health insurance policies, the other selling experience-rated policies. Each side should try to

convince the instructor to buy its policy, first with the instructor as a young, healthy person, then with the instructor as an older person with diabetes. Which policy is the young person more likely to choose, and which the older person?

CHAPTER 3: ACCESS TO HEALTH CARE

1. Describe the two main categories of people without health insurance.

2. Why has lack of insurance been increasing over the past 10 years?

3. Compare access to health care for people with private insurance, for Medicaid recipients, and for people without insurance. Give examples.

4. Compare health outcomes for people with private insurance, for Medicaid recipients, and for people without insurance. Give examples.

5. Describe six categories of underinsurance.

Discussion Topics

1. What are some explanations as to why Ace Banks was healthy at age 48 while Bill Downes died at that age?

2. Women on the average have more visits than men to physicians. Does that mean that women's access to health care is greater than that of men?

3. Discuss possible reasons why minority patients with coronary heart disease receive fewer procedures such as bypass surgery than white patients.

4. What is the relationship between socioeconomic status (including factors such as income, education, and occupation) and health? Why does such a relationship exist?

5. What would be the best strategies to improve the health status of African-Americans in the United States?

CHAPTER 4: REIMBURSING HEALTH CARE PROVIDERS

1. Explain each mode of physician reimbursement: fee for service, episode of illness, capitation, and salary. Explain each mode of hospital reimbursement: fee for service, per diem, episode of illness (diagnosis-related group [DRG]), capitation, and global budget.

Discussion Topics

1. You are a primary care physician (PCP) caring for a young woman with new onset of severe headaches and amenorrhea and a normal physical examination. What are the financial incentives and disincentives that would lead you to order or not to order an MRI in a case in which the need for the MRI was equivocal?

(a) under traditional fee-for-service practice;

(b) under fee-for-service practice with utilization review;

(c) under an independent practice association (IPA)-model health maintenance organization (HMO) in which you receive a capitation payment that places you at risk for laboratory and x-ray studies and specialty referrals;

(d) under a staff model HMO which has a 2-month waiting list for elective MRI scans?

In the case of the staff model HMO, what would you do if you felt you needed to obtain the MRI within 48 hours?

2. You are finishing your family practice residency at a well-known university medical center and looking for the best way to begin your medical career. You are impressed with the dedication of a group of six PCPs, and you join the group. You soon learn that the group has a contract with MiniCare HMO. Under MiniCare, the group receives $35 per month per patient enrolled, a reasonable amount to cover the health care needs of the average patient. Out of this fund, the group pays for laboratory, x-ray, specialty referrals, and outpatient medications. In your first month, you order routine laboratory studies on all your new MiniCare patients, you send 17 MiniCare patients for mammograms, five for CT scans, three for MRIs, eight to specialists, and you prescribe a costly cholesterol-lowering drug for eight MiniCare patients. At the end of the month, the group's business manager meets with you, saying that the group's income from your 100 MiniCare patients amounted to $3500, but that you caused the group to spend $8500 in diagnostic studies, referrals, and prescriptions. You are told that the real world is not like university medicine and that you must reduce the costs of your care. What do you do?

3. You are a hospital administrator, and your hospital is in financial difficulty. You are about to address the medical staff, imploring them to help the hospital financially. In the old days, all you had to say was, in effect: "Admit as many patients as possible and keep them in the hospital as long as you can." But times have changed. For some methods of reimbursement, you want physicians to admit more patients; for others, you don't. For some methods, you want patients to stay long, for others, you don't. What do you tell the medical staff regarding:

(a) Medicare (DRG) patients;

(b) Medicaid (per diem) patients;

(c) HMO (per diem) patients; and

(d) HMO (capitated) patients?

For each of these categories of patients, does it help or hurt the hospital for physicians to

(a) admit more patients;

(b) keep them in the hospital more days; and

(c) order more diagnostic studies?

CHAPTER 5: CAPITATION PAYMENT IN MANAGED CARE

1. How does capitation payment free insurers of risk? How does capitation payment shift risk to providers of care?

2. Describe the flow of money in an IPA-type HMO. In round numbers, How much money per member per month does the HMO receive? How much does the HMO pay out? How much goes for hospital care? How much for primary care? How much for specialty and ancillary care?

3. How does the capitation-plus-bonus mode of reimbursement work?

4. What are the arguments for risk-adjusting capitation payments?

5. If PCPs and specialists are both capitated, what are the financial incentives of each of these physicians regarding the care of patients?

6. How do hospital risk pools function in IPA-type HMOs? Why do these risk-pool arrangements encourage low rates of hospitalization?

Discussion Topic

1. How, as a health care provider, can you resist becoming a homo economicus?

CHAPTER 6: HOW HEALTH CARE IS ORGANIZED—I

Discussion Topics

1. You are 63 years old and you begin to experience chest pain when walking. You do not have a physician. A friend suggests that you need a coronary artery bypass and recommends a cardiac surgeon at the medical school. What do you do

 (a) under a dispersed model of health care delivery;

 (b) under a regionalized model?

2. Give some examples of the statement, "Common disorders commonly occur and rare ones rarely happen." What are the implications of this statement for the ratio of generalist to specialist physicians in the United States?

3. In Great Britain, 65% of physicians are general practitioners. In Canada, 50% of physicians are generalists. In the United States, about one-third of physicians are generalists (general and family practitioners, general internists, and general pediatricians). Assume you are Chair of the Health Subcommittee of the U.S. House of Representatives Ways and Means Committee. What legislation might you propose to increase the proportion of generalist physicians?

4. Discuss the pros and cons of requiring everyone to enter the health care system through a "gatekeeper" health care provider (generalist physician, nurse practitioner, or physician assistant).

5. You are a pediatrician in an HMO, and you provide high quality care to the children whom you see in your office. The medical director institutes a program of community-oriented primary care. What do you do differently from what you did before?

CHAPTER 7: HOW HEALTH CARE IS ORGANIZED—II

1. What are the two generations of HMOs? Give examples of each (if possible, in your community).

2. What is vertical integration? What is virtual integration?

3. What is the difference between an IPA and an integrated medical group?

4. What is the difference between an HMO, a point of service plan, and a preferred provider organization?

Discussion Topic

1. What is the difference between the gatekeeper role in an IPA-type HMO that places the PCP at financial risk, and the traditional gatekeeper role in the British National Health Service?

CHAPTER 8: PAINFUL VERSUS PAINLESS COST CONTROL

1. Give examples of medical interventions that lie on the steeper portions of the cost-benefit curve, and interventions that lie on the flatter portions. Is the elimination of the latter painful or painless cost control?

2. Give examples of painless cost control. Are these painless for everyone?

Discussion Topics

1. CABGville has four cardiac surgery units; one unit performs 300 coronary artery bypass graft (CABG) surgeries each year, the other units perform an average of 40 per year. Cardiac surgeons can schedule a CABG anytime they wish. The small units have an operative mortality of 7% compared with 4% for the large unit. To control costs, the health planning council of CABGville closes the three less productive cardiac surgery units. Elective CABG surgeries now have a 1-month waiting list, and because of tight scheduling, surgeons are less likely to operate; the number of CABGs goes down from 420 to 340 per year; both the overall costs of CABG surgery and the unit cost per CABG operation drop, as does the mortality rate. Did CABGville achieve painful or painless cost control?

2. Total U.S. health care expenditures have been capped and are controlled by a health services commission. Because of tight budgetary constraints, the commission must decide whether to fund an all-out program of mammography or to limit mammography and finance in its place high-dose chemotherapy with autologous bone marrow transplantation for patients with metastatic breast cancer, a regimen whose effectiveness has not yet been proven. Under the first option, several thousand cases

of early-stage breast cancer could be treated with curative surgery each year but women currently suffering from advanced-stage breast cancer would receive no benefit. Which is the more painful cost control option from the point of view of women without breast cancer? From the perspective of women with metastatic breast cancer? From the perspective of society as a whole? Which of these two groups of women should have priority in this decision?

CHAPTER 9: MECHANISMS FOR CONTROLLING COSTS

Discussion Topics

1. Imagine that a managed competition law passes the U.S. Congress and is signed into law by the President. The law does not apply to Medicare, Medicaid, or non–employment-linked health plans. According to the law, employers are responsible to finance employee health insurance in the amount of 50% of the lowest cost plan in the geographic area; any additional employer payments would be taxed. LowCost Plan sets its premium at $100 per month; MidCost Plan's premium is $200 monthly, and HiCost Plan charges $300 per month. How much will the employer and employee pay for health insurance under each plan?

2. Two years after the passage of the managed competition law, nationwide health care costs continue to inflate at rates above 10% per year, and Senators wish to repeal the law. As a Senator arguing for repeal, explain why managed competition has not succeeded in holding down costs. As a Senator arguing against repeal, argue why the managed competition strategy should be given more time.

3. You are chair of the health planning council of CABGville, a town that continues to have a health care cost crisis. The town has 30 physicians, each seeing 30 patients a day at a cost of $30 per visit. Total daily cost is $30 \times 30 \times 30 = \$27,000$. What methods are available to reduce the total cost of physician services? Would it work to reduce the fee per visit from $30 to $20? If an expenditure cap strategy (tying fees to volume) were used, how would it work?

4. The CABGville health planning council changes the mode of physician reimbursement from fee-for-service to capitation: $20 per patient per month to PCPs, with 20 PCPs each having 2000 patients. (PCPs pay specialists from the $20 capitation.) Total cost per month = $800,000 (about $27,000 per day). How could the health planning council reduce the monthly cost? Could physician costs still increase despite this method of cost control? Why or why not?

5. You have finished your residency in internal medicine and have the choice to work at Kaiser or at a private practice that is part of an IPA. You are particularly concerned about your ability to order laboratory tests and x-rays and to obtain specialty consultations. At Kaiser, you learn that you have freedom in ordering tests and obtaining consultations, but that patients may have to wait (except in urgent situations) because of the limited supply of such equipment as MRI scanners and of specialty appoint-

ments. At the IPA, you must request prior authorization for expensive diagnostic studies and for specialty consultations, but once prior authorization has been obtained, waiting periods are fairly short. Which work situation would you prefer, and which do you think has the better chance of controlling costs?

6. You are the President of the United States, and your first term ends in a year. The cost control mechanism you instituted two years ago, based on patient cost sharing and managed competition, has not worked, and the American people are upset about persistent health care inflation. You are preparing for a major television address on health care costs. What will you propose? Can you convince the public that yours is a painless cost control strategy?

CHAPTER 10: LONG-TERM CARE

1. What are activities of daily living and independent activities of daily living?

2. What percentage of long-term care services are funded by which funding sources?

3. Which long-term care services are covered by Medicare and which are not? Which are covered by Medicaid?

Discussion Topics

1. You are president of LTC Insurance Company and are testifying before a Senate committee on long-term care. You are asked two questions: Why do only 4 million people carry private long-term care insurance? How do you answer the complaints that senior citizen advocacy groups make about the terms of private long-term care insurance policies? What do you say to the committee?

2. Your mother's Alzheimer's disease is getting worse; she wanders around the neighborhood, sometimes unable to find her way home; she sleeps during the day and stays up most of the night; and she has become incontinent. Your father died 2 years ago. You and your spouse both work, you have three school-age children, and you have an extra room in your home. The hospital social worker calls and says that your mother needs 24-hour help. Your choices are:

(a) hiring a homemaker to live with your mother at $16,000 per year;

(b) placing your mother in a nursing home whose bill will be paid by Medicaid;

(c) taking your mother home with you. What do you decide?

What reforms in the U.S. long-term care system would have benefitted you in this situation? How should such reforms be financed?

CHAPTER 11: THE PREVENTION OF ILLNESS

1. Why did tuberculosis (TB) decline prior to the identification of the TB bacillus? Why did polio morbidity and mortality decline? Why did Hodgkin's disease mortal-

ity fall in the late twentieth century? From these examples, what are the three major prevention strategies?

2. What are the first and the second epidemiologic revolutions?

Discussion Topics

1. Two people are campaigning for the consumer board of their HMO. The incumbent is running on a platform of charging tobacco users higher premiums than nonusers, because their use of tobacco costs the HMO more money. The opponent believes that society rather than the individual is responsible for tobacco addiction and that the HMO should become involved in social action against cigarette smoking. Conduct a debate between these two views.

2. How do you explain the fact that a large number of heart attacks occur at early ages in people with cholesterol levels below the median level for the United States? That heart attacks almost never occur at these ages in Japan? What is the implication for primary prevention of coronary heart disease?

3. You are named as head of the breast cancer prevention section of the U.S. Centers for Disease Control and Prevention. What primary and secondary prevention programs would you favor to reduce the incidence of and mortality from breast cancer?

4. You have been asked to debate a speaker from the National Rifle Association (NRA). The NRA speaker argues against gun control and ends with the statements, "Guns don't kill people, criminals do. If we outlaw guns, only outlaws will have guns." How do you respond?

5. The Mayor of Chicago has named you as the city's director of AIDS prevention. The incidence of HIV infection is growing rapidly, especially among women and minorities. What primary prevention strategies do you choose to combat the infection?

CHAPTER 12: THE QUALITY OF HEALTH CARE

Discussion Topics

1. Have you ever experienced or witnessed a medical care encounter of poor quality? What did you do about it? What should you have done?

2. In the vignette about Shelley Rush, who do you think was responsible for the error in giving insulin to the wrong patient?

3. In the vignette about Nina Brown, had the physician been working in a fee-for-service environment rather than a cost-conscious HMO, do you think he or she would have admitted Ms. Brown to the hospital?

4. Reread the example of the 23-year-old graduate student whose x-ray report was lost. If you were the administrator of the hospital, what would you do to prevent such

an error from taking place again? If you were the office manager of the internist's office that never received the x-ray report, what would you do to avoid a recurrence of this problem?

5. What is wrong with the malpractice system? What would you do to fix it?

CHAPTER 13: MEDICAL ETHICS & THE RATIONING OF HEALTH CARE

Discussion Topics

1. Pretend that the Lakeberg family discussed in this chapter belongs to an HMO, and that you are the HMO's medical director. The Lakeberg parents want surgery to separate the Siamese twins at the cost of $1 million. The list of benefits covered in the Lakeberg's HMO policy does not either affirm or deny their right to the surgery, so the responsibility to approve or deny the surgery falls on you. What do you decide? If you approve the surgery, who will end up paying for it? Is an ethical dilemma involved or not?

2. You are Dr. Marco Intensivo, as described in the vignette in the section "What is Rationing?" What do you do?

3. In the case of Mr. Olds and Mr. Younger described in the organ transplant section, which patient should receive the donor heart?

4. You are the PCP for Rodolfo, a 58-year-old man who suffered a cerebral hemorrhage and has been in a persistent vegetative state for 18 months. He lives in a nursing home, requires tube feedings and round-the-clock nursing attention, and his care is paid for by Medicaid. Rodolfo's daughter is a nurse in the intensive care unit of your hospital. Rodolfo's wife is deeply religious and has faith that Rodolfo will get better.

About every 6 weeks, Rodolfo develops a urinary tract infection with septicemia and must be admitted to the hospital—often to the ICU—for treatment. Over the course of 2 years, Rodolfo's care has cost $260,000. The hospital ethics committee discussed the case and recommended that tube feedings be withdrawn, or that the next episode of septicemia not be treated, thereby allowing Rodolfo to die. When you discussed the ethics committee recommendations with the family, the daughter agreed but the wife demanded that everything possible be done to continue Rodolfo's life. As Rodolfo's physician, what do you do? Which ethical dilemmas are involved? Autonomy versus beneficence? Autonomy versus nonmaleficence? Autonomy versus distributive justice? Beneficence versus distributive justice? If Rodolfo's care were withdrawn, what would happen to the money saved?

5. Evidence from public opinion polls suggests that people in the United States want the right to health care but don't want to pay for it.

At midnight, a new mother awakens to hear her 2-week-old infant scream. The mother and baby are Medicaid recipients. If she were experienced, the mother would know that the scream is normal, but she is frightened. She phones the emergency room and asks to bring the baby in to be seen. No amount of telephone advice seems to reassure her. Does the right to health care include society paying for her visit to the emergency room? Who is actually paying? Should the mother be advised to come into the emergency room if she was uninsured and wealthy? Uninsured and poor?

6. In Oregon, the Medicaid program was extended to thousands of Oregonians who had previously been uninsured. To help pay for this extension, the breadth of services available to Medicaid recipients was reduced such that recipients lost access to some care that might have been beneficial. You are the Governor of Oregon and you have to testify in a lawsuit alleging that the program is unfair because it deprives Medicaid recipients of certain services enjoyed by privately insured people. What is your response?

7. Should physicians be responsible to serve one master—their patient—or two masters—their patient and the broader needs of society? In your discussion, draw from the examples of the Lakebergs, Dr. Intensivo, and Rodolfo. How has the distribution system for organ transplantation tried to balance these "two masters?"

CHAPTER 14: HEALTH CARE IN THREE NATIONS

1. You are a secretary in a large company in Germany (Canada, UK). How is your health care paid for? You become sick and are forced to retire from your job. How is your health care paid for in Germany (Canada, UK)?

2. If you developed a urinary tract infection, what would you do in Germany (Canada, UK)? What if you needed cataract surgery? What if you had a sudden abdominal pain in the middle of the night? What if you developed leukemia and needed a bone marrow transplant? In each of these cases, which physician would care for you and where would you be cared for?

3. You are a general practitioner in Germany (Canada, UK). How are you paid? You are a specialist in Germany (Canada, UK). How are you paid? You are a hospital administrator in Germany (Canada, UK). How is your hospital paid?

4. How are costs controlled in the three countries?

CHAPTER 15: NATIONAL HEALTH INSURANCE

1. Describe how a government-financed national health insurance plan, an employer mandate plan, and an individual mandate plan would work.

2. What is the difference between a social insurance and a public assistance approach to government-financed national health insurance? Use Medicare and Medicaid as examples.

Discussion Topics

1. You are the speech writers for two candidates for the Democratic presidential nomination. One candidate favors an employer mandate and the other a single-payer

approach. What points would you have your candidate make about the strengths of his or her position and the weaknesses of the other candidate's position?

2. Why do you think that the United States is the only developed nation in the world without universal health insurance?

CHAPTER 16: THE ASCENDANCE OF MANAGED CARE

1. Describe how the payers of health care services increased their power between 1945 and 1995.

2. Describe changes in the relationships between physicians and insurance companies between 1945 and 1995.

Discussion Topics

1. Discuss potential conflicts between the profit motive and the principles of beneficence and nonmaleficence in the following situations:

(a) a private surgeon receiving fee-for-service reimbursement;

(b) a primary physician in a small group practice that receives capitation payments covering primary care, laboratory, x-ray, and specialty referrals;

(c) a physician who is the utilization manager of a large for-profit HMO receiving requests from her employed physicians to authorize expensive MRI scans for their patients;

(d) the administrator of a nonprofit hospital who has calculated that a new cardiac surgery unit will be profitable even if only one surgery is performed each week;

(e) the CEO of an HMO deciding whether to accept Medicaid patients, for whom the state government is paying premiums 30% lower than premiums paid for private patients.

What changes in the organization of health care could be made that would minimize such conflicts?

2. Discuss how health care is organized in your community—who are the payers, insurers, and providers? To what degree has your local health care system moved from a dispersed set of institutions to a small number of vertically or virtually integrated health care conglomerates?

3. Where in the health care system of the twenty-first century would you like to be—as a provider and as a patient? What are your fears and hopes for the future?

Index

NOTE: A *t* following a page number indicates tabular material and an *f* following a page number indicates a figure.